THE POOR DIE YOUNG

40 t

THE POOR DIE YOUNG

Housing and Health in Third World Cities

edited by Sandy Cairncross, Jorge E. Hardoy and David Satterthwaite

EARTHSCAN PUBLICATIONS LTD LONDON

First published 1990 by
Earthscan Publications Limited
3 Endsleigh Street, London WC1H 0DD

British Library Cataloguing in Publication Data
The poor die young: housing and health in the Third World
1. Developing countries. Urban regions. Slums and squatter settlements
I. Hardoy, Jorge E. (Jorge Enrique)
II. Cairncross, Sandy III. Satterthwaite, David
307'.3364'091724

ISBN 1-85383-019-4

Designed by Sandie Boccacci
Production by Bob Towell
Typeset in 10/12 Caledonia by Rapid Communications Ltd, Bristol
Printed and bound by Guernsey Press

Earthscan Publications Limited is an editorially independent and wholly owned subsidiary of the International Institute for Environment and Development.

Contents

MAPS

FIGURES

TABLES

BOXES

Preface

We have many people to thank for helping us to translate our initial idea of a book on the health implications of poor housing and living conditions in urban areas of the Third World into this final product. Our principal debt is to the authors of the various chapters both for the care taken in producing initial drafts and for the diligence in responding to our queries and suggested amendments as final versions were developed. Special thanks are also due to Diana Mitlin for her comments on the drafts for the Introduction and chapters 1, 11 and 12 (which greatly improved the text) and to Neil Middleton and other friends at Earthscan for encouraging us to prepare this book and keeping faith with it, despite the delays. Thanks too to Sian Mills for overseeing its production and Kate Griffin for its promotion.

We are also grateful to Bob Novick and Greg Goldstein at the World Health Organization's Programme on Environmental Health in Rural and Urban Development and Housing (the RUD Programme) not only for their contributions to the text but also for their encouragement and advice. Special thanks are also due to the International NGO Programme of the Canadian International Development Agency (especially its Director, Ron Leger) and to the Dutch Ministry of Housing, Physical Planning and the Environment who funded the research on which chapters 2, 3 and 4 are based.

A considerable part of the text draws from research in which the editors have been involved. Jorge Hardoy and David Satterthwaite have been working on the links between inadequate housing and poor health since 1981, as part of a collaborative programme of research with the Centre for Urban and Regional Studies (CEUR) in Buenos Aires, the Lagos Group for the Study of Human Settlements (Nigeria) and the International Institute for Development Research, Allahabad (India). This work examined the health problems faced by the inhabitants of certain illegal settlements in Allahabad, Buenos Aires and Lagos and considered the extent to which such problems are linked to housing and environment. This research also had action components as researchers worked with inhabitants to seek new ways to tackle the more serious health problems. The Human Settlements Programme of the Instituto Internacional de Medio Ambiente y Desarrollo (IIED-America Latina) in Buenos Aires and the International Institute for Environment and Development (IIED) in London plans to continue and expand its work programme in this subject since the complementarities between programmes to improve housing and living conditions and to improve health are still ignored by many governments and international agencies and the methodologies for establishing these complementarities and operationalizing them within policies, programmes and projects remains poorly understood.

There is a considerable network of individuals and research groups on whose work this book has drawn. We list some of the most useful and accessible books and papers in the section on "Suggested Further Reading". Neither the text nor this list does justice to the many researchers and practitioners who, throughout the Third World, are demanding new approaches to "development" which not only place the health and well-being of people at the centre of the concern but also recognize that any intervention by outside agencies must be shaped by these people's priorities both in its design and in its implementation. We hope this book will help reinforce their efforts.

Sandy Cairncross, London School of Hygiene and Tropical Medicine
Jorge E. Hardoy, IIED-America Latina, Buenos Aires
David Satterthwaite, IIED, London

1st August, 1990.

Foreword

Robert E. Novick, Responsible Officer, Environmental Health in Rural and Urban Development and Housing (RUD), World Health Organization, Geneva, Switzerland.

All constituents of the environment of our planet – rainforests, troposphere, seas and biological environment – ultimately exert an influence on human health and well-being. However, the environment which exerts the greatest and most immediate influence on the lives of people, their health and well-being, is the intimate environment of their home and neighbourhood. A health-promoting home and urban environment embody the fundamental aspirations of the majority of people, where the quality of their lives depends on having a clean, decent, safe home in which to live and raise a family. The title of this book aptly portrays the pervasive implications of degraded living environments for the majority of populations in Third World cities as well as significant numbers of city dwellers in developed countries.

The book is an important contribution to greater understanding and increased awareness about the effects of the home environment on our health and well-being. All factors of the physical environment – air, water, light, space, temperature, land – and many factors of the biological environment are relevant. These are intertwined with social factors such as poverty, educational achievement, the role of women, the right to property, nutrition, migration and democratic governance.

We know that poor housing is always associated with high rates of morbidity and mortality. The complexity of the relationship has obscured precise epidemiologic expression of the health burden. This, in turn, has hindered understanding on the part of the general public and governments of the relative importance of housing to human health and well-being. For this, and other reasons, housing generally is not high on the list of societal needs and governmental priorities.

The attention paid to health in housing by the media and by

governments is largely directed towards the issue of "protection", in other words protecting residents from unwarranted disease, injury and discomfort. This entails the provision of adequate and safe water supply, the disposal of human and other wastes, the provision of drainage, the control of insect and rodent vectors of disease, controlling indoor and outdoor air quality, the use of safe building materials, protection against climatic extremes and controlling noise. These and many other safeguards are regulated by means of building codes, housing occupancy codes, plumbing and electrical codes, air and water pollution regulations, zoning laws and land subdivision regulations. These types of legally promulgated protection are a common feature of national and local government in Europe, North America and Australasia where they are more or less well enforced. In many Third World countries, these safeguards either do not exist, or they are based on obsolete colonial legal/technical concepts. But even where they exist, enforcement is ineffective. WHO has estimated that if all housing could be brought to minimum acceptable standards there would be five million fewer deaths and two million fewer permanent disabilities annually on a global basis.

Approaches to health in housing must always maintain a central focus on people. The way in which people *use* their housing environment is intimately interwoven with both negative and positive influences on their health. The best safe water system and facilities for safe disposal of excreta will do little to protect against the spread of communicable disease unless properly used for personal and domestic cleanliness. No amount of land-use planning and zoning can ensure a pleasant and safe neighbourhood if the residents allow it to deteriorate. There are, however, limits to what the people can achieve with good intentions and conscientious effort. Societal and governmental responsibilities are the other side of the coin. This is readily exemplified in such matters as refuse removal and provision of water supply in cities where large populations and high population densities make it impossible for individual residents and families to provide satisfactory services for themselves. In such situations, satisfactory services depend upon institutional arrangements.

There is, however, a further dimension to health in housing. This pertains to consideration of the home as a positive contribution to, and reinforcement of, human health and well-being. It is a subtle relationship. The World Health Organization has defined health as a state of complete physical, mental and social well-being and not merely the absence of disease or infirmity. The importance of housing is sometimes questioned, taking into account that there is no human function which requires a house for its performance. However, in the context of WHO's definition, the significance of the home environment to health assumes much greater importance and meaning. A home is essential as a place for contemplation, comfort and leisure; for learning and socialization of the young; a place for security and sleep; for eating and personal hygiene; a place for nurturing the family – the fundamental building block of society. These are values which are familiar to us all and yet cannot be defined in technical terms.

I propose a goal, as a practical step towards health-promoting housing. It is a goal which goes beyond the concept of protection to include the positive values of health. The goal is phrased in terms of the ideal community in which any person would wish to live in order to raise a family and progress through life. Such a community would have the following characteristics:

1. Clean, decent and safe housing of ample size for the family, together with pleasant surroundings, facilities for recreation and social intercourse.
2. Satisfying employment providing an acceptable standard of living and a sufficient quantity and variety of food.
3. An environment where people would not be subject to local health hazards, whether from communicable diseases, including water and food borne infections and those spread by poor sanitary conditions and insect and rodent vectors; chemical hazards such as air pollution, adulterated or contaminated foods; or physical hazards such as excessive road traffic, earthquakes or floods.
4. Efficient health and social services including: *preventive health services* to safeguard against environmental hazards, but also provide for immunizations, maternal and child health care, health education and occupational health; *medical services* for outpatients and an adequately staffed hospital; and *social welfare services* ensuring financial provision for sickness, unemployment and old age and including care for handicapped people.
5. Participatory government arranging essential physical infrastructure, police and fire protection services, education and judicial services and responding to the desires of the citizens for enjoyment of life, the development of personality and freedom from undue stress and anxiety.

This health goal is neither revolutionary, utopian nor unfeasible. Each provision is a current objective of health workers and society in general. It should be recognized that most communities currently have acceptable experience with at least some of the listed provisions, and the shortcomings, although enormous in a global sense, are also within humanity's long term capability.

The short term outlook for health in housing is bleak. Conservative estimates indicate that more than one billion people in cities throughout the world live in grossly inadequate housing bordering on squalor, and more than one hundred million have no housing whatsoever. The major developmental trends which could influence this situation are also unfavourable i.e. global population growth, rapid urbanization and debilitating debt in many Third World countries. These are times which call for courage and determination on the part of all people working for social and economic development and improvement of the living environment. Over the years I have found a note of encouragement wherever I had the opportunity to visit low-income communities. It seems that no matter how desperate the economic or environmental situation, there are always a few resourceful individuals and families who are able to make a clean and welcoming human refuge, and that groups of people, working together, can create a pleasant community. There is always something that can be done by conscientious self-reliant people to improve their home environment. Governments and societies in general can and must do more to support the natural inclinations of people everywhere to improve and use their housing environment so that its health potential can be realized to the full.

This book is a substantial contribution to the literature on health in housing. It achieves its aims of clarifying the relationship between selected factors of the housing environment and health and also of contributing to much greater awareness of the importance of health in housing to the human family.

INTRODUCTION

Sandy Cairncross, Jorge E. Hardoy and David Satterthwaite

The scale of the problem

Most poor people die young in the Third World. Half of all deaths are infants or children; in many poor communities, half of all deaths are children under five years of age. In western Europe, North America and other prosperous regions, 80 per cent of the population live for over 65 years; in the South, only a quarter live to this age.[1] In the Third World, poor people's lives are characterized by almost continuous ill-health; a high proportion are also disabled (for instance by polio or from injuries arising from household or workplace accidents which receive inadequate treatment).[2]

Certain statistics give an idea of the severity of these problems. In many Third World nations, a child born today is 15–20 times more likely to die before the age of five than a child born in a prosperous western nation.[3] Among many poorer households in Third World nations, the child is 40–50 times more likely to die before the age of five than a child born in the West.[4] A woman born poor in the Third World is 150 times more likely to die in pregnancy or childbirth than a woman in Europe or North America.[5] Infants and children in the Third World are several hundred times more likely to die from diarrhoea, pneumonia and measles than those in Europe or North America; these are the most common causes of child death in the Third World. In 1986, an estimated 14.1 million children under five years of age died; 98 per cent were in the Third World.[6]

In many of the poorest Third World nations, between a quarter and a third of all children die before the age of five; among the poorer families within these nations, one child in two may die before the age of five. This compares with a rate of less than 1 child in 100 dying before the age of five in the richest nations.

For the rich, rates of infant and child mortality in Third World nations are often as low as those in western nations. But amongst poor families, for every child who dies, many more live on in hunger and ill-health; on average, children in these families under five have survived ten attacks of diarrhoea.[7] Around a quarter of the Third World's children are malnourished, which reduces their energy, stunts their growth, lowers their resistance to disease and impairs their intellectual attainments.[8] Their nutritional weakness is often exacerbated by parasitic worm infections which afflict more than a quarter of the world's population.

Other statistics give an idea of how many people suffer. One estimate suggests that some 2.2 billion people live in poverty in the Third World.[9] Nine out of ten of them have no access to safe drinking water, most have no primary health care service and one child in four is of low birth weight.[10] In the absence of sophisticated equipment and highly trained medical personnel, a high proportion of low birth-weight children die before the age of one. Fewer than half the mothers receive adequate care from qualified personnel during their pregnancy and only one child in seven will receive vaccinations which protect them from such common childhood killers as diphtheria, tetanus and whooping cough.[11] Some 500,000 women die each year from pregnancy-related causes, 99 per cent of them in the Third World.[12] More than 750,000 newborn babies (and many of their mothers) die of neo-natal tetanus each year – virtually all of them in the Third World. A measure as simple as immunizing women against tetanus would considerably reduce both infant and maternal deaths.

Poor people in Europe and North America also suffer more ill health and premature death than richer groups. But in the Third World, the problem is of a much larger scale and severity; a far higher proportion of the population are poor and their health problems are much more severe. In around two-thirds of all Third World nations, the poor are the majority as a result of their lack of income, capital resources or productive land. This means that they use virtually all their resources on daily necessities (especially food) and have a very limited capacity to pay for housing or basic services (including health services). But even in most of the wealthier Third World nations, between a quarter and half the population are also too poor to be able to spend much on such necessities. If the government does not ensure that there is an effective preventative and curative health care system – and that everyone can find accommodation with piped water, sanitation, cooking and washing facilities and sufficient space – the poorer groups will continue to suffer from easily preventable disease, disablement and premature death.

Table 1.1: The world's most prevalent diseases

Diseases	Number of People Infected
Vaccine-preventable diseases	
Tuberculosis*	1,700 million
Measles*	49 million
Whooping cough (Pertussis)*	46 million
Tetanus*	1.5 million
Polio*	200 thousand
Diphtheria*	›23 thousand
Tropical diseases	
Malaria*	270 million
Schistosomiasis*	200 million
Filariasis*	90 million
Chagas' Disease*	15–18 million
River Blindness*	18 million
Leishmaniasis*	12 million
Leprosy*	10–12 million
Guinea worm*	5–10 million
African sleeping sickness (new cases)	›20 thousand
Diarrhoeal diseases	
Amoebiasis*	480 million
Giardiasis*	200 million
Typhoid*	1 million
Cholera*	›40 thousand
Sexually transmitted diseases (new cases)	
Trichomoniasis	120 million
Genital Chlamydia	50 million
Genital Papillomavirus	30 million
Gonorrhoea	25 million
Genital herpes	20 million
AIDS virus	5–10 million
Syphilis	3.5 million
Endemic Treponematoses	2.5 million
Chancroid	2 million
Other Infectious and parasitic diseases	
Hepatitis B	2,000 million
Ascariasis*	700 million
Hookworm*	700–900 million

Diseases	*Number of People Infected*
Trichuriasis*	500 million
Dengue*	30–60 million
Toxoplasmosis	420 thousand
Rabies*	35 thousand
Yellow Fever*	10-25 thousand
Endocrine and nutritional diseases	
Iodine deficiency*	200 million
Diabetes (Third World)	40 million
Vitamin A deficiency*	40 million
Others	
Cardiovascular diseases (deaths)	12 million
Pneumonia (deaths)*	4.8 million
Anaemia*	1,500 million
Mental disorders	200 million
Drug abuse	›85 million
Trachoma*	6-9 million
Cancer (new cases)	6.4 million
Meningococcal Meningitis	›65 thousand
Brucellosis	›80 thousand

Source: World Health Organization, 1990, see note 13. Note that many people are infected with multiple diseases; tuberculosis infects 1.7 billion but only 20 million are sick. From the 5–10 million people infected with the AIDS virus, only some 400,000 are sick with AIDS.

Table 1.1 lists the 48 most prevalent diseases worldwide while Table 1.2 lists the most common causes of death. Those marked with an asterisk could be enormously reduced at a relatively low per capita cost through improved housing and living conditions, better nutrition and comprehensive coverage of primary health care. For instance, vaccinations could radically reduce the number of deaths and infections from tuberculosis, measles, whooping cough, tetanus, polio and diphtheria – together saving each year several million lives and tens of millions of people from ill health. Improved water and sanitation and the wider availability of simple, inexpensive oral rehydration salts would cut enormously the number of people who die or suffer regularly from diarrhoeal diseases. Improved water and sanitation would greatly reduce the incidence of most parasitic worms – including schistosomiasis, hookworm and roundworm – especially if combined with treatment (it is common for half or more of the population in low income settlements to have one or more intestinal parasite). Pneumonia, one of the main causes of child death in the Third World, can be reduced with better nutrition, immunization against other childhood diseases (since these often combine with pneumonia to cause death) and by equipping mothers with the knowledge of how to diagnose it.[14] If no action is taken to address these most serious health problems, in the next ten years 200 million people may die prematurely from preventable causes.[15]

With few exceptions, the causes of diseases and death in the Third World are no less a factor in urban areas than they are in the countryside. While average rates of disease, malnutrition and death for many cities are lower than in the surrounding rural areas, they are held down by the presence in such cities of a high proportion of the nation's middle and upper income classes who enjoy a relatively good standard of health. By contrast, the poor in urban areas generally live in overcrowded tenements, cheap boarding houses or illegal housing and usually suffer comparable or even higher rates of disease and death than their rural counterparts. The close proximity of large numbers of people, in an environment which provides no protection from the pollution caused by their own and other city wastes creates conditions very favourable to the rapid spread of a variety of infectious diseases, often in disastrous epidemics.

The focus of the book

This book highlights the very high levels of ill-health and premature death among lower-income groups in urban centres of the Third World and further it examines their links with housing and living conditions. It seeks to highlight the fact that a substantial proportion of such ill-health and premature death can be prevented by relatively inexpensive health care systems combined with other projects and programmes, whose initiation and running is not necessarily the responsibility of trained medical personnel.

The book concentrates on the roles and responsibilities of people other than health specialists in promoting good health: architects, planners, engineers and teachers, community leaders, and local and national government departments concerned with housing, building, planning and public works. It also concentrates on the physical infrastructure needed in all residential areas for good health (piped water supplies, drains, roads, all-weather paths), and on the services – in addition to health services – their inhabitants need (for instance the regular collection of household wastes and emergency services to respond to accidents). It is often forgotten that the remarkable decline in mortality rates and improvements in health in Europe and North America in the late-nineteenth century and early-twentieth century owe more to improved nutrition and improvements in water supply, sanitation and other aspects of housing and living conditions than they do to medical establishments.[16]

Table 1.2: The world's most common causes of death from disease

Diseases	*Annual Deaths*
Vaccine-preventable diseases	
Tuberculosis*	3 million
Measles*	1.5 million
Whooping cough (Pertussis)*	500 thousand
Tetanus (neo-natal)*	775 thousand
Tropical diseases	
Malaria*	1-2 million
Schistosomiasis*	200 thousand
African sleeping sickness*	20 thousand
*Diarrhoeal diseases**	5 million
Other infectious and parasitic diseases	
Hepatitis B	1-2 million
Hookworm*	50-60 thousand
Others	
Cardiovascular diseases	12 million
Pneumonia*	4.8 million
Chronic obstructive lung disease	2.7 million
Cancer	4.8 million
Maternal mortality*	500 thousand
Aids virus	200 thousand

Source: World Health Organization, 1990, see note 13. Note that the cause of death is often a result of several factors – for instance malnutrition weakens the body's defence against disease and death from pneumonia is often caused by a body weak from measles or diarrhoea or malnutrition.

The authors of the different chapters all have long experience working in the Third World; most are themselves citizens and residents of Third World nations. The urban context is discussed in Chapter 1: the scale of the Third World's urban population, the deficiencies in the provision of basic infrastructure and services and the reasons why these deficiencies demand more attention. It also outlines the links between housing problems and health problems and the reasons why, to date, the health aspects of housing have been ignored. It ends by proposing a new framework for understanding and identifying health problems.

Chapters 2, 3 and 4 describe the housing and health conditions faced by poorer groups in certain districts in very different cities – Buenos Aires (Argentina), Lagos (Nigeria) and Allahabad (India). They illustrate the conditions under which poorer groups live; housing and health conditions in these districts are not dissimilar to those in many other districts in each of these cities. The lack of basic services and infrastructure is not dissimilar to that suffered by most other low income groups in other urban areas of the Third World. The scale and nature of housing problems in any city are influenced by many factors which differ from city to city – for instance, the prosperity of the city's economy, the distribution of income among the population, the pattern of land ownership and laws concerning land ownership rights, government policies and the attitude of government and the judicial system to illegal settlements and to political struggles around the issue of shelter.[17] But what is more uniform and comparable in each city is the inadequate standard evident in housing used by poorer groups, the indoor space available per person, the quality of basic infrastructures and the availability of basic services.

Chapters 5 to 10 describe the infrastructure and services which are essential for good health: safe and sufficient supplies of water; sewers or other means for the removal of excreta and households' waste water from the human environment; drainage; regular removal and disposal of household garbage; technical and financial support for households and community organizations to remove disease vectors from their living environment; and emergency life-saving services with an emphasis on reducing risks and people's vulnerability to accidents. Each chapter outlines the needs and considers how they can be met.

These chapters include many examples of innovative projects which have met local needs, despite the limited resources available to local governments and the limited capacity of local people to pay for services. Many can be judged as successful in comparison to what had been done before they were implemented. But these are not proposed as models for replication elsewhere. They are given as illustrations of how and in what form solutions were sought which were more appropriate to the local context, making best use of local resources and overcoming local constraints. Each has relevance to other districts, cities and nations but more in how new solutions were sought and who was involved than in what was actually done.

Chapter 11 considers two kinds of urban future for the Third World: a future in which no changes are made in the current approaches of governments and aid agencies or the future which unfolds if lessons are drawn from current failures and new solutions sought.

Chapter 12 is about new attempts to achieve more healthy cities. It discusses the new alliances between local governments, professionals and community organizations. It also discusses the role of privatization and of NGOs within this new approach, as well as the role of national governments.

This book is one of three volumes published by Earthscan which seek to summarize conditions, trends and problems in urban areas of the Third World. This volume does not dwell in detail on such questions as the scale, nature and distribution of urban change in the Third World and on the effectiveness of governments' response to such changes; those are covered in more detail in *Squatter Citizen: Life in the Urban Third World* by Jorge E. Hardoy and David Satterthwaite, published in 1989 (this book also includes a detailed discussion of the effectiveness of governments' housing policies and an overview of environmental problems in Third World cities). Nor does *The Poor Die Young* consider in detail the issue of urban land and the extent to which poor people's housing problems are rooted in their exclusion from the legal land market; this and other legal aspects of improving housing and living conditions are the subject of *Urban Land and Shelter for the Poor* by Patrick McAuslan, a new edition of which is to be published later in 1991.

Chapter One

THE URBAN CONTEXT

Sandy Cairncross, Jorge E. Hardoy
and David Satterthwaite

Urbanization without health

In recent decades, most Third World nations have experienced a very rapid growth in their urban populations without the needed expansion in public provision. The result is that in virtually every urban centre – from the large cities to regional centres and small market towns – many people live in neighbourhoods with little or no provision of the infrastructure, services and facilities that are essential for health. In addition, many live in cramped, overcrowded dwellings such as tenements, cheap boarding houses or shelters built on illegally occupied or sub-divided land.

Some 1.3 billion people live in urban centres in the Third World;[1] there are now more urban dwellers in the Third World than in Europe, North America and Japan combined. In most Third World nations, the number of rural inhabitants still outnumbers those in urban areas (in many nations by a factor of three or more), but there is a long term, well-established trend towards increasingly urban societies. In most nations, the economic, social and political factors which drive urbanization are unlikely to stop before a majority of people live in urban areas.[2]

Virtually all Third World governments have failed to ensure that rapid urban growth has been accompanied by investments in services, especially in the poorer areas. As will be discussed later, few national governments gave any priority to increasing the resources available to the city and local governments which were meant to cope with this growth. The result was an escalation in the number of people living in very overcrowded conditions and in illegal or informal settlements. Chapters 2 and 4 illustrate some ways in which poorer groups sought to solve their own housing problems. In Buenos Aires, this took the form of a well-organized invasion of vacant land on the city periphery by over 20,000 people. In Allahabad, poorer people built illegal settlements on small pockets of vacant land and sought through negotiation to be allowed to stay there. Chapter 3 illustrates the development of tenements: In Olalaye, the landowners in what had been a peripheral village to Lagos developed shacks in which individual rooms were rented out to households, as the village became engulfed by Lagos's expansion.

There are hundreds of such case studies describing the development of the different illegal or informal settlements where most new housing has been developed in Third World cities over the last 30–40 years.[3] These case studies reveal the ingenuity with which new settlements have been built at a low monetary cost and with scarce resources; they often demonstrate a sophisticated capacity among poorer groups to organize and plan.[4] But individual ingenuity and collective organization among low-income households cannot address problems of no paved roads, drains and sewers, no piped water and no services to collect garbage and treat accidents, injuries and illness in the absence of outside support. Even where community organization does seek some solution to some of these, as described in Chapter 2, this is often undermined by the hostility of the public authorities to the settlement's very existence. Nor can we expect such examples of collective organization to multiply to the point where they make a major impact on solving shelter problems for poorer groups, within the current economic climate and when such groups have so little possibility of access to cheap credit and technical support.

It is impossible to estimate with any precision what proportion of the 1.3 billion urban dwellers live in inadequate housing with inadequate provision for water, sanitation and other basic needs. Case studies of specific cities show that it is common for between 30 and 60 per cent of the population to live either in illegal settlements or in tenements and cheap boarding houses. But most of these case studies are of large cities, when in fact a high proportion of the urban inhabitants in most Third World nations live in relatively small urban centres. Estimates for 1990 suggest that less than 2.5 per cent of the Third World's urban population lived in cities with 10 million or more inhabitants and less than 25 per cent live in cities with 100,000 or more inhabitants.[5]

In most small urban centres – and in many of the larger cities in the poorest Third World nations – the proportion of people living in illegal settlements may be less than that suggested by case studies of large cities. Part of the reason would be less monetized land markets. In addition, in many of the least-urbanized nations, traditional land tenure systems limit an individual's right to own, buy and sell land and this has made it easier for poorer households to obtain land for housing.[6] Despite smaller proportions of people living in illegal settlements in such urban centres, the proportions living in areas with inadequate infrastructure and services may be as high or higher than in the largest cities in richer Third World nations – the inadequacies stemming less from their illegal status and more from lower incomes and weaker local governments.

Drawing from estimates made by the World Health Organization, in 1985 a quarter of the Third World's urban population had no access to adequate, safe water supplies and half had no adequate sanitation system. While there has been considerable progress during the 1980s (designated the International Drinking Water Supply and Sanitation Decade) in increasing the number of people reached with better water and improved sanitation, these figures certainly understate the number of people inadequately served. First, the criteria used to define an "adequate" water supply are open to question. For instance, the availability of a water tap within 100 metres of a house is often considered adequate yet as Chapter 5 describes, this is not necessarily adequate for good health.

In addition, figures for the proportion of people adequately served come from statistics supplied by governments – and governments are known to exaggerate these figures. For instance, they may assume that all those with water taps in their settlements are adequately served – but there are often so few communal water taps that people have to wait for a long time in queues. This acts to cut water consumption below volumes needed for good health. In addition, piped water systems in many tropical cities function only intermittently, for a few hours each day, which makes it especially difficult for households relying on communal taps. The water in piped systems is often of doubtful quality due to the risk of contamination in old and leaky distribution pipes by groundwater and sewage. Many households and settlements judged by governments to be adequately served by public systems may resort to other water sources because of the problems mentioned above or they may not be able to afford to purchase the water they need. Official figures for many of the poorer Third World nations claim that over 80 per cent of the urban population had access to safe water in the mid-1980s including 100 per cent coverage in Nigeria and Liberia and 99 per cent coverage in Togo.[7] Local specialists find it hard to reconcile these figures with the reality in the urban centres in which they work.

We estimate that at least 600 million people living in urban areas of the Third World live in what might be termed life and health threatening homes and neighbourhoods. Perhaps as many (if not more) have inadequate access to effective health care – although again, official statistics provided by governments claim much better coverage (some as much as 99–100 per cent) than that known to exist in reality.[8]

Virtually all the homes and neighbourhoods of poorer groups share two characteristics with serious impacts on health: the presence in the environment of pathogenic micro-organisms (especially those in human excreta) and crowded, cramped housing conditions.

A lack of readily available drinking water, of sewerage connections (or other systems to dispose of human wastes), of garbage collection and basic measures to prevent disease and provide health care ensure that many diseases are endemic: diarrhoea, dysenteries, typhoid, intestinal parasites and food poisoning among them. These combined with malnutrition so weaken the body's defences that measles, pneumonia and other common childhood diseases become major killers.

Most urban centres in Africa and Asia – including many cities with a million or more inhabitants – have no sewerage system at all.[9] As later chapters will describe in more detail, rivers, streams, canals, gullies and ditches are where most human excrement and household wastes end up, untreated. For those cities with a sewage system, it is rare for more than a small proportion of the population – typically the richer, residential, government and commercial areas – to be served. Garbage collection services are inadequate or non-existent in most residential areas; an estimated 30–50 per cent of the solid wastes generated within urban centres is left uncollected.[10] It accumulates on streets, open spaces between houses and wasteland, causing or contributing to serious health problems. And it is poorer households who suffer most since it is overwhelmingly the poorer areas where there are no services to collect garbage or where service levels are very inadequate. Box 1.1 illustrates these inadequacies in water, sanitation and garbage collection in different cities.

Box 1.1: Inadequacies in water supply, sanitation and garbage collection

BANGKOK: About one-third of the population has no access to public water and must obtain water from vendors. Only two per cent of the population is connected to a sewer system; human wastes are generally disposed of through septic tanks and cess pools and their effluents – as well as waste water from sinks, laundries, baths and kitchens – are discharged into stormwater drains or canals. In 1987, around a quarter of solid wastes generated in the city remained uncollected and were dumped, mostly onto vacant land or in canals and rivers.

CALCUTTA: Some 3 million people live in "bustees" and refugee settlements which lack potable water, endure serious annual flooding and have no systematic means of disposing of refuse or human wastes. Some 2.5 million others live in similarly blighted and unserviced areas. Piped water is only available in the central city and parts of some other municipalities. The sewerage system is limited to only a third of the area in the urban core. Poor maintenance of drains and periodic clogging of the system have made flooding an annual feature.

DAKAR AND OTHER SENEGALESE TOWNS: Senegalese towns have no provision for the removal of household and public waste. Of the five urban centres with sewage systems, generally only the inner urban population has access to these facilities. In Dakar, the capital, a survey in 1980–81 found that 28 per cent of households have private water connections while 68 per cent rely on public standpipes and 4.2 per cent on buying water from carriers. A survey in Pikine, the outer part of Dakar, found an average of 696 persons per standpipe with 1,513 in one neighbourhood. In Dakar, nearly one-sixth of all human faeces are dumped outside proper toilet facilities.

DAR ES SALAAM: From a survey of 660 households drawn from all income levels in 1986–87, 47 per cent had no piped water supply either inside or immediately outside their houses while 32 per cent had a shared piped-water supply. Of the households without piped water, 67 per cent buy water from neighbours while 26 per cent draw water from public water-kiosks or standpipes. Only 7.1 per cent buy water from water sellers. The average water consumption is only 23.6 litres per person per day. Only 13 per cent of the dirty

Box 1.1: (continued)

water and sewage produced is regularly disposed of. Of the 660 households, 89 per cent had simple pit-latrines. Only 4.5 per cent had toilets connected to septic tanks or sewers. Most households have to share sanitary facilities. Overflowing latrines are a serious problem, especially in the rainy season, and provision to empty septic tanks or latrines is very inadequate. Only a quarter of the city refuse is collected.

JAKARTA: Less than a quarter of the city's population has direct connections to a piped water system; some 30 per cent depend solely on water vendors with water costing five times that of piped water. The city has no waterborne sewerage system. Septic tanks serve about 25 per cent of the city's population; others use pit-latrines, cesspools and ditches along the roadside. Much of the population has to use drainage canals for bathing, laundering and defecation. Around 30 per cent of the garbage is not collected and ends up in canals and rivers and along the roadsides where it clogs drainage channels and causes extensive flooding during the rainy season.

KARACHI: Potable water has to be brought more than 160 kilometres from the Indus and is available for only a few hours a day in most areas. One-third of households have piped water connections and most slum dwellers and squatters must either use public standposts or buy water from vendors at inflated prices. Only one-third of the solid wastes produced in the city are being removed.

KHARTOUM: The systems of water supply, sewage disposal, refuse disposal and electricity supply are all inadequate both in the coverage of the urban area and the maintenance of the service. The water supply system is working beyond its design capacity while the demand continues to rise. The coverage is poor, with the low-income groups in squatter settlements suffering the cost of all through paying the most for water, often bought from vendors. Breakdown and cuts in the supply system are common. The municipal sewerage system serves only about 5 per cent of the Khartoum urban area. Even that system is susceptible to breakdowns when waste is discharged either directly into the river or onto open land. For most people in the low-income areas, there is no system of sewage disposal.

KINSHASA: There is no sewerage sytem in Kinshasa. Around half

Box 1.1: (continued)

the urban population (some 1.5 million people) are not served by a piped-water network. High income areas are often 100 per cent connected while many other areas have 20–30 per cent of houses connected: essentially those along the main roads. The sale of water flourishes in areas far from the network – in these areas water is usually obtained from wells or the river. Household waste is only collected from a few residential areas. In the rest of the city, household waste is dumped on roadsides, on illegal dumps, in stormwater drains or buried in open spaces.

MADRAS: Only 2 million of the 3.7 million residential consumers within the service area of the local water supply and sewerage board are connected to the system. On average, they receive some 36 litres per capita per day. The rest within the service area must use public taps which serve about 240 persons per tap. Another million consumers outside the service area must rely on wells – but supplies are inadequate here too because of falling groundwater levels. The sewerage system serves 31 per cent of the metropolitan population and raw sewage flows freely into the metropolitan area's natural watercourses at many points.

MANILA: Only 15 per cent of the population of Metro Manila is served with sewers or individual septic tanks. Some 1.8 million people lack adequate water supplies – as well as educational, community, health and sanitary services. Inadequate collection of domestic wastes also means that garbage blocks canals and drains and makes flooding problems much more serious.

SAO PAULO: Of the more than 13 million people living in the metropolitan area, 64 per cent lived in households not served by the sewage system in 1980, and very little sewage was treated. One-third of the population live in areas with no service to collect household wastes.

SOURCE: Jorge E. Hardoy and David Satterthwaite, *Squatter Citizen: Life in the Urban Third World* (London: Earthscan Publications, 1989), see note 11 for a full list of references.

A second characteristic common to most of the homes and neighbourhoods of poorer groups is crowded, cramped conditions. This ensures that diseases such as tuberculosis, influenza and meningitis are easily transmitted from one person to another – their spread often being helped by low resistance among the inhabitants due to malnutrition. Many of the households whose living conditions are described in Chapters 3 and 4 have less than one square metre of space per person in their homes. In the most extreme cases, even small rooms are subdivided to allow multiple occupancy, as in Hong Kong where many people live in beds stacked three high in dormitories, with each bed surrounded by a cage (for privacy and protection against robbbery). In one dormitory, 130 persons were found living in this way.[12] In Calcutta, in the "hotbed" system, bunks stacked one above the other in tiny rooms are available for rent by the hour, with two or more persons renting the bed within any 24 hour period.

Household accidents are also common in overcrowded conditions (see Chapter 10). This is hardly surprising when many people live together in one room and there is little chance of giving the occupants (especially children) protection from fires, stoves and kerosene heaters.

Health risks from overcrowding and lack of infrastructure and services are often further exacerbated by dangers from the sites on which houses are built. Large clusters of illegal housing often develop on steep hillsides, on floodplains or in desertland. Poor groups build on such sites because they are cheap or because their illegal occupation of such sites is less likely to be threatened since the land is unsuitable for commercial developments. Storm and surface water drains are rarely installed in most new residential developments. Frequent flooding, water-logged sites, lack of paved roads or paths and damp housing all take a serious toll on health. For most low-income groups, house sites, structures and surrounds increase the risk of falls, burns, scalds, cuts, bites and injuries in and around the house.

The impact of such injuries is further magnified by a lack of provision for first aid and the difficulties in transporting a sick or injured person to hospital (and, of course, ensuring that the person will receive rapid treatment once they arrive). A lack of paved roads and inaccessible sites also mean that in the event of fires or other emergencies, neither fire engines nor ambulances can reach the settlement, at least not without long delays (see Chapter 10 for more details).

The current economic crisis is reducing the purchasing power of poorer groups and diminishing even further their capacity to pay for improved housing or services. During the 1980s, average incomes are reported to have fallen by 10 per cent in most of Latin America and over 20 per cent in sub-Saharan Africa while in many urban areas, real minimum wages have declined as much as 50 per cent.[13] Field studies from many different areas suggest that malnutrition is increasing which in turn means that lower income groups are more vulnerable to diseases.

The economic crisis is also forcing most governments to cut social expenditure; the result is often a decline in what were already very inadequate levels of investment in water, sanitation, garbage collection and health care. The per capita expenditures on health in Third World nations were already very low at the beginning of the 1980s: an average of US $4 per person per year in 92 Third World nations compared to an average of $220 per person per year in 32 rich nations. In this same year, in a third of the Third World nations, spending per person per year was less than $2.[14] Even the meagre resources allocated to health care often went largely to curative-based hospitals in one or two major cities which provided services for a very small proportion of the national population and represents one of the least cost-effective ways of improving health.[15]

Health spending per person has declined in most nations since 1980. The 1990 edition of *The State of the World's Children* reported that a decline in health spending per person has been documented in more than three-quarters of the nations of Africa and Latin America in recent years and that the decline is almost certainly more widespread than the statistics suggest: "Hundreds of health clinics have been closed down, and many which remain open are understaffed and lacking essential supplies".[16] This report also stated that infant mortality is known to have risen in parts of Latin America and sub-Saharan Africa and the incidence of low birth-weight (a sensitive indicator of women's well-being) had increased in 7 of the 15 nations for which recent information was available.[17] Cuts in governments' social expenditure are often demanded by outside agencies before aid (or balance of payments support) is given.

It is a truism to say that what unites poorer groups everywhere is an inadequate income. But it is this inadequate income which underlies the housing and health deficiencies they suffer. Higher incomes would allow more to be spent on housing (so poorer groups could afford to rent, purchase or build better quality accommodation). More could also be spent on health services. The higher the proportion of city-dwellers unable to afford adequate homes and private health care, the higher the proportion that will die young. This fact has led many specialists to stress the need for income-generating projects as a higher priority than the improvement of housing and health services. Higher incomes for poorer groups, it is argued, would mean that they could find their own housing solutions in the private market and pay for private health care.

In practice, there are many reasons why a concentration on improving poorer groups' incomes is only a very partial solution. First, it is difficult to increase these groups' incomes to the point where they can meet their own housing and health needs within the private market. To do so implies not only ensuring an increasingly prosperous city economy but also that it should fundamentally change so that a much higher proportion of the benefits flowed to the poor. For most urban centres in the Third World, this would demand a scale and level of intervention far beyond the means of governments and outside agencies. Secondly, even if poorer groups' incomes do improve, it does not mean that their housing conditions necessarily do so. Landowners and landlords may be the main beneficiaries as the price of land for housing and rental accommodation rises to reflect the increased capacity to pay.

But the most relevant argument against concentrating only on improving incomes is the fact that well designed and implemented government actions to improve housing, infrastructure and services are not expensive and a high proportion of costs can be recovered by charges that even many of the poor can afford. The poor may lack sufficient income to represent a profitable market for private sector enterprises in the provision of good quality housing and basic services. However, governments can achieve economies of scale in the provision of many kinds of infrastructure and services such that the costs of their provision are not beyond most households' capacity to pay. Governments need to be flexible to achieve this – the quality of infrastructure and services in different areas can be linked to capacity to pay but with everyone entitled to certain minimum standards. Later chapters will present examples of innovative approaches which greatly improved the provision of infrastructure and services, but at much lower per capita costs than in conventional projects. Ironically, it is often the richer households and businesses in cities – not the poor – who are paying far less for the publicly-provided infrastructure and services they use than the real cost of their provision.[18] One of the most important untapped sources of funds for government investment in infrastructure and services could come from charging the rich more realistic rates – although the political difficulties in doing so are obvious.

This book is about developing new approaches to improving housing, infrastructure and services which reach a far higher proportion of those in need at a cost which is affordable both to the users and to the government. As the final two chapters elaborate in more detail, to achieve this demands two preconditions. The first is developing the capacity within local government to work with local populations in identifying local problems and devising the most appropriate local solutions. The second is for local governments to develop new ways of working with the community organizations formed by low-income groups in their settlements to ensure that basic levels of infrastructure and services are provided and maintained and that health care provision meets the most pressing needs.

Justifying a concentration on urban problems

This book concentrates on housing and health problems in urban areas of the Third World. Although some of the techniques and organizational innovations described in Chapters 5 to 12 are drawn from rural examples or are urban examples which have relevance to many rural settings, the concentration remains urban. As in the two other books published as companion volumes to this,[19] in choosing to concentrate on the needs of urban inhabitants and the failure of government to work with these people in meeting their needs, we do not imply that the needs of rural inhabitants are less pressing. We do not suggest that housing and health problems are in general worse in urban areas than in rural areas although there are almost always important qualitative differences between the two within each national context and some health problems are often worse in urban than in rural settings. Nor do we pretend that there are more poor people in urban areas than rural areas or that the poor in urban areas are worse off than the poor in rural areas.

The justification for this book is the very large and growing urban population in the Third World whose housing and health needs are not being met. Furthermore, major improvements are possible at relatively low cost, if existing resources are used in different ways. The health problems faced by poorer groups in rural areas also deserve much greater attention, as do the links between improving their health and improving housing and living conditions.

Different means are generally needed in rural and urban areas to meet poorer groups' housing and health needs. For instance, acquiring a house plot and building materials are generally far more difficult for poorer groups in an urban area (and much more expensive); in many urban centres, this leads to many poorer households building on unsuitable sites which bring new kinds of health risk. The fact that many urban dwellers live in illegal settlements and are subject to a constant threat of eviction also has serious health impacts; the proportion of rural dwellers subject to threat of eviction is generally much smaller, although in many nations there are the special problems of insecure housing faced by plantation workers and seasonal migrants.

Urban houses are usually subject to far more government regulations in regard to their location, size, materials and structure. Urban settlements usually have much higher densities than rural settlements which means different techniques are needed for excreta disposal. Poor urban households often live in much more cramped conditions which exacerbates the transmission of communicable diseases. Many urban dwellers face far more serious health problems arising from industrial pollution than rural dwellers. Alternatively, farmers and agricultural labourers face serious health problems from biocides which are less of a problem in urban areas, except where they come to contaminate urban water supplies. Governments will also face greater difficulties (and higher costs) in reaching many rural dwellers with schools and health care and emergency life saving services because the population is far less concentrated.

There are instances where rural innovations can prove appropriate for certain urban situations (as in the case of certain kinds of latrine, developed first in rural areas and then applied in some peri-urban areas as described in Chapter 6) and where urban programmes can be transferred to more concentrated rural settlements (for instance mobilizing community action within villages to identify the most common insect and rodent disease-vectors and to reduce their numbers). In general, however, the differences between rural and urban areas suggest the need for different approaches to promote better health through improved housing.

It is often suggested that urban inhabitants already receive priority in government expenditures and policies – that they benefit from "urban bias". If this were the case, it would seriously weaken the justification for more attention to urban areas. It was largely as a result of the idea that there was urban bias in government policies that in recent years, many governments and most aid agencies have justified giving more attention to rural poverty than to urban poverty. For instance, most investment in primary health care by governments and the official aid agencies has been in rural areas.[20] But the idea that there is urban bias in the expenditures of Third World governments is increasingly questioned. For instance, most of the evidence presented to support the fact that there is an urban bias in the provision of health services relates to large hospitals in capital cities (or other large cities). But most Third World urban citizens live in relatively small urban centres, as noted earlier. This suggests that perhaps it is only citizens in capital cities or large cities who might benefit from this bias in health service provision. Moreover, Chapters 2, 3 and 4 are among the studies which show that the existence of health services in a city does not mean that the poor can actually use them.

There may be urban bias, or large city bias, in investments by governments or aid agencies in public housing, water supplies, sewers and drains – but again, few if any of the poor majority of urban (or large city) inhabitants benefit from this. In virtually all Third World nations, public housing programmes have been on such a small scale in relation to need that only a small proportion of urban dwellers have benefited – and it is often not the poorer groups who received the subsidized units.[21] Similarly, in most cities, public investments in infrastructure do not benefit the poor majority since the settlements in which they live do not receive piped water, sewers and drains and benefit little (if at all) from investments in ports, airports, power stations and roads.

In addition, the extent of disease, disablement and premature death among the poor in urban areas has almost certainly been underestimated because of the lack of studies carried out in poor communities. As a recent book published by the World Health Organization points out:

> The facts about the urban poor are hidden because figures for their health and nutritional status are often omitted from the statistics or presented as aggregated data, along with the figures for more prosperous neighbourhoods. For the rapidly increasing numbers of urban poor, health conditions may in some respects be even worse than they are for the rural poor, and deteriorating. In any attempt to deal with the needs of the urban poor, better information is required, since its absence makes it difficult to know the extent of their problems, to persuade people that these problems exist and to formulate effective responses to them.[22]

Many case studies within specific cities have highlighted the fact that those living in poorer districts face much more serious health problems than those living in richer districts (see Box 1.2); in a review of such case studies published in 1977, S.S. Basta pointed to the far higher infant mortality rates among poorer households within cities, compared to the city average.[23] These and other subsequent studies also suggest that the health problems of the poor majority in these cities is generally understated because so many of the poor are not included within health statistics or health studies. Some studies show that the health problems among poorer urban groups are qualitatively different from those among poorer rural groups – and poorer urban groups may in some instances face more serious health problems than their rural counterparts, especially in nutritional levels.[24] But a debate as to whether the rural or urban poor suffer most is one which for most nations cannot be settled and in many ways is a misleading debate. There may never be sufficient precise, accurate data to allow this question to be settled. This would demand detailed studies for relatively large samples of poor people drawn from a diverse sample of rural and urban areas for a large number of Third World nations. Such a study is likely to reveal major differences in the scale and nature of health problems suffered by the inhabitants of different rural areas and different urban areas, so no generalized urban or rural health picture would emerge for comparison. But there is sufficient hard evidence to suggest that hundreds of millions of poor urban dwellers have very serious health problems which could be greatly reduced with new approaches and this is the reason for this book. We also suspect that more detailed studies would show that ill health, disablement and premature death were far more closely associated to people's age, gender and household income than to whether they lived in large cities, smaller urban centres or rural areas.

Box 1.2: Comparisons of health problems between rich areas and poor areas within cities

BOMBAY and DELHI: In some low-income settlements (*bustees*) in Delhi, the child mortality rate was 221 per 1,000 but reaches nearly twice this rate among poorer castes within these settlements. In Bombay, the crude death rate on Bombay island (the central city area) was twice as high as that of the suburbs and three times that of the extended suburbs.

BANGLADESH: In 1978, the infant mortality rate in "urban slums" was 208.5 per 1000 (live) births, more than twice the rate for "non-slum" urban areas.

URBAN AREAS IN GUATEMALA: Infant mortality rates for different population groups in urban areas vary from 113 per 1,000 for the children of illiterate women in the poorest socio-economic group to 33 per 1,000.

KARACHI: In three low-income areas, between 95 and 152 infants per 1,000 live births died before the age of one; in a middle class area, only 32 per 1,000 died.

MANILA: A series of surveys in the mid-1970s revealed the disparities between health problems in a large squatter settlement (Tondo) and other non-squatter areas of the city. In Tondo, the level of severe malnutrition among infants and young children was three times the level for non-squatter areas. Tondo's infant mortality rate was 210 per 1,000 live births compared to 76 for non-squatter areas in Manila. The proportion of people with tuberculosis in Tondo was nine times the average for non-squatter areas while diarrhoea was twice as common. In Tondo, anaemia was twice as common and typhoid four times as common.

PANAMA CITY: A study in 1979 found that of 1,819 infants with diarrhoeal diseases, 68 per cent came from those living in slums or shanties with zero infection rates observed among children in better quality housing.

PORT-AU-PRINCE (Haiti): In the slums, one in five infants die before their first birthday while another one in ten die between their first and second birthdays; this is almost three times the mortality

Box 1.2: (continued)

rates in rural areas and many times the rate in the richer areas of Port-au-Prince where infant and child mortality rates were similar to those in urban areas of the United States.

PORTO ALEGRE (Brazil): In 1980, a study examined differentials in health between those living in shanty towns (one fifth of Porto Alegre's population) and those living elsehwere. Infant mortaltiy rates among residents of shanty towns were three times as high as among the non-shanty town residents. Neo-natal mortality rates were twice as high and post-neonatal mortality more than five times as high. Mortality from pneumonia and influenza was six times higher in shanty towns and from septicaemia eight times higher.

SAO PAULO: Infant mortality rates can vary by a factor of four, depending on the district. In the core area, 42 infants die before the age of one for every 1,000 born alive while in one of the predominantly-poor peri-urban municipalities, the rate was 175 per 1,000 live births. Infant death-rates from enteritis, diarrhoea and pneumonia on the city's periphery were twice as high as in the core area.

SOURCES: Most of these examples are drawn from Chapter 4 in Trudy Harpham, Tim Lusty and Patrick Vaughan (Editors), *In the Shadow of the City: Community Health and the Urban Poor*, (Oxford University Press, 1988). See Note 25 for a complete list of sources.

The above statistics suggest that infant mortality rates or the incidence of some of the most serious, common diseases are several times higher in poor districts when compared to city averages or to richer districts. Most of these figures certainly understate the health problems faced by poorer groups because they rely on averages within districts or cities. Most highlight the health problems of poorer groups because they contrast average health statistics for districts with a majority of poor inhabitants with averages for the whole city or for districts with a majority of rich inhabitants. Contrasting health statistics for poorer groups and richer groups would probably reveal an even greater disparity.

For instance, a study in India found a tenfold difference in infant mortality rates between the poorest families (180 infants dying, per 1,000 live births) and the richest families.[26] In the example given in Box 1.2 of Delhi, the infant mortality rate among the poorer households within the *bustee* was twice the average for the whole *bustee.*[27] There may also be serious disparities between different household members. The fact that children are especially vulnerable to diseases associated with poor housing and living conditions is evident from the above statistics. Women's vulnerability during pregnancy and childbirth is also evident in the very high levels of maternal mortality in most Third World nations. In many low-income settlements, there may be a significantly higher incidence of certain diseases among women, linked to the fact that they are taking most of the responsibility for child rearing and spending more time within the settlement and its contaminated environment. For instance, they may suffer more from the diseases associated with inadequate water and sanitation, or the respiratory problems associated with smoky living environments because they spend more time inside the house where cooking or heating is done on open fires or cheap stoves, using coal or wood.

The complexity of housing problems

A better understanding of links between housing and health demands an understanding of the housing problem which goes beyond the inaccurate stereotype of poor people living in slums and squatter settlements. Each city has its own unique range and mix of different housing sub-markets which present their inhabitants with serious health risks. This range and its relative importance changes over time. It usually includes some form of inner-city tenements, cheap boarding and rooming houses, squatter settlements and illegal subdivision developments with *de facto* owner-occupiers and renters. The range and the form each sub-market takes is influenced by factors such as the city's employment structure, income distribution, structure of land ownership and government attitudes to different kinds of illegal housing development. The range of housing options open to lower-income groups can change rapidly in any city, as in the case of Santiago de Chile when the military coup in 1973 brought large-scale repression of community organizations and the removal of the possibility of obtaining land on which houses could be built.

Different health risks are evident in different housing sub-markets. For example, the health problems of a family renting one room in an inner-city tenement with one kitchen, bathroom and WC shared among 30–40 people are likely to be different from those of a family who have built their own shelter on illegally-occupied land where there is no public provision of infrastructure, services and facilities. Similarly, different settlements will have different demographic structures. Particular areas within a city may have a high concentration of old people with very low incomes renting rooms, while others may have developed as centres for cheap boarding houses for newly-arrived migrants who are generally young. Improved services and facilities are needed in virtually all instances but the actual form in which these are needed and the way in which they should be provided must relate to the particular circumstances of each area and the needs of its residents. Improving conditions in rented accommodation can prove more problematic than in settlements where most occupiers are owners (or *de facto* owners, in illegal settlements). Landlords may be the main beneficiaries and the tenants the losers, as they are pushed out by higher rents as public programmes improve conditions there.

There are three generalizations relating both to housing and health which are valid for the low-income majority in virtually all Third World cities. The first is the fact that the accommodation in which they live is inadequate in protecting them from health risks. The second is that through lack of income they have very little chance of obtaining a more adequate (or healthy) house, with sufficient space, security, services and facilities. The third, almost as universal as the previous two, is insecure tenure. Fear of eviction is a constant worry for most tenants, temporary boarders in cheap rooming houses, *de facto* owners in illegal settlements or renters of land on which a house has been built.

Why has the impact of poor housing on health been ignored?

The most obvious reason why the health problems inherent in many residential areas in Third World cities have not been addressed is that the professionals and specialist agencies who work in housing do not recognize that promoting health is an essential part of their work. The architects, planners, engineers, social workers or other professionals working in housing may recognize that their work has important links with health, but they rarely have a clear idea of the health problems that low income groups face in different neighbourhoods and housing sub-markets, or of their potential role in helping to tackle such problems. Government agencies or ministries concerned with housing, building and planning, or with public works, also have important responsibilities in regard to promoting good health. But these responsibilities are rarely made clear and explicit.

If housing, or "the built environment" is viewed too narrowly in terms only of physical structure, the health–housing links may not seem so important. The most important health–housing links only become apparent when considering the impact on health of the physical environment provided by the house, the services and facilities it contains, and its surrounds. A false separation between these has led some specialists to dismiss the importance of housing to health while at the same time linking health with a sufficient, safe, domestic water supply, attention to water and food storage practices, washing and personal hygiene and the hygienic disposal of human wastes. But all these factors are intimately related to housing. So too is the site on which the house is located. It is a housing problem if children playing outside the house contract diarrhoea through ingesting pathogens from fecal matter which contaminates the land on which they play. A high incidence of respiratory diseases may owe much to smoky fires or stoves within the houses. A high incidence of burns and scalds may be largely the result of small, overcrowded huts in which occupants cook on open fires or unguarded stoves.

In looking at housing and health, to consider only the house's structure is to miss the point. It is the house – and whether it has piped water and provision for washing, cooking, laundry, food storage and the removal of human wastes and waste water – together with the neighbourhood within which each house is located, which should provide much of the defence against injury and disease. A large part of the task of improving housing and living conditions is reducing or eliminating the most serious health hazards present within poor quality housing. Indeed, an upgrading programme for inner-city tenements or squatter communities could be one of the most effective ways to improve health and reduce accidents.

Another reason why the professionals and agencies working in housing have not been active in addressing the health problems in low-income housing developments is because institutional structures have not responded to the multiple causality of disease. The idea of multiple causality has become more widely accepted since the Alma Ata Conference in 1978, when the concept of primary health care was defined and endorsed by all participating government representatives.[28] In the vast majority of urban areas, it has not been acted on.

Figure 1.1 illustrates the great diversity of factors which influence health. This helps place into context the role of housing improvements. It also illustrates the complexity of the issues involved. Drawing from this figure, it can be seen that each individual's health is influenced by a set of underlying factors such as different aspects of the physical environment or socio-economic factors like income, form of housing tenure, type of work and level of education or, the availability of health services. These factors may have a profound influence on a person's health status in the nations where public provision is most limited.

Figure 1.1: Examples of the many factors which influence a person's health

BACKGROUND

1. The strength and prosperity of the national economy
2. National society, political structure, laws and the ways and means by which they are enforced
3. Distribution of income and capital assets within the society

These set the context for any individual's possibility of obtaining adequate income and the possibilities for government to provide infra-structure and services

UNDERLYING FACTORS

1. Physical/environmental – including characteristics of the house (e.g. amount of space, physical materials) and the workplace (including quality of indoor environment and degree of protection from injury by machines, toxic chemicals etc.) characteristics of the house site (e.g. risk of flooding, landslide or other natural disaster) and location (especially in relation to health services)
2. Infrastructure and service provision – quality and quantity of water, provision for sanitation and drainage, garbage disposal, health care, emergency services, public transport etc.
3. Socio-economic characteristics of person concerned – diet, income and kind of work; also time available to cook nutritious food, take care of children, work to improve or extend housing and other health promoting activities. Legal status is also important, as is location within the society which influences whether help can be obtained when faced with economic or health problems or an emegency
4. Age and gender (e.g. infants, young children and adolescents each particularly vulnerable to certain health problems; women more vulnerable to certain health problems than men)

INTERMEDIARY FACTORS

1. Knowledge of health-enhancing behaviour at the individual/ household level
2. Knowledge of health-enhancing behaviour at community level and level of community organization
3. Use made of health-care system and other public services and facilities

LEVEL OF HEALTH

As indicated by:
1. Frequency and type of ill-health
2. Duration and severity
3. Mortality

The underlying factors are, in turn, influenced by the laws, codes, norms and practices of national, city and municipal governments. The priority given by a government to basic service-provision is obviously one factor. They are also influenced by such factors as the level of prosperity within the national or regional economy which in turn is influenced by the working of the international market. The broad economic context has a strong influence on whether the government has the trained personnel and resources to allow it to become more effective at addressing health problems.

For some of the poorest nations, the main constraints to improved health lie here. Many Third World nations can never, under current conditions, achieve a level of development which allows the elimination of poverty. They lack a stable, viable economic base to allow them to function as nation states. They have very little that the world market wants which cannot be produced more cheaply elsewhere and they lack the resources and trained personnel to provide adequate living standards for their citizens, using only their own internal resources. Their future is bleak without a worldwide redistribution of resources in their favour and a more equitable deal from the world market (the main exports of most such nations are primary commodities whose price within the world market has fallen steadily, in comparison to manufactured goods). In such nations, more can be done to improve health using existing resources, but achievements will always be limited by economic constraints and, in most instances, by political instability which is much exacerbated by economic problems. In such cases, background and underlying factors will always limit the level of health the population is likely to achieve.

Background variables also influence underlying factors such as the quality of housing, living and working conditions. A rapidly growing national economy increases the possibility that incomes for some poorer groups will rise and that more public resources can be devoted to infrastructure and services but in itself it is not sufficient; political and socio-economic structures often limit this and ensure that most of the benefits are concentrated in the hands of a small elite. By contrast, a stagnant economy will limit the possibility of improved health although there are examples of changes in government policies which improved the level of health, despite economic stagnation.[29]

A person's level of health is also influenced by intermediary factors. These relate to the knowledge and behaviour of a person, household or community in addressing their own health problems. One example of an important intermediary factor is the level of education of a mother; the proportion of children who die young tends to be lower, the better educated the mother.[30] The precise reason for this may be difficult to ascertain but a mother's ability to read and to make use of health education materials which advise on how to prevent child illnesses and how to treat them is obviously an advantage. The extent to which women have access to education links back to certain underlying variables (for instance, the extent to which the society supports women's education) and the background (for instance, the level of priority given by the government to education and the extent to which the national economy generates the resources to allow this to be funded).

Not surprisingly, it is difficult to determine the precise mix of reasons – and their relative importance – for someone's illness. Consider, for instance, the case of the workforce in a particular factory in a Third World city which sells much of its output to Europe or North America. They may have their work hours (and wages) cut because of a fall in demand for that factory's product. This may in turn be the result of a protectionist barrier created by the European Commission or the government of the United States, or the result of their government's economic policy which increased the value of the national currency against those of their main export markets. Lower incomes for the workforce can mean poorer quality diets for some of their children who then become more vulnerable to diseases so deaths from diarrhoea or measles may increase. We suspect that too little weight is given to the influence of background and underlying factors on poor health in urban areas of the Third World.

Figure 1.1 does not include a complete list of factors which influence a person's health status. Other factors may be important for low-income groups. For instance, health may be influenced by the degree of cohesion and mutual self-help within such a group. It is certainly influenced by the form that their housing tenure takes. Those renting houses or rooms are likely to be less movitated to improve their house than owner-occupiers – for obvious reasons. Squatters who fear their houses may be bulldozed not only lack any incentive to improve their housing but also face strain and anxiety caused by the possibility of forced eviction. Thus, it would be expected that the relative importance of different variables in the frequency and duration of illness and in mortality will differ considerably from area to area within one city – and, of course, between cities and between nations.

Most research into health problems to date has been done by health professionals. This has meant too little attention given to the health impacts of many of the underlying and intermediary factors, including those relating to housing conditions. Research has concentrated on the incidence of diseases or on their biological processes. Policy recommendations are oriented towards the role of health professionals in disease prevention, control or treatment. Although most health professionals recognize that national health budgets dominated by building and maintaining one or two large city-based hospitals are ineffective ways of addressing health problems, there is still a strong bias towards the role of health professionals. As John Briscoe has pointed out, this is illustrated in the idea of "selective primary health care" through which non-medical activities such as community water-supply, sanitation and nutrition supplementation – critical parts of the original primary health care package – are rejected as less cost-effective than medical interventions such as oral rehydration therapy (ORT) for diarrhoea in children and immunization against the major infectious diseases.[31] The much increased availability of ORT has meant great improvements in the treatment of child diarrhoea. But its-long term impact is limited if risks of contracting diarrhoea again through contaminated water, lack of facilities for washing, housing sites contaminated with faecal matter and lack of adult supervision (since all adults have to work to earn enough to survive) are not addressed. Many of the deaths caused by diarrhoeal diseases are the result of persistent diarrhoeas and dysenteries rather than the dehydration brought on by acute diarrhoeal attacks. Those cannot be prevented by ORT.

There are signs of changes in professional and public attitudes. For example, within the last ten years, some Third World governments have laid increasing stress on the importance of clean water and improved sanitation. The concept of upgrading slums and squatter settlements has become more accepted, in the hope that such upgrading will improve conditions there, even if it is rarely undertaken with a clear idea as to how it can tackle the inhabitants' most serious health problems. Site drainage and the collection of household refuse have become more common as components of water and sanitation projects. There is an increasing interest among both health and housing researchers in links between health status and socio-economic factors. Examples include the research whose findings were noted earlier and recent research on the effect on child mortality of mothers' educational level[32] and on the impact of the physical environment on health and nutrition.[33] An increasing volume of research is revealing how the housing needs and priorities of women have been constantly misunderstood or ignored with serious impacts both on their health and on the health of infants and children.[34] Too little attention has been given to developing the capacity within each locality of the Third World to determine the most effective and cost effective ways to address housing and health problems. Virtually no progress has been made in thinking through the institutional implications of new approaches: how to ensure that government at national, city and district (or municipal) level has the power, trained personnel, knowledge and resources to take up its responsibilities in addressing the housing and health problems of the low-income majority.

Chapter Two

COMMUNITY ACTION TO ADDRESS HOUSING AND HEALTH PROBLEMS: THE CASE OF SAN MARTIN IN BUENOS AIRES, ARGENTINA

Beatriz Cuenya, Hector Almada, Diego Armus, Julia Castells, Maria di Loreto and Susana Penalva

Introduction

Greater Buenos Aires is one of the world's largest urban agglomerations; in the 1980 census, it had 9.8 million inhabitants within an area of 3,880 square kilometres. At its core is Buenos Aires Federal District, the 200-square kilometre area which, as the name implies, is the capital city of Argentina and which had 2.92 million inhabitants in 1980. The concept of Greater Buenos Aires developed during the 1930s, as the city's built up area spilled over the Federal District boundaries. Initially, Greater Buenos Aires included the Federal District and seven surrounding municipalities but over time, as the built up area expanded and other existing urban centres were engulfed by this expansion, Greater Buenos Aires came to include 19 municipalities. Table 2.1 below presents basic data about population growth in Buenos Aires.

Table 2.1: Population growth in Greater Buenos Aires

Year	*Population (thousands)*
1869	234
1895	781
1914	2,034
1947	4,724
1960	6,739
1970	8,353
1980	9,766

Source: Derived from census data

While Greater Buenos Aires remains the dominant industrial, financial and commercial centre in Argentina, its rate of population growth has declined in each of the last four inter-census periods. The proportion of Argentina's national and urban population living in Greater Buenos Aires is also declining; in 1947, Greater Buenos Aires contained 46.3 per cent of the national urban population, while in 1980 it contained 42.9 per cent. In 1970 it contained 36.1 per cent of the national population, while in 1980 it contained 35.0 per cent.

Background to the invasions

While Argentina has long been one of the richer Third World nations, the last two decades have seen a considerable weakening in its productive capacity, a fall in real income for most people and a rapid increase in the number of people living in extreme poverty. Large proportions of the population are now facing economic problems and health risks which to a considerable extent had seemed to be overcome in previous decades. With a very large external debt and a stagnant economy, government ministries and agencies at all levels face severe constraints on all social expenditures.

Greater Buenos Aires is one of the urban areas where the growth in informal-sector enterprises and a process of de-industrialization have become evident. As a result, there has been a serious decline in real income, the availability of adequately paid employment and living conditions for a large proportion of the population. Findings from the 1980 census suggest that a quarter of all households in Buenos Aires lack basic needs. Ever since the onset of rapid population growth in the late-nineteenth century, there have been large deficits in the number of adequate-quality housing units, in basic urban infrastructure such as piped water, paved roads, drains and sewers, and in services such as schools, child-care centres and health centres.

Conditions for poorer groups in Argentina worsened considerably, after an authoritarian military regime took power in 1976. The regime's economic plan led to a decline in real income for a majority of the population and reduced standards of living. In addition, the channels for popular protest were suppressed since there was no Congress, political parties were banned and labour unions' actions repressed. In addition, popular organizations (for instance those formed by the inhabitants of low-income areas) were also repressed. Meanwhile, public spending on measures to improve conditions for poorer groups was cut.

Rent control was abolished in the hope that this would stimulate private investment in rental housing but very little low-cost housing was built. With little investment in new housing, rental prices increased. With no legislation to protect them, as their incomes fell and rents rose, many tenants were evicted. The number of people seeking cheap accommodation grew rapidly but the supply of such accommodation fell; many people who once had sufficient income to rent reasonable quality accommodation now found themselves evicted and competing with poorer groups for a diminishing supply of cheap rental accommodation in tenements or cheap boarding-houses.

Meanwhile, the Military Government initiated a major campaign to demolish the *villas miserias* (the Argentine term for squatter settlements),[1] especially those in the Federal District. These destroyed one of the few kinds of centrally-located housing that was available to poorer groups, including most of the cheap housing close to jobs or sources of income. Representatives of the Military Government could claim that they had greatly reduced the number of people living in *villas miserias* in the central city (Federal District) but these people had simply been forced to find accommodation in the counties around the Federal District. Thus, the numbers in need of cheap accommodation grew substantially while the supply of legal accommodation fell.

The number of people with access to health services also declined in the second half of the 1970s. Economic stagnation and the drop in real wages for a high proportion of the workforce also affected the private and semi-private suppliers of health services – especially the social welfare funds. As one commentator noted:

> While the drastic fall in real wages affected the support (of the workers) for these social welfare funds, the dislocation of the job market also meant a decline in the number of people who were members. At the same time, the costs of medical equipment and the fees requested rose very rapidly; most of these funds suffered serious financial difficulties as a result.[2]

State provision of health services worsened, despite the large and growing numbers of those who were not members of these social welfare funds or who could no longer afford to maintain payments to them. The coverage of state-provided health services was severely limited by three factors: reduced public spending (the number of beds per inhabitant in Buenos Aires fell); charges introduced for hospital care which had previously been free; and the decentralization of responsibility for hospitals to provincial agencies who lacked the resources to allow them to fulfil this responsibility. This decentralization was not accompanied by a decentralizing of funds or of fund-raising powers.

This was the background for the emergence of new forms of housing provision for lower income households. One important new form was the large-scale, well-organized invasion of undeveloped land. This produced a different kind of settlement to the earlier *villas miserias* which had grown more slowly and gradually, without prior organization and violent confrontation. The first of these invasions took place in Quilmes county.

Quilmes is in southern part of Greater Buenos Aires, in the industrial belt. It is on the periphery of the built up area and, like many other peripheral areas, is made up mainly of densely-occupied working-class residential neighbourhoods interspersed with industries and large plots of undeveloped land. Quilmes county covers 125 square kilometres, with a population of 445,662 in 1980. It began to urbanize in the 1950s, when factories were built in the area and attracted a workforce. Public provision of infrastructure and services grew much slower than population; by 1980, almost half the population lacked a water supply and more than 60 per cent lack sewers. Health and education services are poor in the county, with a shortfall of 3,000 hospital beds. Furthermore, only 22 per cent of the beds are run by the public sector, hence the lowest income sectors have even less access to health services (1978 estimates).

In 1970, Quilmes had some 25,000 people living in *villas miseria*. By 1980, estimates suggest that it had grown to 35,727 in 16 different settlements, four of which had populations of over 1,000 inhabitants. This represented over eight per cent of its total population – although many people think that the number of people living in precarious settlements at this date was much higher than this. Quilmes has a long history of community action where inhabitants of a particular neighbourhood work together both to lobby the government for some public services and to organize some minimum level of infrastructure and services themselves. Many child-care centres, nursery schools and first aid centres have been developed by neighbourhood (*barrio*) Development Centres and the first school to open in the areas "was built with the work and sacrifice of the squatters: it began with two wooden rooms and later the Education Council made improvements."[3] In Quilmes and in many other low-income areas, church-based community organizations proved very important in providing the institutions around which community action – including land invasions – was organized. They also provided the network of friendships through which news about the initial invasions and the possibilities for more people to join in the invasions were spread.

The land invasion

In late-1981, some 22,000 people invaded 211 hectares of undeveloped private land (see Map 2.1). These invasions began in September with an initial, relatively small and well-organized squatter invasion by a group of families living close by in what after the invasion came to be called *barrio viejo* (old *barrio*). This prompted many other people to join in. Towards the end of November 1981, as word spread, in just five days about 3,000 people entered the settlement with their belongings; the local parish and its priest helped both in spreading the news and in the organization of the land occupation. The invaded land was sub-divided in a pre-determined plan which followed the basic rules of urban planning regulations.

The priest explained what happened in these early days:

> A lot of people said "I would like land". Then there were about 20 or 30 people who were told "all right, those who do not have land yet step to the side and those that do have land over here to organize yourselves". So 20 or 30 went to the side, signed up [for a plot of land] and were told "all right, come here next Saturday because we are going to give you land". So, they did everything and with the Committee, we started giving out land. Then more people came; we met there: "All right, those without land over here" ... and they were around fifty in number. "All right, go to this place because we are going to invade it and take the land" ... and that is how we went on taking and in around one week, 1,000 persons arrived ....

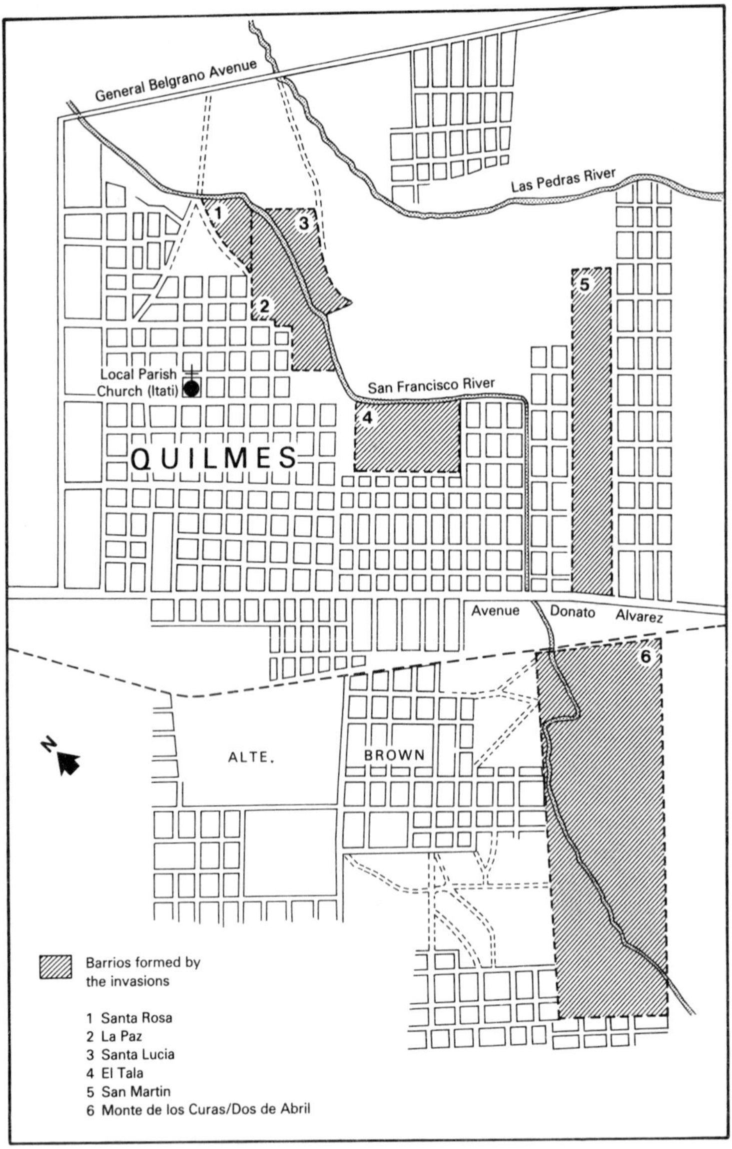
General Belgrano Avenue
Las Pedras River
San Francisco River
Local Parish Church (Itati)
QUILMES
Avenue Donato Alvarez
ALTE. BROWN
N
1
2
3
4
5
6
Barrios formed by the invasions
1 Santa Rosa
2 La Paz
3 Santa Lucia
4 El Tala
5 San Martin
6 Monte de los Curas/Dos de Abril

Map 2.1

> We told them to come on Friday or Saturday morning and we took El Tala (El Tala being one of the settlements within the invasion) with between 700 and 900 families .... We started to put them there, to give land out through the same Committee ... and later, during that same week, about 5,000 people came .... We told them to come at midnight. Most [of the small land invasions] were in the morning but that time, we planned it for the night .... In San Martin [another of the settlements], around 5,000 people showed up at 11 o'clock at night ... and 200 trucks! They were asked to bring everything that was needed to build homes.... So, those in San Martin went about 15 blocks, walking at midnight with their kids, with sticks, with scrap material .... That was something worth filming!

The government tried to bulldoze the first settlement to be formed but was successfully resisted – largely by women and children and the local priest who stood in front of the bulldozers. Support for the squatters soon grew, especially from priests, church groups and certain lawyers.

The police then tried to isolate the new settlements by forming a cordon around it with 300 vehicles and 3,000 men. One of the squatters described how they got around this:

> We worked at night. On the houses too. We knew that the police did not have the authorization to tear down the houses; their function was to keep us from building them. The people who were going to enter the settlement waited outside the police cordon; when it relaxed a bit, because they were asleep and there were fewer of them, we would slip in through the first gap and carry with us the metal sheets and planks of wood. All the neighbours helped. In two hours, we built one house; later the neighbour who just arrived helped to raise others. By morning, when the police entered, five or six houses had been built.[4]

Box 2.1 tells the story of how the Castillo family obtained their land in the invasion.

Many of those taking part in the invasion were having similar problems to the Castillos in affording rented accommodation. Most of those who took part were long-time residents of Buenos Aires, not recent migrants to the city. The local priest estimated that 70 per cent of the households who came to join the invasion were having problems in affording the steep rise in rents.

Box 2.1: The Castillo Family.

The Castillos are a couple with two children. He is 31 and from Uruguay but has lived in Argentina for over ten years. She is 29 and from Chaco Province, in the northwest of Argentina; she came to Greater Buenos Aires as a child. Both children attend a school in the area. Before moving to San Martin, the husband had a stable job working in a café but he lost this job because of the time he had to spend in San Martin in the early months to secure a housing plot there. He now does odd jobs and helps his wife run a grocery store from the front room of their house.

The family moved to San Martin because they were threatened with eviction from the small room and bathroom they shared in Solano, nearby. The husband learnt of the possibility of obtaining a building plot from someone at work who had obtained a plot in one of the other five *barrios* formed in the Quilmes invasion. He visited the local parish offices and paid a nominal amount for a number and immediately went to visit some relatives to obtain metal sheets so that a rudimentary structure could be put on the new building plot. He then went to San Martin but found that all the plots had already been staked out with string. He then marked out a plot for himself next to a factory, put up a shack and returned to the parish office for guidance. The priest said that the people in each block must work out plot allocations themselves. So the husband returned to San Martin and slowly, an organization developed. Some people had marked off more than one plot and built a small shelter on each but if these plots were not occupied, the organization re-allocated them. The husband then obtained a new plot and moved his shelter there.

At first, the husband occupied the shack on their new plot while the rest of the family stayed in their rented room in Solano. This was during the police cordon around the settlement and the husband told of the need to keep constant watch against the possibility of eviction. Later, the wife and children joined him and bit by bit, they built their house. At first, they made building blocks themselves. They

Box 2.1: (continued)

also managed to acquire some 2,000 bricks and building rubble from a neighbour who was leaving, although they had to borrow the money to allow them to do so. The Castillos also tell of the help provided by her brother who put a lot of work into the house, without charging them anything. They also borrowed money from a neighbour to purchase 30 fibre-cement sheets which they were offered at a good price – with this same neighbour then taking 20 of them and the Castillos retaining ten for their roof. Having lost his job at the café, the husband sold newspapers and did odd-jobs; during the Malvinas war, there was a high demand for newspapers and the extra income this brought helped to pay for additional building materials.

Initially, their only source of water was to walk with buckets into the housing areas next to the land sites which had been invaded and asking those living there if they could use their taps. The full buckets then had to be carried back to their shelter. Later, a pump was installed to serve those in their block but there were problems with its cleanliness; later still, the people in the block collected enough money to buy pipes and connect them to the public water system to distribute the water around the block. The Castillos now have a tap on the plot but no connection into the house; they explained that the tap remains outside because many other people use it.

They have a chicken coop on their plot (made with the sheets that served as the walls in the first rudimentary shack) and a small vegetable patch, though the earth is not very good. They run a small grocery store from the front of the house, selling milk, cold meats and such but the income from this is only enough to survive and he must look for work. The Castillos say that the *barrio* has improved since they first moved in and they like living in the settlement. They would like to make many improvements to their house (more rooms, better facilities, better materials) but what they now have is far better than what they previously rented. The husband resigned from his work as a block delegate because it was taking up too much time. They also told of how it had been quite a difficult job, especially in trying to get people to collaborate, to give money and to organize to make improvements which brought benefits to

Box 2.1: (continued)

everyone on their block: the installation of a water pump and pipes to distribute water, the construction of pavements and hook-ups to the electricity supply.

The story of the invasions was widely covered in newspapers and magazines but not by radio and television. One commentator reported that

> ATC Channel 7 (one of the television channels) sent a team of reporters. They looked around, listened and then went back to the channel. Nothing ever got on the air. Television, drowning us daily with its irrelevancies, did not consider as worthy of interest the plight of 20,000 persons lacking a roof. Is it that the sight of families living in tents and cardboard shacks would have shown the social failure of a rich and powerful Argentina?[5]

In the autumn of 1982, the security forces gave up their attempt to maintain the cordon. One reason was the Malvinas War with the United Kingdom; another was the consequent weakening in the confidence and power of the military government.

Some months after the initial invasion of Quilmes, one of the residents explained what had happened:

> We are here today, this is the result of a lot of time, many struggles which led us to make the decision to come to find land for our children .... Perhaps for the world, for the people around us, it was something unbelievable because it was the first time 20,000 people, driven by hunger, driven by high rental costs and unemployment searched for abandoned lands ... and that is why, today, thank God, we are able to be here, to be organized, to be united.... The only thing the authorities provided was a police cordon which frightened our children and hindered our progress. So we had to struggle, clandestinely, any way we were able; we had to suffer and that suffering, although the law may say otherwise, is what gives us the right to be here.[6]

San Martin was one of six new settlements (*barrios*) formed by this invasion. Despite the illegality, the new settlers were determined not to live in a *villa miseria*; the motto was "create a *barrio* worthy of our families". To avoid this, they organized the site so that space was left for access roads and for community facilities. A democratic system of planning and organizing the settlement soon developed. At the lowest level – the level of the block (*manzana*) – inhabitants elected block delegates (one representative and two deputy representatives) who served for six months on the Board of Delegates. Committees were also elected to supervise and co-ordinate activities and petitions for larger units. Each neighbourhood had a co-ordinating committee which was represented on what came to be called the "Co-ordinating Committee of Neighbours of the West Quilmes Settlement".

This organization developed soon after the invasions. As one settler remarked:

> the organization did not come already planned... the need was there for a filter against all those people who wanted to slip in; against criminals, against the dictatorship, against the police... the only way of keeping them out is to be well organized... that is why meetings were held here at four or five in the morning during the first days. The local parish priest was an important supporter right from the initial invasion and he helped in the organization.[7]

The Co-ordinating Committee published a newsletter, *Nuestra Esperanza* (Our Hope), and quickly took charge of negotiations with public agencies for electricity, health care and public works. Initially, they had little success. Illegal connections were made to the electricity grid and to the mains water supply; the electricity company had agreed to supply the settlement but the police kept the company out. The need for piped water was particularly pressing, since the nearby stream, a possible alternative source, was contaminated with wastes from local paper, weaving and meat packing plants.

Conditions in San Martin and the other *barrios* remained very poor since the local government refused to pave the streets or install sewers or drains or provide health care. Diarrhoea epidemics were especially serious in the summer months which led to the community organizing a campaign to demand health care. When this failed, the inhabitants organized for themselves a basic level of health care and built a health centre with help from the local Catholic parish. They also built their first school.

In the run up to democratic elections in 1984, each political party made promises to the inhabitants of San Martin; offers such as the services of a physician or the supply of medicine were made by both the main political parties while a former military junta member promised a totally-equipped dispensary. The Co-ordinator's response was: "To the political party that came to tell us 'we have four physicians, we have milk and medicine to distribute' we answered 'fine, bring them, leave them at the parish, we will take them to the barrio'".[8]

With the election of a democratic government in 1984, the municipal authorities became more sympathetic to the squatters' needs and there are no longer fears of eviction. Some medicines have been provided and vaccinations made available; on occasion, garbage has been collected – although the longer-term problems of no drains and sewers and no paved roads and pathways remain.

The case of San Martin

San Martin is one of six *barrios*, formed by the invasion, which make up the Quilmes Settlements (see Map 2.1). It covers 30 hectares of lowland in an area prone to flooding alongside the Francisco Solano River. Its urban structure follows the traditional Buenos Aires pattern of a grid-iron lay-out and its physical make-up is one of constant change as the slow process of urbanization and housing construction takes place bit by bit.

San Martin houses 807 families. At the time of the invasion, their principal objective was legal and secure land-ownership, so that they could build their own houses; this is illustrated by comments made by squatters, during interviews:

> We don't want to live in villas or abandoned areas… we ask for help to build respectable homes, nothing else, because we're working-class people who can't possibly pay the high rents they're charging us.

> We're fleeing from other villas because we're afraid of being forcefully evicted and feel that here we can get the land. We're workers, we only want to live with our families in a respectable home.

> The idea was to mark off 10x30-metre plots so as not to lead to another villa… since the start our motto has been to keep the streets, blocks, plots well-ordered.

San Martin was divided into 20 blocks (*manzanas*) with streets and sidewalks dividing them. Blocks were sub-divided into plots except for two plots reserved for the first aid centre and a child-care centre which the inhabitants hoped to develop.

For many of San Martin's inhabitants, moving there meant a drop in living conditions, poorer access to schools and health centres and fewer basic services; however, the opportunity to own a piece of land and build their own house and the freedom from landlords that this represented outweighed these disadvantages. A survey of the inhabitants' own priorities showed that secure land-tenure remained top priority; services, infrastructure and communal facilities and housing improvements were of secondary importance.

Even before the land invasion, the area had very inadequate public services: "there are no first aid rooms, the post office is two kilometres away, there's no public telephone or high school".[9] With the influx of 20,000 new settlers into the area, water, electricity and medical and health attention all became pressing problems. Few resources were available and the problems were further exacerbated by the fact that state agencies could refuse legitimate demands for help because the inhabitants were "illegal". Self-help and mutual assistance characterized the way in which the settlement organization tackled the problems: "the people organize themselves, they are setting up communities with delegates by block to negotiate the titles to the land, to keep order, to request some authorization for the supply of drinkable water and the installation of a medical tent".[10]

Water was a problem from the start. Initially, each family obtained water as best it could, mainly from those living in existing neighbourhoods, next to the sites invaded. Then pumps were installed with the tools and materials needed to set them up smuggled past the police cordon. One resident recalled the way that the first water pump was installed:

> We could not bring in any material past the [police] cordon In a large bread basket, we brought in drill bits to drill the well by hand. A cart selling *choripan* (a popular cheap snack of bread and a sausage) smuggled in the pipes and the pump.

> We worked all night by hand. When the police came in the next morning, the first pump was already installed.[11]

Some-blocks decided to make illegal connections direct to the public water-supply network and gradually the network distributing water from the illegal connection grew to serve most of the settlement.

Electricity comes from illegal hook-ups. *Barrio* leaders approached SEGBA (the Electricity Board) to request meters and to arrange proper connections. This Board agreed, but when their staff came to do the work, the police prevented them from doing so. The settlers then made their own illegal connections. Resolving the land issue would legalize the connections, though at present most blocks have electricity, and there is even some street lighting.

Initially, there were no health services and no medical assistance. The water shortage and great heat of the first summer, with the possibilities of epidemics and diarrhoea, concentrated the inhabitants' minds on health problems and the dangerous sanitary conditions. Repeated requests to government agencies for help and advice were ignored during the last two years of the military regime. The settlements' relations with the nearby San Francisco Solano hospital (the only public-sector hospital or health centre in the area) were almost non-existent. The settlers were not treated if they couldn't pay and, initially, they were discriminated against because they came from the illegal settlements. This lack of state involvement and the dangerous lack of basic services encouraged the settlers to establish links with outside organizations such as religious groups, political groups, activists and popular organizations.

The struggle for health care was initiated by the settlers themselves. They started to set up first-aid rooms in each of the *barrios*. They managed to obtain some medicines from social welfare funds, unions and medical organizations and some volunteer doctors and nurses offered their time free. One doctor who was one of the first to do so reported that he examined between 80 and 100 children per week who were showing signs of diarrhoea and other health problems related to unhygienic living conditions.[12] After these initial measures came the idea of building a first-aid centre. It also became a focal point for the battle for the settlements. Its construction would consolidate the *barrios* and further the struggle for the land:

> We knew perfectly well that the central issue was the land;

> that was the political part. But we also knew that creating a solid and ordered structure within the site would mean fewer possibilities that they would throw us out. That's why the [health] centre was considered from the start as a strategic move of great importance for the organization and also as a place where the people would be provided some benefit, a place with medicine, where things are resolved that can't be resolved individually.[13]

Unlike the land issue which focused on the settlements as a whole, the first-aid centre became an issue for the *barrio* alone. The co-ordinator supported the idea of a single health-centre, but *barrio* leaders disagreed. It was agreed that each *barrio* would fund and build its own centre and be responsible for obtaining its own medicine and doctors.

In the case of *barrio* San Martin, health action had been a bit haphazard. Settlers' homes had been used as first-aid rooms where a volunteer doctor attended once a week and medicines were dispensed. In an effort to formalize the centre, the *barrio* organization decided to pay a doctor as best it could, start a membership system and begin construction of the health centre.

A voluntary association scheme was set up to raise funds for building and running the centre, whereby inhabitants paid a monthly contribution for the right in the future to free use of medical services. Those not joining this association would have to pay for health services as they used them.

The construction of the centre began in July 1982. The local parish donated 5,000 bricks – as it had done to other *barrios*. This, together with funds already collected allowed a start on laying the foundations, following a plan devised by an architect. Problems soon emerged as the design proved too ambitious for the funds available and construction was halted. This led to people who had joined the association no longer paying their contributions so no more funds became available. However, due to the initiatives of some political activists and some Internal Committee members, construction resumed in January 1983 (the community organization was too preoccupied with the land question). Building materials were donated – some bricks, a roof, some panelling. Membership cards for the association were printed and receipts issued to those who began or resumed payment. The centre was built by the settlers themselves, and consisted of one room, a cement floor, plastered walls, zinc roof and very basic furnishings. By mid-1983, the centre had been completed to the point where the room was used and medical attention available on Mondays and Thursdays. Members of the association did not pay; others were charged at a price comparable to other centres.[14]

However, the health care provided was still fairly limited and it was up to the squatters to provide continuity to the doctor's care. There was no strong preventive health element, although this was much needed. Many of the settlers (mainly the women) learned to dispense medicine and administer basic health care. In this way, they tried to keep the centre open each day. Membership quotas paid for the centre's costs, though there were problems in collecting these from some of the members. Initially, medicines were obtained from contributions; after the end of the military regime in 1984, they were supplied by the new (elected) municipal administration.

After 1983, the health care centre did not develop much, although foundations for its expansion had been laid. One reason is the existence of other sources of health services such as the social welfare funds, the public hospital, private medicine, popular healers and home remedies. The choice of which is used is dictated by many factors including the level of income, current employment situation (the person may or may not belong to a welfare fund run by their union), what's available nearby and seriousness of illness. Another reason for lack of the centre's development was limited resources to guarantee an efficient health care service. There was also the state of uncertainty due to the illegality of the land occupation and the continued hope that the state might assume the responsibility for health care.

During the military regime, little if any aid was forthcoming from the government authorities. With the arrival of a democratic government, some awareness of the problems of the settlement has been achieved, but provisions are still very inadequate. Palliatives, such as the provision of some materials and medicine, have been provided rather than concrete solutions to problems. There are discussions about trying to integrate the health centre's activities with other health units, with the Solano hospital as the central point. This has some support from *barrio* leaders except that they want to retain control of the centre. Their preference would be for the municipality to provide doctors, equipment and medicine, and to let the *barrio's* own internal committee run it. This suggests that the health centre provides a meeting place for the settlement and is almost its headquarters, a place where people can gather to discuss issues and to try and resolve problems. Furthermore, since mid-1984, the centre has also become a distribution point for nutrition packages for the National Nutrition Plan, which is promoted by the national government and affects over 80 per cent of those living in San Martin.

The inhabitants of San Martin

Although most people in San Martin had been living in Buenos Aires before joining the invasion, relatively few were born there. Of 986 persons surveyed, most had been born in urban centres outside the province within which Buenos Aires is located: 36 per cent from the northeastern provinces, 16 per cent from the northwest provinces and 16 per cent from the Pampas. Although 20 per cent were from Greater Buenos Aires, only 4 per cent were from the central city area (the Federal District).

Most household heads are males, under 40 years of age; only 10 per cent of households were headed by women. Two-thirds of all household heads had lived close to San Martin before joining the invasion (in the San Francisco Solano area) while 28 per cent had moved from other parts of Greater Buenos Aires. Only 8 per cent had moved from other parts of Buenos Aires province. Most inhabitants had come to San Martin at the end of 1981 or early 1982; 60 per cent had come in November/December 1981.

Infants, children and young people make up most of the population; half of the sample were under the age of 12 and nearly a third were under five years of age. Only 3 per cent were over 50.

Educational levels were generally low; almost half of the household heads and their partners had not completed primary school and five per cent had never gone to school. Of the rest who had completed primary school, only two per cent had completed secondary school. There was little variation in the education levels of household heads and their partners except that three per cent of the partners had completed secondary school compared to only one per cent of household heads.

Most household heads make a living working in manufacturing industry or construction, although over two-thirds of their partners who are employed work as domestic helps. Household incomes are generally very low; when the survey was undertaken, 57 per cent of all households were earning less than the legal minimum wage.

Of the potentially economically active population (those of 10 or more years of age) 41 per cent are employed with 28 per cent as students and 21 per cent as "housewives". Only five per cent were unemployed – that is to say without work but seeking it at the time of the survey. Virtually all household heads were economically active and 89 per cent were employed; 23 per cent of their partners were also employed.

Table 2.2 summarizes the job categories of household heads and partners. Three-quarters of employed heads of household and spouses are wage-earners, as opposed to the rest who are self-employed labourers. Many of the wage-earners (those working for a private or public employer and receiving a salary or a wage) do not receive social benefits such as unemployment compensation, payment during holidays, annual bonuses and pensions on retirement, despite working for a firm; these work on a contract basis or are domestic workers (except women who work by the hour and consider themselves self-employed) or are those who described themselves as wage-earners but could in fact be classified as self-employed. Table 2.2 highlights how a much higher proportion of partners have precarious jobs when compared to household heads.

Table 2.2: Job categories for employed household heads and partners

Job Category	*Percentage of*		
	Household Heads	*Partners*	*Total*
Workers or employees with precarious jobs	30	64	34
Rest of workers/employees	43	22	39
Self-employed labourers	27	14	24

Examples of precarious jobs: workers or employees who receive no social benefits from their employers such as pay for vacation, unemployment compensation, pension, etc. Examples include people working in bakeries, construction or carpentry, meat packers, domestic help, night watch staff, leather workers, bus-drivers.
Examples of jobs where employees receive social benefits: metal workers, dockers, railway workers, people working in glass and paper works.
Examples of self-employed: shop keepers, brick-layers, plasterers and painters, porters, barbers, domestic helps who charge by the hour.

If conditions for households in San Martin are compared with the average for the district (San Francisco Solano) and the county (Quilmes), San Martin households are generally worse off. Table 2.3

presents figures on the percentage of households in San Martin, San Francisco Solano and Quilmes suffering from overcrowding (households with three or more occupants per room), inadequate housing (for instance, made of temporary materials), poor sanitary conditions (houses with no latrines), low school-attendance (a household with some member between 6 and 12 years old who does not or never did attend school) and high dependency ratios/low educational level (households with four or more persons per employed member, and whose household head has two or less years at primary school). Nearly 90 per cent of San Martin households suffered from one or more of these compared to 31 per cent in San Francisco Solano as a whole and 24 per cent in Quilmes County as a whole. However, these differences may be smaller because the data for Quilmes and San Francisco Solano comes from the 1980 census while those for San Martin come from the survey in 1984 and conditions certainly worsened in Quilmes and San Francisco Solano between 1980 and 1984 because of the rapid growth in the number of impoverished households in the district or county in these four years.

Table 2.3: Proportion of households with unmet basic needs

AREA	*Households with unmet basic needs*	*Percentage of households with*				
		Over-crowding	*Inade-quate housing*	*No latrine*	*Low school at-tendance*	*High depend-ency ratio*
San Martin	88.6	42.6	82.5	27.9	3.3	8.5
S.F. Solano	31.1	13.1	12.1	5.0	3.6	7.0
Quilmes	23.6	9.0	14.1	2.9	2.3	4.8

Basic services and infrastructure in San Martin

The land sites the squatters invaded had no infrastructure and no services. The squatters were responsible for any improvements but inevitably, their achievements are financially and technically limited.

All homes have electricity but electric connections and installations are make-shift and dangerous. In 16 of the 20 blocks within San Martin, drinking water is obtained from the official district water-pipe network, but through an illegal connection and distribution system. The other four blocks obtain their water from wells with hand operated pumps. But the water distribution system is not of sufficient quality to guard against the water's contamination.

Generally, ground-water quality is good but there are risks of contamination at the first level from latrine residues and thus, this should be avoided as a source of drinking water. The quality of water in the San Francisco stream is also good when it enters the district but it is contaminated along the way by untreated or inadequately treated industrial wastes. Water tests show varying degrees of bacterial contamination and salt levels depending on the source.

Sanitary conditions are very poor. There is no system for the collection and safe disposal of excreta and there are no plans for the installation of sewers because of the scale of work involved and the high cost. Households simply dispose of excreta in latrines which are usually no more than holes in the ground. Nearly three-quarters of all households have unsafe outdoor latrines, with 29 per cent claiming rudimentary flush toilets and 31 per cent non-flush toilets. Thirty per cent of households have no latrine at all, implying the use of a neighbour's facility.

There is no public system to collect household wastes. Dwellers either have to pay a private collector or bury and burn trash in their own backyards with smoke, fumes and smells polluting the neighbourhood – Box 2.2 gives an example.

Box 2.2: The Garay Family.

The Garays are a married couple with three children; both parents come from provinces in the northwest of Argentina. Their eldest child is 11 years old and attends a public school near the *barrio* while the other two (aged three and a half and two) stay at home with their mother. He has been working at the port as a stevedore for 13 years; she would also like to work but finds it difficult because of the children. The husband completed primary school, is one of San Martin's block deputy delegates and is involved with the National Nutrition Plan; the wife dropped out of school at first grade.

Before coming to San Martin, the Garays had lived in a "room and kitchen" they built themselves on a lot belonging to her brother. They moved to San Martin because of the chance of owning their own house and land site; they were looking for new accommodation at the time of the invasion because the owners wanted the land back

Box 2.2: (continued)

to accommodate a growing family. They tried to obtain a land-site in another *barrio* where lots were apparently to be given out but in the end the land was not given out. They moved to San Martin in 1982, after the police cordon had gone. To obtain a plot, they had to present their case to existing residents in block meetings. The plot they were allocated had already been occupied and a room had been built; they purchased this building off the man who was leaving. The present house is built of wood (from the port) and sheet metal (bought a little at a time) and consists of a kitchen-dining room, bedroom, storage room and bathroom. They have a connection to the public water system and have three taps on the plot, one of which is inside the house. There are often water shortages, particularly in the summer, and they try to keep a full tank of water. The tank is also cleaned regularly.

The Garays tell of the year they spent having to fetch and carry water from a faucet in the middle of the block. They usually went to collect the water in the early morning to try and avoid the long queues. The queues were particularly bad in summer and they told of having to queue for "hours and hours". The husband feels that block inhabitants should work together to lay a proper network of pipes and give all the houses proper connections. They have a vegetable patch and garden. They have make-shift electrical connections which they feel are dangerous and they worry about falling cables, particularly during storms. They pay to have the garbage removed three times a week; a man comes with a cart three days a week and collects garbage which has been bundled in small bags from those households who pay him to do so. The Garay's ideal would be to build a house with permanent building material, bit by bit as money allows and the cement foundations have already been laid. They still have reservations about improving their house because of the uncertainty of their tenure of the plot; they don't want to invest in improving the building and then be turned off the land.

For health care, they use both the first-aid centre and the social welfare clinic in Constitucion. The wife prefers the clinic for the children, who were born there and she takes them there for regular check-ups. They worry about the cold in winter, about poor nutrition

Box 2.2: (continued)

and diarrhoea, though they say that they are well fed and dress warmly. They make some use of herbal remedies and home cures dispensed by some women in the *barrio*. The family would like to have a doctor available 24-hours a day and a proper clinic built in the settlement, not just first-aid centres in the *barrios*; but they feel that there would be arguments as to where it should be situated and it would be difficult to get the *barrios* to come to some agreement.

Drainage for both rain and household waste is very inadequate. The only form of drainage in much of the site is open, unlined dirt ditches along the streets and pavements and these create ideal breeding grounds in the summer for disease-carrying insects. Furthermore, inadequate provision for drainage, along with the proximity of the river, means that San Martin is often flooded.

Most streets are still dirt-tracks which rapidly become mud-tracks in the rain. The settlement has only two paved roads. Government schools provide primary education, but it was left to the community to provide day-care centres, first-aid centres and nursery schools with help from their development centres and grass-roots religious communities.

The development of the first-aid centre was discussed earlier. It is basically a few rooms, built by the settlers themselves with donated building materials. Approximately 30 per cent of families make a monthly payment to the centre and benefit from its services free of charge.

Shelter

In general, housing conditions in San Martin are poor with inadequate water supplies, inadequate provision for washing, food preparation and personal hygiene, very inadequate provision for sanitation and high levels of overcrowding.

For any household invading land, the most important thing is to build a dwelling on this land as quickly as possible; this establishes their claim to that plot. This meant that most shelters in San Martin were erected very rapidly, using temporary building materials such as cardboard, sheet metal, canvas and even branches. Households plan to build more solid houses using more permanent building materials later. But two and a half years after the land invasion, the majority of settlers still live in their provisional dwellings. One reason is simply the inhabitants' lack of funds to allow them to improve the quality of the house. Another perhaps more fundamental reason is their uncertainty over whether they will acquire the legal right to occupy the land; there is no point in investing time and money in improving the house if you might be evicted from the land. There is little incentive to build until the issue of land tenure is resolved (see Box 2.3 for an example).

Box 2.3: The Frias Family.

The Frias are a married couple with two children and they are expecting a third. The husband comes from Chaco province from the northeast of Argentina, adjacent to Bolivia and Paraguay, while the wife is Paraguayan. He had worked in the construction industry, but now works as a bakery worker, and she runs a small goods store from the front room of their house. He has recovered from tuberculosis, but now suffers from Chagas disease (a very debilitating disease, transmitted to humans by a blood sucking insect) for which he is receiving medical attention.

Before coming to San Martin, the family had rented a room of just two by three metres in a house in Ezpeleta, but their income could not cover all their needs. They heard about the land invasion and decided to take part. They moved to San Martin with the help of a cousin who had a pick-up truck. They built their house very quickly at night, using scrap sheet metal. Little by little they have enlarged and improved it and put in a concrete floor. But it is still largely made up of panels which can easily be taken apart and moved, if they are forced out of San Martin. There are two bedrooms, a kitchen, small dining area, grocery store at the front and small washbasin and bathroom outside which they share with a neighbour. The husband said that he would like to build a brick house and see a housing co-operative develop in San Martin but this would only be possible if they receive legal tenure to the land on which their house is built. They obtain water from the network the inhabitants installed, illegally connected to the district system but they do not

Box 2.3: (continued)

have a connection into their house – only a tap in their garden. They try to avoid drinking the water from this system whenever possible (for instance, by purchasing bottled water).

For health care, they usually go the Del Plata clinic. This is a clinic funded by a social welfare fund and although the Frias family are members of the San Martin health centre, they hardly ever use it. Their children were born at the Del Plata clinic and the wife seeks medical advice from there, whenever she feels that any of the children are ill. They claim to be happy with the medical treatment they receive.

The quality of dwellings in San Martin reflect both the uncertainty about land tenure and also the economic possibilities and needs of each household. Most plots are 200 – 500 square metres, with a temporary dwelling in the centre and with a garden or vegetable patch. Most dwellings have one or two rooms for living, sleeping and preparing food and a separate area for a latrine, garbage cans and, in some cases, a shower. Some houses have connecting, covered passages which are also used for washing, cooking or as living rooms, and most have a solid surface area outside for outdoor activities. Three-quarters of all households have an average of two or more persons per room while more than a third have four or more persons per room.

The physical quality of the housing is poor. Four-fifths of the houses surveyed use light-weight materials (sheet metal, cardboard, wood) for exterior walls and interior partitioning. Only 20 per cent use brick or cement blocks. Two-thirds of the roofs are made of sheet metal or fibre-cement while virtually all other roofs are made out of cardboard or scrap material; only two per cent are made of reinforced concrete tiles. Just over half of the dwellings have dirt floors and these obviously present problems of hygiene, especially with flooding being common and very inadequate provision for drains for storm and surface water and for domestic waste-water; most of the rest have cement or brick floors.

Sixty-one per cent of households are connected to a water supply system installed by the inhabitants, drawing from public water mains but only a small proportion have water piped into their homes. Many households have no tap on their plot and so water has to be collected daily from elsewhere (see Table 2.4). Tests for water quality showed that water taken from the public

Table 2.4: Water supply

Type of supply	*Percentage of households*
Precarious connection to public system	
tap on plot but not piped into the shelter	20
tap on plot, piped into the shelter	6
tap but not on the plot	35
Water pump drawing from ground water	
Piped into the shelter	7
Not piped into the shelter	28
Purchase from water carriers or some other source	4

system had little bacteriological contamination and that this could be enhanced by improving the connection and distribution system (eliminating the possibility of dirty water seeping into the distributions system and better maintenance of the taps) and introducing sodium hypochlorite into the water until the bacteria level was lowered. Water drawn by pumps from the first-level ground water had a very high bacteria content and this should not be used. Pumps that drew from deeper wells, sunk to the second level of ground water, provided much better quality water although wells here should also be treated with sodium hypochlorite.

The houses have very few windows and those that exist tend to be small and close to the cooking area. There are few windows in the sleeping quarters, resulting in poor ventilation and inadequate light. External openings are deliberately kept to a minimum in order to conserve heat during the winter, when it can get very cold.

Half of the dwellings have a refrigerator (a low figure by Buenos Aires standards); 92 per cent use bottled gas for cooking and food storage facilities are inadequate.

Health

Three factors were assessed to give a picture of health conditions in San Martin: inhabitants' access to health services and coverage of primary health needs; levels of risk in contracting a disease as a function of the health care given; and proportion of people showing symptoms of disease, when subject to physical examinations and simple clinical tests.

Access to Health Services: Nearly three out of five household heads turn to the public hospital or first-aid centre as the first health service. A third look to health care provided through the social welfare funds to which they contribute (a benefit only available to those legally employed). However, 35 per cent of workers with the right to use social welfare fund services still prefer to use the public hospital or the first-aid centre as the first service to which they turn (see Table 2.5).

Table 2.5: The health service to which people turn first

First health service sought	*Per cent who use it and who are entitled to social welfare fund coverage*	*Per cent who use it and who are not members of social welfare fund*	*Percent (total for each group)*
Household heads			
Hospital or first aid centre	31	80	58
Business or insurance	9	5	7
Social welfare fund	56	–	25
Don't know/no response	4	15	10
Spouses/partners			
Hospital	25	33	29
First aid centre	42	60	52
Social welfare fund	22	–	10
Other	11	7	9
For children			
Hospital	47	68	57
First aid centre	31	30	30
Social welfare fund	16	–	7
Other	6	2	6

Note: figures for children include responses by household head or spouses/partners and are for all infants and children under 15 years of age.

The proportion of partners or spouses who have the right to use social welfare fund services but do not use these as their first option is even higher than that for household heads. Social welfare funds usually provide health services for members' families. However, legal marriage may be a prerequisite for other family members receiving services and the fact that many couples in San Martin are not legally married might explain the low usage of these health services.

For 52 per cent of women, the San Martin first-aid centre that the inhabitants built themselves is the first service to which they turn. Considering the lack of resources at this centre, this reflects the inadequacy of health care coverage. The local health centre is preferred to public hospitals because of the lack of help to look after their children while they visit the hospital, and the high cost of transportation.

The first choice of treatment for children is the public hospital (57 per cent), however costly or distant. This probably reflects the fact that mothers know the hospital if the child was born there; that the child may have been going to the hospital since infancy; and that a particular hospital has better paediatric services.

Many of the inhabitants of San Martin are not covered by any insurance scheme for work-related injuries. Employers cover medical costs for 37 per cent of full-time workers and social welfare funds run by workers unions cover 23 per cent of personnel. One-third of wage-earners have no job injury protection at all, a figure related to the number of people in precarious employment, where there are no social benefits.

Risk of Illness and Level of Preventive Health Care: Three factors which help determine the risk of illness and the level of preventive health care are: the regularity of health check-ups for mothers, pregnant women and children; the proportion of children immunized against the most common, dangerous diseases; and the nutritional status of infants.

Medical check-ups for children are a basic part of preventive medicine. Seventy-three per cent of mothers polled said they took their children under three years of age for regular check-ups (although post-survey interviews with 20 mothers suggest that this figure is too high). Most of the mothers interviewed said that they took their infants and young children to check-ups once or twice a year which is well below the national norm. The interviews suggest that mothers usually take their infants and young children for check-ups only when there is some symptom of illness. Mothers who recognize the need for regular check-ups pointed to the lack of services available to them and the high cost of transport as the reasons why regular check-ups are not common.

For school-age children (6 – 12 years), immunization and dental and medical check-ups are normally performed at school. Three-quarters of all mothers were aware of the check-ups while the same proportion of mothers who were aware of them thought they were a good thing. The fact that 25 per cent did not think they were a good thing suggests a lack of communication between school health-programme officials and parents. Three-quarters of the mothers showed an interest at being present at check-ups.

In a survey of 198 women, about 75 per cent sought medical care during pregnancy, though not suspecting any problems. This figure rises to 89 per cent if women seeking help after suspecting some problem are included. Three per cent refused any help. About 12 per cent had too few check-ups during their first pregnancies (only one or two), about 50 per cent had a good number (6 or more), and 20 per cent an acceptable number (3 to 5). In the good and acceptable cases, check-ups began within the first three months of pregnancy, while those women with few check-ups sought assistance much later on and then probably only because of the onset of complications. Hospital care for childbirth was preferred in 90 per cent of cases.

Family planning is either completely unknown or only partially known to 40 per cent of the women. This lack of knowledge is probably due to the lack of government services promoting family planning. Of those who are aware of it, 27 per cent feel that the methods are either harmful or useless. The negative responses could be due to misinformation or bad experiences.

In regard to child immunization, only 28 per cent of all households had all their children under seven years of age fully immunized against the most common and dangerous childhood diseases (diphtheria, whooping cough and tetanus, polio and measles). In 36 per cent of households, some of the children have received the necessary immunization while in the remaining 36 per cent, all children are only partially vaccinated. This represents a very low level of immunization, as the required level to protect a population is between 80 – 95 per cent depending on the disease. Also worrying is the fact that 15 per cent of mothers feel that the vaccine might endanger the child or make it ill.

In considering the nutritional state of the children, three factors were looked at: the type of food given to infants (aged 0 to 1 years); the use of foods considered important (milk, meat, cheese, fruit) in 1 – 9 year olds; and weight – height measurements; the results are summarized in Box 2.4. These suggest an inadequate protein intake for children and below average heights and weights.

Box 2.4: Findings from the nutrition survey

In a group of 54 infants, most were on an exclusively milk-based diet up to the age of six months: 91 per cent of 0 – 2 month olds had milk only (82 per cent mother's milk alone or complemented by dairy milk, nine per cent dairy milk only); as did 78 per cent of 3 – 6 month olds (56 per cent and 22 per cent respectively) and 40 per cent of 7 – 12 month olds (12 per cent and 28 per cent).

In the 1–9 year old group, despite the limitations of a one-day survey which looked at the food they consumed, the findings suggest an inadequate consumption of protein. Only 49 per cent of the 1–4 year-old group and 54 per cent of the 5–9 year-old group had eaten meat on the day of the survey; 64 per cent and 39 per cent respectively had drunk milk. Fifteen per cent of both groups had eaten eggs; four per cent and one per cent cheese; 24 and 28 per cent fruit. For more than half the children surveyed, the diet was mainly carbohydrate.

A group of 10 infants, 50 children of between 1 and 4 years, and 43 children of between 5 and 9 years were examined, using height–weight charts. Using the official Buenos Aires Province Public Health Ministry charts, both average heights and weights were below that expected for healthy infants and children, especially among children of between 1 and 4 years.

Diseases Detected: The research team lacked the resources to undertake a comprehensive study of health problems arising from physical examinations and laboratory tests. However, physical examinations for a relatively large sample (99 infants and children, 21 adult males and 44 adult females) and laboratory tests for smaller sub-samples give some indication of the diseases which most seriously affected the population at the time of the field-work. The findings are summarized in Box 2.5.

Box 2.5: Findings from physical examinations and laboratory tests

INFANTS AND CHILDREN (0 – 14 years): Physical examination of 12 infants less than one year old; 51 1 – 4 year-olds; 60 5 – 9 year-olds and 21 10 – 14 year-olds. The main health problem evident was the inflammation of the upper respiratory tract. This was evident in 41 per cent of infants, 15 per cent of 1 – 4 year olds, 10 per cent of 5 – 9 year olds and 19 per cent of 10 – 14 year olds. Blood and urine tests for 56 infants and children showed:

– two cases of haematuria (presence of blood in the urine)
– 10 cases with pyuria (suggesting urinary infection)
– 15 cases with iron-deficiencies (anaemia)
– One case of probable diabetes
– 35 cases of eosinophilia (which with other clinical tests, suggests intestinal parasites).

ADULT FEMALES: Physical examinations for 44 women showed the following as the most common health problems: varicose veins in lower body (18 per cent); spinal column afflictions (14 per cent); dental problems (14 per cent); arterial hypotension (11 per cent); upper breathing tract infections (11 per cent); chronic bronchial infections; urinary infections (9 per cent). Blood and urine tests found haematuria and/or microscopic pyuria in 32 per cent and slight anaemia in ten per cent.

ADULT MALES: Physical examinations for 21 males showed the following as the most common health problems: dental problems (38 per cent); alcoholism (24 per cent); chronic bronchitis (24 per cent); varicose veins in lower parts of body (24 per cent); cardio-vascular disease (10 per cent); haemorrhoids (10 per cent); upper respiratory tract infection (10 per cent). Blood and urine tests found haematuria and/or microscopic pyuria in 29 per cent of males.

In addition, 63 per cent of adults tested showed evidence of intestinal parasites. Thirteen people were tested for Chagas' Disease – a particularly debilitating infection; three of the tests proved positive and all three persons had originally come from Chaco Province where Chagas' Disease is very common (see Chapter 10 for more details of Chagas' Disease and its links with housing).

Some Conclusions

This chapter has provided a sketch of how a very large group of people, most of them with low incomes, took action and worked together to solve their own housing problem – and the difficulties they faced in doing so. It also outlines the social, economic and political context of this invasion and its cordination (even if they did not succeed in obtaining legal recognition for their land occupation). The initial organization began during a period of severe economic crisis and political repression. Once the land invasion had been effected, the invaders also felt that they had the right to make legitimate demands on the state for basic infrastructure and services. In addition, the invaders formed their own democratic and non-hierarchical organization to defend what they had achieved, to negotiate with the government and to organize (mostly at neighbourhood level) collective action to address some of the most pressing health and habitat problems. The chapter illustrates both the considerable potential that low-income communities have to address their own housing and health problems and, at the same time, the limitations they face in doing so, especially in the absence of government support. New partnerships forged between local governments and community organizations formed by low-income groups may greatly improve housing conditions and health status at relatively low cost, but local governments must have the resources and expertise to respond much more effectively to low-income groups' needs for secure tenure, basic infrastructure and services. Central to the improvement of health would be better equipped health-care centres, easily accessible and open for those hours which best suit working parents.

Chapter Three

Housing and Health in Olaleye-Iponri, a Low Income Settlement in Lagos, Nigeria

Tade Akin Aina

Introduction

Lagos is the largest urban agglomeration in sub-Saharan Africa; although no accurate statistics exist as to its current population, estimates suggest that these were over 4.5 million inhabitants by the mid-1980s.[1] Its current size owes much to its role as capital of Nigeria, sub-Saharan Africa's most populous nation. Although in the mid-1970s construction began on a new federal capital (Abuja) in the geographic centre of Nigeria – and Abuja is now the capital – Lagos had been the national capital for over 50 years from 1914 when the British colonial government joined together what had previously been two separate protectorates of Southern and Northern Nigeria. Lagos had also been a key administrative centre, port and railway terminus before 1914.

Lagos had little importance in the pre-colonial period; in the late-eighteenth century, it was a relatively small and unimportant Yoruba fishing and farming settlement on what came to be known as Lagos Island. It owes its current name to the Portuguese, being named after a southern Portuguese port, and it became first a centre of the slave trade and later a centre of agricultural commerce. Once under British rule (commencing in 1861) it developed as the centre of the colonial bureaucracy and then as the port and railway terminus serving western Nigeria. Lagos also became a centre for repatriated emancipated Yoruba slaves returning from Brazil, the West Indies and Sierre Leone. Estimates suggest a population of some 5,000 in 1800, 74,000 in 1911, and then, within an expanded metropolitan area, 303,500 in 1952, 726,600 in 1963 and over 4.5 million by the mid-1980s. In 1901, it covered no more than 4 square kilometres, centred on Lagos Island. By 1978, it covered some 879 square kilometres and had long since spread over large areas of the mainland.[2] It remains the nation's pre-eminent industrial, commercial and financial centre; enterprises located there benefited greatly from the large revenues generated by oil exports in 1973 and for some years after that. But investments in basic infrastructure and services never kept up with the rapid growth in economic activities and population and the deficiencies have not been addressed during the 1980s, when the economy has been much less buoyant.

Housing and health conditions and policies in Nigeria

That part of the West African coast on which Lagos is located has never had a good reputation for health among Europeans. The early writings of colonial officials confirm the precarious health and habitat conditions, particularly in Lagos. According to Peter Marris

> all European descriptions of Lagos in the nineteenth century harp wearily on squalor and disease. Sir Richard Burton, when made British Consul in the area commented "They are trying to kill me, but I shall live, just to spite them". He considered Lagos, "certainly one of the most unhealthy spots on these malarious shores" and recommended street widening, drainage and public health regulations. At the end of the century, the death rate amongst the European population was worse than ever. A grim item in the Lagos Standard protested that "it was time that something should be done to relieve the grave diggers from the strain of work to which they are continually subjected – they are working a twelve-hour day, Sundays included. Drainage and swamp reclamation, scavenging and fresh wells, seemed to make little difference: the grave diggers were still overworked".[3]

Although very few studies of Nigeria have directly tried to link health and habitat conditions, there is still some mention in the literature on the health problems associated with uncontrolled urbanization and poor housing.[4] The most consistent sources of information on conditions during the colonial period refer to Lagos. Around 1900, the fact that Lagos was located on an island (at this time with no bridge to the mainland) – and its unplanned beginnings – made it highly susceptible to serious overcrowding.[5] There was very poor sanitation and periodic outbreaks of epidemics. These epidemics contributed to the high infant mortality rate, estimated to be 41.4 per thousand population and 450 per thousand live births, around the beginning of the twentieth century. In response to this problem, the colonial governments set up health boards to begin projects for the improvement of sanitation, sewage disposal and the supply of pipe-borne water to the city population. There were also various anti-malarial projects and vaccination campaigns to check the constant outbreaks of smallpox epidemics.[6]

By 1950, housing standards were still very poor. Most houses had neither piped water nor connection to a sewage system. Marris notes the appalling conditions and inadequacy of services such as water, drainage, toilet facilities, the low standard of housing and the serious overcrowding. He points out that the conditions create serious problems for health. "The commonest serious illnesses in the city ... are infective and parasitic diseases especially malaria, bronchitis and pneumonia, dysentery and diarrhoea, and skin complaints. The first three groups caused nearly half the deaths registered in 1947."[7]

Records show that colonial officials recognized the connection between controlling these diseases and improving the urban environment and housing conditions. The annual report of the Federal Medical Services for 1957 noted that "the eradication or diminution, of pneumonia and dysentery as causes of death are long-term projects involving such social advances as slum clearance, better housing, waterborne sewage and, not least important, the education of the public in the proper use of these amenities..."[8]

It was this kind of reasoning that must have inspired the Lagos Slum Clearance Scheme begun in 1955. But, as has become obvious, slum clearance schemes alone are insufficient guarantees either for good environmental sanitation or the improvement of health and habitat conditions. The ineffectiveness of such schemes was shown by a study conducted in the immediate post-independence years (Nigeria achieved independence in 1960). Investigators looking at the core area of Lagos wrote in 1967 that "the area is overcrowded, congested and modern sanitary facilities are lacking. Generally, those who live there are susceptible to any onslaught of epidemics. Ignorance and economic deprivation are characteristics of the people living in this area."[9]

Until the 1970s, governments in Nigeria had not concerned themselves in any major way with the provision of mass-housing. This neglect originated in the colonial period, when government housing schemes concentrated on the provision of housing in exclusively non-Nigerian neighbourhoods for expatriate staff of both the colonial service and commercial companies, and tiny working-class row houses for African civil servants. The main attempts at public intervention in mass housing during the colonial period – through the creation of the Lagos Executive Development Board and the subsequent Lagos slum clearance scheme, swamp reclamation and rehousing programmes – were initially motivated by reactions to epidemic outbreaks such as that of bubonic plague in Lagos between 1924 and 1930. The essentially elitist colonial government's policy on housing was inherited by the post-colonial governments under which more exclusive Government Reservation Areas and heavily-subsidized housing estates for civil servants were built.

In the early post-colonial period, the national government showed little interest in trying to improve housing conditions; little was allocated to public housing except for funds allocated to housing for government staff. In the early 1970s, some new initiatives were taken including setting up the National Council on Housing in 1971 and an increase in the government's equity share in the Nigeria Building Society in 1972. In 1973, the federal government announced a programme to build 59,000 housing units of which 15,000 were to be built in Lagos. The same year, a Federal Housing Authority was established to implement federal housing programmes.

The Third Plan period, 1975–1980, saw the emergence of housing as a separate sector in development planning, with a very substantial independent allocation of 1,837 million *naira*; this was later increased to 2,256 million in the revised 1975 – 80 plan, which at 1977 exchange rates was equivalent to some US $3.5 billion. Government revenues had increased very considerably as a result of the growth in oil exports. Government policy towards housing became more explicit: it became "part of its social responsibility to participate actively in the provision of housing for all income groups and it will therefore intervene on a large scale in this sector".[10] However, only 19 per cent of the original target was completed in the Lagos Metropolis and only 13 per cent in the rest of the country.[11] In addition, many of the units built in this public housing programme were not allocated to poorer households.

The Fourth Plan Period, 1981 – 1985, saw a return to civilian electoral politics. The different political parties in control of the federal and state governments tried to outdo each other by placing housing as a major issue on their election programmes. Each set ambitious targets – for instance the party controlling the federal government set up a Federal Housing Scheme under which it proposed to build a total of 200,000 housing units at the rate of 2,100 per year in each of the 19 states of the federation. The same government in 1982 also set out a national housing policy which attempted to combine the direct provision of housing with other elements to facilitate home-ownership through private initiatives. But the goals of both the national housing policy and the public attempts failed for several reasons. These included the fact that targets for the number of housing units were never met; the housing projects were over-subsidized; many of the projects were never completed owing to the inefficiency and corruption of the contractors; some of the units were allocated on the basis of political patronage, nepotistic and other sectionalist considerations; and, in a lot of cases, people did not want the houses because they were either too expensive and/or were built on inaccessible and undesirable sites.[12] By 1984, a military take-over saw the emergence of a new regime which re-evaluated previous housing policies and which, facing the economic recession, shifted its position from the direct provision of housing to an emphasis on sites and services.

No recent figures give a detailed picture of housing conditions in Lagos. An official survey of Lagos State in 1976 showed that conditions had changed little in the previous ten years; only nine per cent of houses were in what it termed "good sanitary conditions" and about 53 per cent were in "poor sanitary conditions". Over two-thirds of all houses had poor drainage facilities, and only about 34 per cent were connected to pipe-borne water supply. Flush toilets were used by only about 18 per cent of households; one-third used bucket latrines while 29 per cent used pit latrines and about 18 per cent had no toilets at all.[13] Although no more recent statistics are available on the proportion of people living in adequate quality housing units with basic infrastructure and services, the proportion of people in Lagos State or the Lagos urban agglomeration adequately served is unlikely to have increased from the 1976 figures and has probably declined. In 1980, the governor of Lagos State summarized the problem in the introduction to a new state interim masterplan:

> a notorious feature of the territories now comprising Lagos State over the years has been haphazard development. Many of the popular towns and districts in the State – particularly in Metropolitan Lagos – were unplanned. They sprung up as contraventions and the Government of the day, rendered helpless by the sheer quantity of the contraventions, eventually accepted them as de facto towns.... there are no infrastructural services in most of them and such as exist are grossly inadequate.[14]

Although made over ten years ago, this statement remains accurate today.

These examples indicate what seems to be the state of health and habitat conditions in Nigerian urban areas, particularly within their low-income settlements and the core areas of traditional towns. The deprived urban conditions complicate and erode the effectiveness of hospital-based medical care to which governments' policy and spending have been geared over the past 30 years or so. The result is that indicators of the health conditions of the population continue to show tremendous deficiencies.

Table 3.1: Major notifiable diseases in Nigeria, 1968, 1973 and 1977 (thousands of cases reported)

	1968	*1973*	*1977*
Malaria	266	724	1,223
Dysentery (all types)	129	227	242
Measles	50	109	283
Pneumonia	28	69	97
Gonorrhoea	42	70	65
Whooping Cough	19	21	42
Chicken Pox	10	19	39
Filariasis	7	20	25
Schistosomiasis (all types)	9	25	24
Tuberculosis	9	14	15

Note: Other major causes of morbidity in Nigeria (diseases or disease conditions not notifiable to medical authorities but in the top ten) are protein malnutrition and motor traffic accidents.

Source: ILO/JASPA, *First Things First: Meeting the Basic Needs of Nigeria*, 1981, p. 60

Table 3.1 presents a picture of this deficiency through the distribution of major notifiable diseases for selected years. It is significant that nothing much seems to have changed since 1947 in terms of the prevalence of diseases. The three top killers identified by Marris for 1947 (pneumonia, malaria and bronchitis) are still important,[15] as are dysentery and other diseases pointed out by investigators as being important in 1958 and 1967.[16] It should also be noted that Table 3.1 does not present an accurate picture of health conditions. Many serious health problems are not notifiable. In addition, many of the diseases in Table 3.1 will be under-reported, especially by people who do not go to health centres and who have parasites such as schistosomiasis, filariasis and ascaris. What Table 3.1 suggests is that in spite of all the development-planning efforts since 1946, and the improvements in education and increase in financial and human resources in the country, there is no apparent diminution of these diseases. It is also notable that many of the most prevalent diseases are ones which are associated with poor quality housing and living conditions and lack of basic services.

Olaleye-Iponri

In the years 1984–6, a study was undertaken in Olaleye-Iponri, a densely- populated, predominantly low-income settlement in Lagos with around 20,000 inhabitants. The study examined in detail the history and socio-economic, spatial and political structure of the settlement and the community life, activities, health conditions and needs of its inhabitants. The sources of data included: structured interviews with 438 heads of households; extended unstructured interviews with government officials such as physical planners, community-development officers, local-government administrators, health officials, police officers and waste-disposal agency officials and with community leaders, religious leaders, market women, tenants and landlords; life-histories and health–habitat profiles for selected informants living in the settlement; and documents such as official reports, maps, title deeds, conveyances, newspaper reports, minutes of meetings, court summons and letters. This and subsequent sections are a summary of the research findings; readers wanting a more complete and detailed report of the findings should refer to the longer research report.[17]

Olaleye-Iponri originally consisted of two independent communities lying next to each other on a site of some 35.3 hectares (see Map 3.1). They are located primarily within the jurisdiction of the Lagos Mainland Local Government. The communities in their present location make up highly compact settlements whose expansion is limited by a series of natural and human-made barriers. To the northwest is the Western Avenue, a major road linking Lagos Island through Eko bridge with the rest of the mainland. On the west and south, expansion is hindered both by the railway track and the extensive property of the Roman Catholic Church which includes schools, living quarters and a convent. Towards the east, there is a natural boundary made up of a stretch of swampy terrain and an earth drain referred to as the "canal", and in the northeast there is the highly-priced high- to medium-income settlement of Alaka Estate. To the south Olaleye-Iponri shares boundaries with a police station and barracks and the highly-built up low-income settlements known as Abule-Nla and Apapa Road. Olaleye-Iponri's central location within metropolitan Lagos and its contiguity to Alaka Estate makes it a valuable site for its inhabitants, despite the deficiencies of the site and infrastructure and service provision there.

Olaleye and Iponri, although considered one settlement, were originally separate. Olaleye is believed to have been founded less than 150 years ago when the (then) Oloto of Oto (a major land owning Lagos chief) gave the parcel of land to a certain Ajao Olaleye for use as farmland. Since the area was dense forest and uninhabited, Ajao Olaleye could not live on the farmland. He invited a man known as Baba Egun, to settle on and farm the land. Baba Egun was both a farmer and a herbalist who specialized in treating psychiatric disorders. He farmed both his own allocation and the plots of Olaleye who resided instead in Oto. Baba Egun invited another man, Sadiku, to live with him on the land. They invited others onto the land and these became the first generation of settlers. Most engaged in agricultural pursuits such as palm-wine tapping, palm-oil processing, fruit planting, market gardening, fishing and trapping.

When Baba Egun died, Sadiku was the oldest man in the village and became the *Bale* (the traditional head of village). In this capacity, Sadiku was asked by Olaleye to bring more people into the village. According to our informant, this accounted for the upsurge in the population of the village and its development.

Olaleye-Iponri contains a complex mix of tenants, landlords who own buildings but rent the land on which they stand and landowners (most of them living elsewhere). Most inhabitants of Olaleye-Iponri are tenants. Most of the land in both settlements belongs to a small group of absentee landowners. Families usually live together in

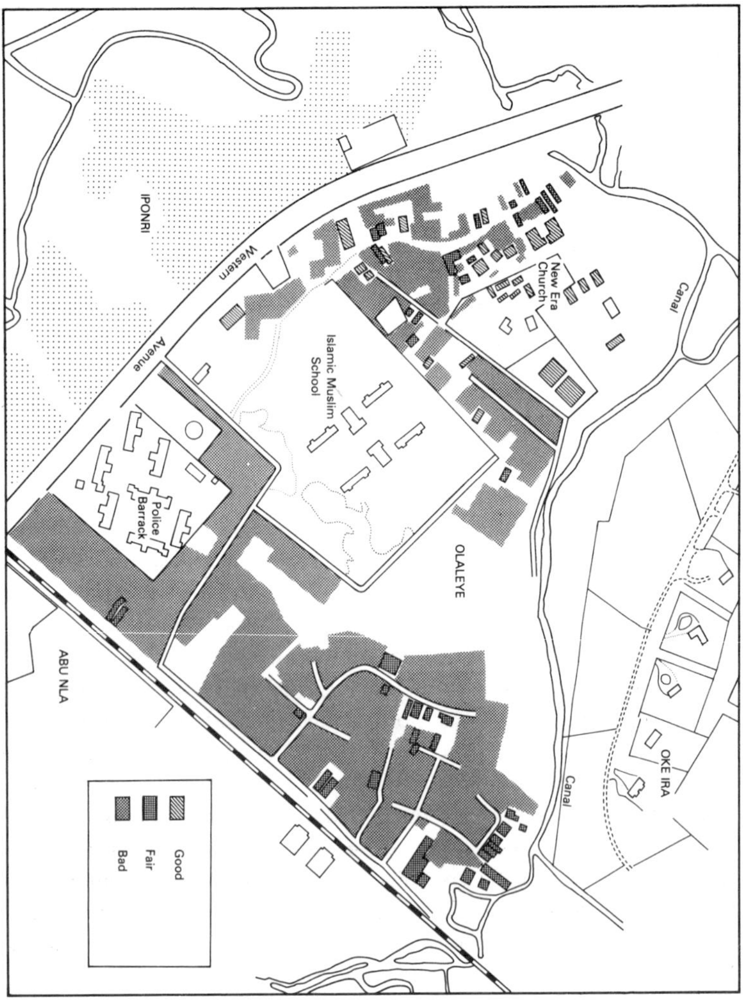
IPONRI
Western
Avenue
Islamic Muslim
School
Police
Barrack
New Era
Church
Canal
OLALEYE
ABU NLA
OKE IRA
Canal
Good
Fair
Bad

Map 3.1

one rented room. There are also many small landlords living in Olaleye-Iponri who own the buildings but are also tenants in that they lease the land on which their building stands. Today almost three-quarters of the landlords hold lease tenancy agreements and receipts issued by the Olaleye family.[18]

Olaleye's initial growth began with the construction of various phases of the railway line, particularly the extension to Apapa (Lagos's main port) during the 1940s and early 1950s. It is with this that the first wave of migrants arrived to work as construction workers, labourers and staff of the railways and the petty traders. Estimates suggest approximately 2,500 persons in Olaleye village by 1967. These lived in 270 buildings on 31.6 acres (12.8 hectares) and in the words of the officials consisted mainly of "labourers, vagrants and many people of the low-income group".[19] The settlement has grown rapidly since the end of the Nigerian Civil War in 1970 and the beginning of the economic boom caused by the rise in petroleum oil earnings. This period has been identified as a second phase of rapid urbanization in Nigeria and there was a major influx of migrants from the eastern parts of the country to Olaleye Village.[20] In September 1983, the population was estimated to be 16,590.[21]

Iponri Village is believed to have been founded by a certain Abegundoko who came from Niger State in 1878. Although our informants were not sure, Abegundoko must have acquired the land from the Oloto family who owned virtually all the adjoining lands in these parts of Lagos Mainland. Abegundoko farmed the land, planting cashew, mangoes and apples. As his farming thrived, he was joined by many other settlers from areas such as Badagry, Apapa-Elemu and Gbotifa (all of which are now settlements on the outskirts of Lagos). These different settlers created adjoining settlements such as Agegunle Village, Caterpillar Village, Good-U-Morning and Saro Garden Villages. Most of these have now disappeared as separate settlements.

Iponri's community has grown in response to the same conditions that account for the expansion of Olaleye. But it has been greatly affected by government land acquisitions for various projects ranging from the building of roads and bridges (a new express highway now forms its western border) to the construction of offices, and housing and shopping estates. In more recent times both Iponri's and Olaleye's population has grown in response to specific needs within the socio-spatial system of Metropolitan Lagos. These include serving as a residential and business base for both low-income, self-employed and casual labour. An official estimate puts the joint population of the two villages at 20,090 in 1984. Iponri is clearly the smaller of the two communities.[22]

On entering Olaleye Village, either across the railway line from Apapa Road or through its main access road from Western Avenue, one gets the impression (at least before the spate of demolitions that occurred from mid-1984) of a vibrant and lively economic life, despite the prevailing nation-wide economic recession. This is because both entrances into the village go past the market and the various stalls on the railway line. Apart from the buzz of voices coming from the market women bargaining or quarrelling with each other and purchasers, there is also the insistent and deafening blare of music from gramophones in the shops on the railway line selling textiles, patent medicines, auto spare parts, electronic goods and records. There is also the larger concentration, particularly in the evenings, of petty traders with their wares on trays either on the railway line or in front of the market stalls on the road that leads into the village. These sell foodstuffs like pepper, vegetables, oil, dried and fresh fish. Others sell products such as tinned milk, sugar, beverages, matches, cigarettes, sweets and kolanuts.

On the same route leading into the village (which forms its central business district) are two beer-parlours, a beer-parlour/night-club/brothel, another brothel, and a make-shift cinema whose walls are built of corrugated iron-sheets and which usually shows popular Indian movies. Further evidence of economic activity can be seen in the women who sell a wide range of cooked food products such as rice and beans, fried and roast plantains, fried yam chips, fried meat, fried bean balls (*akara*), bean cakes (*moin-moin*) and corn-flour paste. Particularly in the evenings, all of these come to life creating an atmosphere of an intensely vibrant, candle and lamp-lit bazaar. Normally in the daytime life within the village is less lively but this picks up on Saturdays when the market and the village are busy both day and night.

Apart from the petty producers, Olaleye also contains several activities in the area of craft production and artisanal activity. Tailors (both male and female) abound. There are shoe-makers, blacksmiths, tinkers, watch-repairers and knife-sharpeners. Others include washermen (personal laundry-services), mechanics, battery-chargers, shoe-shiners and itinerant beauticians (pedicuring, manicuring and barbering).

As for Iponri, the picture is that of a decaying residential area. It contains its own share of beer parlours, provision shops and pools-betting shops. But the climate of the bazaar that greets one on entry into Olaleye in the evening is missing. Iponri contains some visible informal–sector activities in its own shops – and household producers of various goods – but lacks the equivalent of Olaleye's central district with its hotels, cinema, nite club and brothels.

Box 3.1: Michael And Josephine's family:

Michael and Josephine are both from the same village in Bendel State. Michael, 51 years-old, is a retired railway locomotive driver with the Nigeria Railways. Josephine is 31 years-old. They have six children who live with them (aged 13, 10, 7, 4, 2 and 6 months); Michael has three children by a previous relationship but they are 24, 22 and 20 years-old, and do not live with them.

The family rents one room in a "face to face" building with 15 rooms and ten other households. Their room itself is not big (about 3 by 2.4 metres) and is stuffy, poorly lit and poorly ventilated. There is only one window and no ceiling. Nothing reduces the heat of the sun that falls directly on the corrugated iron sheets making up the roof. There are two toilets and two bathrooms in the building but the landlord who also lives there has exclusive use of one each of these so the other 10 households share the remaining bathroom and toilet. Josephine does her cooking in the corridors with a small kerosene stove. The house has no internal source of water supply; water is purchased for drinking and cooking from hawkers. At times, they also use the public taps in the settlement and fetch water from a nearby well for other purposes. They store their drinking water in a plastic container.

The main health complaints for the adults are coughs, malaria fever, headaches and joint aches. This is not surprising in the case of Michael considering his previous occupation. For the children, the main complaints are diarrhoea and malaria. The main source of health care is the Railway Hospital and occasionally the chemists in the settlement. One of their children died, some six or seven years ago, of a urinary tract infection – "he could not urinate properly". The parents claim that they have recently vaccinated all their young

Box 3.1: (continued)

children at the Desalu health centre. On being asked what was the major health problem in the settlement, Michael and Josephine answered that it was malaria fever.

On its outskirts, and bearing little or no direct relationship to life within Iponri, are some structures devoted to more developed economic activities. There is, for instance, a petrol station on Western Avenue and a multi-storey building owned by a Lebanese family a few metres away on the same road as the petrol station. This building, with its own security guards, houses a few federal government and private ventures, and is also the residence of the current Lebanese landlord. Iponri is a little more developed than Olaleye in terms of the standards of buildings and the socio-economic status of some of its residents. One of them has a plastic shoe moulding factory within his premises. This enterprise, whose employment varies between nine to 20 employees, is an example of a small-scale industry in the settlement.

Socio-economic characteristics

The fieldwork in Olaleye-Iponri and official sources show that this is a low income, predominantly working-class, settlement. Official planning estimates for January 1984, suggest a total population of 20,090 with 2,979 adult males, 2,995 adult females and 14,116 children.[23] Large households are the norm. In Olaleye, households of between five to eight constitute just less than half of respondents, while households with between nine to 11 persons account for another one-fifth. For Iponri, half the sample are from households of between five to eight persons, while about 13 per cent are in households of between nine to 11 persons. Three-fifths of all respondents have three or more children in their household while a third have six or more children.

Most of the workforce are employees of the civil service, private-sector enterprises or parastatals (partly government-owned enterprises providing commercial and other services, including the railways). Of these, the civil service is most important in Olaleye employing over a third of all respondents (see Table 3.2). A considerable proportion are also self employed, especially in Iponri.

Table 3.2: Sources of employment

Source	*Olaleye*	*(percentages)*	*Iponri*
Civil service	35.9		24.8
Parastatals	6.4		10.5
Private sector	25.4		18.1
Self-employment	31.9		46.7
Other	0.3		–
Number	295		105

Table 3.3 shows respondents' occupations. Office workers, factory workers, petty traders, petty artisans and craftworkers predominate. Workers are the most important grouping among Olaleye respondents of which office/clerical work is the leading category followed by factory/general work. Other categories of importance among Olaleye inhabitants working for an employer include the occupational groupings listed as messengers/drivers, security workers and construction workers.

Table 3.3: Main categories of occupation

Occupation	*Olaleye*	*(percentages)*	*Iponri*
Petty trading	12.5		14.8
Petty artisans/ craftworker	10.4		17.6
Domestic/catering	3.5		1.7
Construction trade	2.1		5.5
Security	5.6		4.6
Factory/general work	19.5		15.7
Office work/clerks	21.9		12.9
Teacher	1.4		2.8
Contractor/business representative	8.7		11.1
Preacher	0.7		–
Priest/healer			
Retired/pensioner	1.4		1.9
Messenger/driver	9.4		12.9
Others	2.8		–
Number	287		108

Among the self-employed, petty traders, artisans and those engaged in crafts are also important categories in Olaleye, followed by contractor/business representatives. In Iponri, a higher proportion of the workforce is engaged in each of these self-employed categories: petty trading, artisans/craftworkers and contractor/businesses representative with a lower proportion in factor/general work and office work/clerks.

Further information was collected which considered the location of residents' employment and the location of customers for the self-employed. Both are helpful in understanding the relationship of Olaleye-Iponri to the wider city of Lagos. Relatively few residents of Olaleye work in the village and most businesses there draw more on customers from outside the settlement than from the settlement itself. However, most residents do not travel far to work and most customers for businesses located in Olaleye-Iponri also live closeby. Only Iponri's self-employed find much custom from those living outside the settlement. This is likely to be related to the fact that it is in Iponri that one finds the main location of workers dealing with automobiles and electrical goods, which few residents can afford.

Olaleye-Iponri's location provides a short journey time for its residents going to and from work. For most, this reduces the ordeal which Charles Abrams, Otto Koenigsberger and others pointed out in 1964 when they noted that "thousands of workmen in Lagos travel more than two hours to get to their work.... We found cases when 10–15 per cent of the family budget went on fares at the expense of other essentials like food or education for children."[24] Serious traffic congestion and very inadequate public transport remain major problems today.

Most of those interviewed had very low incomes; more than 85 per cent earned less than 300 *naira* per month (at the time of the study, one Nigerian *naira* was worth around US $1; by June 1989, the exchange rate was N7.5 to $1). Seven out of ten respondents in Olaleye and about three-fifths of those in Iponri, earn between N60 and N240 per month. These income groupings, if evaluated by the current pattern of public sector remuneration, are based within the broad category known in Nigeria as "junior employees".[25] Further evidence that the settlement is predominantly one of low-income dwellers is provided by an unpublished official survey in 1984 which established that 82 per cent of the population earn less than N2,000 per annum, while only 18 per cent earn between N2,000 and N6,000 per annum.[26]

Box 3.2: Akinwande and Elizabeth's family.

Akinwande is a 47 year-old technician with the Federal Ministry of Industries who lives in one room with his wife Elizabeth, 46, and five children. They are from Ondo State. The children, three males and two females, are aged 21, 20, 16, 12 and 10 years-old. Elizabeth is a petty trader with a stall where she sells provisions at Oyingbo Market, a "not-too-far distance" away. Akinwande went to a Government Technical School while Elizabeth spent four years at, but did not complete, secondary school. All their children except the youngest who is in the final year of the primary school have secondary school education. They live in a rented room in an 11-room house shared with ten other households. Although their room is reasonably clean, it is poorly-lit, poorly-ventilated with only one window, crowded and cramped. Beds, furniture, a fridge, a black-and-white television set, a tall standing fan, suitcases and trunk box are all crowded in. There is scarcely space to move. The family share one bathroom and toilet with the other ten households. There is a communal kitchen but Elizabeth does not use it, preferring to cook in the passage. There is pipe-borne water into the house and they store their supply in plastic buckets.

The children suffer mainly from malaria, cuts and insect-bites which occasionally give rise to rashes on their feet and legs. They are taken to a private clinic whenever there is a serious problem. Two of their children have died; the parents said that the causes were malaria, a very high temperature, and convulsion. Elizabeth said that poverty was also partly to blame because they had no money to buy proper drugs. Akinwande interjected that the children who died had a natural orientation or "proneness" towards convulsion. On each occasion, the high temperature had occurred suddenly and without warning with devastating effects for the children. They claim that they have taken advantage of all government campaigns on immunization and have innoculated their children. They feel that the most serious health problems are the lack of a health clinic and the fact that the bucket latrines they have to use are very unhygienic and not emptied regularly. The buckets are often full and the waste usually spilt on the floor causing the place to be infested with flies

Box 3.2: (continued)

and maggots. They also complain of the poor sanitation in the settlement, that the water supply is inadequate even though they have pipe-borne water in the premises, and that the accommodation is overcrowded.

Housing, land and land-tenure

The nature of the land site, the conditions under which it is used, the nature of the relationship between residents and land owners and the quality of infrastructure and services are central to the type and standard of shelter that is available. All these factors contribute to the conditions of housing. All have implications for health in terms of problems of sanitation, and the control and spread of communicable and other diseases. For example, the type and age of buildings, the density, the building materials utilized and the proximity of each building to the next, all can constitute potential health and fire hazards. The effectiveness of basic infrastructure and services such as water, roads, drainage and waste-disposal have implications for health. The environment is also of great importance. The swampy, flooded terrain common in the tropics is a fertile habitat for vectors of various water-borne diseases and others such as malaria. In short, the physical and social environment of housing is central to the health conditions of residents. These features are examined below.

As noted earlier, Olaleye-Iponri covers about 35.3 hectares. At every point in the settlement, structures combine commercial, residential, religious, educational and even small-scale industrial use; in each case, the particular function or functions is dependent on what the owners and users of the structures see fit. Land-uses are hardly affected by the prevailing official regulations, bye-laws and building codes. Thus houses and compounds contain shops, beer-parlours, typing schools, food-stores, churches and mosques, and even brothels, all within the same spatial setting. At the same time, shops and market stalls double as sleeping quarters and dwelling places.[27]

Land plots are typically 25 by 18 metres, 18 by 18 metres, 18 by

12 metres and, at times, 12 by 6 metres. However, the standard size of plots prevalent in low-income settlements of this type is 18 by 12 metres. The most common form of building is a one-storey bungalow type structure (square or rectangular, depending on the shape of the plot) with a central corridor. Most buildings have nine or more rooms. Nearly half the sample in both Olaleye and Iponri had between 9 and 15 rooms while 21 per cent in Olaleye and just over 25 per cent in Iponri had 16 or more rooms.

As noted earlier, most inhabitants are tenants who live within a household, sharing one small room, while most other inhabitants are small-scale landlords who have built the dwellings they rent out on land they have rented from absentee landowners. Traditionally in Nigeria one of the main ways in which people acquired shelter was in a family compound or communal house with the right to live there deriving from descent. But only four per cent of respondents stated that this was the basis for their housing tenure. It is often assumed that customary land-tenure relations still predominate in many sub-Saharan African cities but the evidence from this study points to the intense commercialization of both housing and land and the replacement of customary tenure by commercial transactions and relationships.[28]

Most land-users lease their land on relatively short leases; over half of the landlords in the survey have leases of less than five years. One reason is the extensive practice of sub-letting. Many landlords who own buildings which they rent out have no direct link with the actual landowner but pay a rent to an intermediary landlord who holds the lease on the land site from the landowners or their agents.

A second reason for the prevalence of short-term leases is the fact that some large landowners avoid investing in buildings for fear of government expropriation of their land but at the same time, they dare not leave their land vacant for fear that squatters will occupy it illegally. One particular family, apart from being landlords (they have developed a medium-income estate of six or seven bungalows), have let out a large portion of their land-holding on a monthly basis to tenants who are explicitly instructed not to construct permanent or durable structures. The result is a line of shanties and shacks built of corrugated iron sheets, zinc sheets, wood boards and planks. The land owner is thus protecting the land from both government acquisition and squatters through keeping it occupied by tenants, but the emphasis on non-durable structures ensures that the family can respond rapidly to speculative bids for their land through their capacity to give very short notice for repossession of the land.

Another related aspect affecting the nature of housing in Olaleye-Iponri is a general insecurity of tenure that affects all property owners. Since the 1950s, most of the area has been the subject of threats of government acquisition. The intention was shelved because the area was considered to be too swampy. But the issue was reopened in the late-1960s and early-1970s, and then again in 1983. The experience of most low-income settlements that have come up for redevelopment is that these schemes almost invariably include a process of evictions, demolitions and resettlement. The residents of the settlements are quite familiar with this because much of the land on which Iponri originally developed has been expropriated and developed by the government for public projects such as the highway, the flyovers, the shopping centre and the new residential estate.

Box 3.3: Pa Ogun and Damola's family:

Pa Ogun is a 70 year-old tailor who lives with his 48 year-old wife Damola, who is a typist. They have three children living with them and two relatives of Damola. Pa Ogun has six children in all by this marriage and a previous relationship but the eldest three all have jobs and families and do not live with them. Pa Ogun did not complete primary education but his wife finished primary schooling and then went on to typing school.

They live in two rooms in a six-room house partially demolished to make way for a road-widening project. They are tenants but Pa Ogun is also the caretaker to this and a few other buildings. There are four other households in the building. One of their rooms also doubles as a workshop, show-room and reception area for Pa Ogun's tailoring business. This outer-room has only one window. It is stuffy and cramped, containing the two sewing-machines used by Pa Ogun and one of his journey men, some benches, a small narrow bed tucked into a corner, clothing materials and finished clothes. The house has cement walls and, perhaps as a result of the partial demolition and rebuilding, is freshly painted. There is a piped water supply to a tap in the compound. All five households share a bathroom, toilet and kitchen. The kitchen, though an outhouse, is built of concrete

Box 3.3: (continued)

materials and close enough to the main building to be convenient to use. The space between the house and outhouse is cemented and there is an internal drainage (open gutter) that runs from the kitchen, the bathroom, and the tap in the yard, by the side of the wall-fence to the main gutter outside. This internal gutter is clean and well-maintained.

Health problems of the children in the Ogun family include malaria fever, sores, colds, burns and other minor stomach complaints. The family uses the military hospital at Yaba, because Pa Ogun's eldest son is a sergeant in the Nigerian Army. Occasionally they use the chemists' shops in the settlement for minor ailments. Pa Ogun claims to have lived in Olaleye-Iponri for over 30 years. Two of their children have died – one was stillborn, the other died of convulsions after an attack of malaria. Pa Ogun claims that he lost four or five children in his previous relationship due to fevers, convulsions and cholera. The family says their younger children have all been immunized. To them the main health problems include lack of good toilet facilities, garbage dumps at backyards because of no service to remove garbage, drainage problems and the burning of rubbish.

There is very serious over-crowding in Olaleye-Iponri. The predominance of large households and the small sizes of rooms means that many households must live with less than one square metre per person in their rooms and less than two square metres per person for the whole plot. More than half of all households live in one room. Households occupying between two to three rooms account for about one-third of all responses. The most common room-size is between 2.4 by 1.8 metres and 2.4 by 2.4 metres. Occasionally larger rooms are 3 by 3.6 metres and 3.6 by 3.6 metres. Thus a common feature is to have households of five or more persons all living in a 2.4 by 1.8 metres-room.

According to the 1983 survey, the settlement is an area of poor housing by current standards of urban housing in Metropolitan Lagos. The survey reported that 88 per cent of dwellings are in poor condition with 7.8 per cent in fair condition (which can be improved with some basic repairs) and only about 3.8 per cent in good condition.[29] Internal and external walls are mainly built of cement. Next in importance is zinc, corrugated iron sheets or wood planks. These are the most common materials for walls amongst those who built makeshift and other non-durable structures. Other materials such as mud and sandcrete account for about 7.5 per cent of the walls in Olaleye, while they are virtually non-existent in Iponri.

Zinc and asbestos sheets emerge as the most popular types of roofing material while cement is the most common material used for floors. The use of predominantly modern construction materials does not point at any direct health hazards (except in the case of asbestos sheets), but when put together with the state of buildings, the regular flooding in the settlement and other negative environmental features, they constitute a health hazard. A related element is that some of these materials are flammable. Combined with the proximity of the structures to each other, and the kind of equipment used for cooking and lighting, this creates another serious health hazard.

Services and Facilities

An important aspect of housing conditions with far-reaching implications for the health status of dwellers in low-income settlements is the nature and state of basic services and facilities in houses. These include toilet facilities, bathrooms, kitchens, water supplies, electricity, type of cooking fuel and provisions for drainage and sewerage. Availability or non-availability of these, their current state, the pressure on them in terms of number of users and whether they are adequate in number, are all central to the existence and maintenance of basic hygiene and consequent prevention of diseases and ill health.

About 15 per cent of Olaleye respondents and 12 per cent of those in Iponri have no bathroom. Only 6 per cent of the Olaleye sample and 7 per cent in Iponri claim exclusive use of such facilities. Thus, 93 per cent of those with access to a bathroom share with other households and it is not unusual for 30 to 50 persons to share one bathroom. A typical "bathroom" is an outhouse, built of non-durable materials – four poles stuck into the ground, with wooden boards or corrugated iron sheets, zinc sheets or any other recycled metallic or flat material fixed on three sides. The 'doorway' is often covered by another detachable object, either a plank board, or zinc sheet. In many instances, users are obliged to provide cover either with their towel or a piece of cloth. The outdoor bathrooms often have no roofs and rarely have a cement floor. The waste water is often drained via the use of an open drain or gutter which runs through the whole compound or, in some cases, into a cemented ditch from which the water is then emptied by residents using a bucket. In a few cases, waste water is simply allowed to sink through the floor of the bathroom. This is often an uncemented floor covered either with gravel or stones. Such water could become stagnant and smell for days; it can also provide a breeding ground for mosquitoes.

In regard to excreta disposal, 28 per cent of respondents have no access to toilet facilities. Most of those with toilet facilities only have access to the outhouse type and, with this, the use of bucket-latrines is predominant. About 88 per cent of Olaleye respondents and 72 per cent of Iponri respondents use bucket-latrines. Next in importance is the use of pit latrines (or *salgas*), which account for about 12 per cent in Olaleye and 7 per cent in Iponri. Toilet facilities, as with bathroom facilities, are extensively shared; over 90 per cent of respondents with access to toilets share these facilities. The pressure can be imagined particularly in cases where there is only one toilet serving a house with six or more households with an average household size of not less than five. It is not surprising that human waste is disposed of as a matter of routine in both the gutters around the houses, near-by bushes, the railway line and any other available discreet corner.

Box 3.4: Evie's family.

Evie is a 47 year-old cleaner who lives with her four children, a much younger sister and niece. She lost her husband who was a soldier during the Civil War (1967–70). Her eldest child, a male, is 25 years old while the youngest, also male, is 19. She has three boys and a girl.

The seven of them live in one room they rent in an 11-room house with nine other households. The landlord who lives in the house has a room and a parlour with his family. Evie's room is reasonably large compared to others in the settlement – it is about 3.6 by 3 metres. It is reasonably ventilated, has two windows and more natural light

Box 3.4: (continued)

than most. There is a wood board ceiling and the house is built of concrete. The room is crowded with furniture and other household property. There is no source of water supply within the house and the family obtains drinking water from nearby public taps which they then store in plastic buckets under a cover.

There are two toilets, two bathrooms and two kitchens in the house but the landlord's family makes exclusive use of one of each of these, while all other tenants have to share the other facilities. The family does its cooking in the passage using a kerosene stove. Health problems include malaria fever, cuts, colds and sores for the children when they were younger. Evie suffers from headaches and other aches and body pains. She feels this is related to her job. The family uses the military hospital, a benefit they are entitled to since her husband died in active service. She also uses her company clinic. Health problems identified include the poor state of the toilet and drainage and flooding in the settlement.

In regard to cooking facilities, over half of all respondents cook in their corridors; only a small percentage (seven per cent in Olaleye, four per cent in Iponri) cook in their rooms. This is hardly surprising given the extreme overcrowding noted earlier with many households having less than one square metre per person. Most houses have places specifically designated as kitchens but these tend to be either another outhouse or a makeshift structure in the compound where many families live. Only eight per cent of Olaleye and 19 per cent of Iponri residents have exclusive use of a kitchen. Residents often do not use them because there is little space. Another problem is that they are outside the main house and tend to be either too far away or difficult to use during the rains, late at night or the very early morning. The corridors are not only more convenient and closer, but more exclusive.

The type of equipment used for cooking and the fuel used also has major implications for safety and fire hazard. The passages and corridors of houses, which is where over half of respondents cook, are often built of inflammable materials such as wood boards and zinc sheets. Over 90 per cent of respondents cook on kerosene (paraffin) stoves. It was evident, when undertaking the survey, that these contribute to indoor air pollution; many stoves do not have efficient burners and are often smoky, and produce a strong kerosene-fuel smell. There is also the fire hazard kerosene stoves present. Residents told of a few major fires – for instance one in 1970–71 in Iponri, another in the Old Olaleye Market area in 1983 and another in Iponri near the community-hall building in 1982. They also told of countless cases of "minor" fire mishaps in which a whole house or some rooms have burned down. Fires which seriously damage or destroy one or two houses appear to be common. They are said to be caused usually through carelessness during the preparation of meals or use of candles as the main source of lighting.

In regard to sources of water, only a small proportion of residents have water piped to their living quarters. In Olaleye, 36 per cent of respondents have water piped directly into the building in which they live but only 21 per cent have it piped into their own living quarters. Another 15 per cent rely mainly on water from wells in their buildings, while nearly a third purchase their water from water-hawkers who obtain the water either from wells or piped sources. For Iponri, about 71 per cent of respondents claim they use piped water but only 36 per cent have it piped into their living quarters; about 15 per cent purchase water from private hawkers.[30] Sources such as springs, streams and wells are not important (they are used by about four per cent of the respondents). For those who obtain water from outside their living quarters, 52 per cent of Olaleye respondents and 45 per cent of those in Iponri claim they get water within 100 metres of their living quarters. The rest either use other means or get water from distances over 100 metres.

In regard to electricity, virtually all houses have direct, legal supplies, even though a public supply only became available for the first time in 1975. But the residents of Olaleye-Iponri, like other residents of Lagos, suffer regular power cuts and loss of power after 1979. Most residents have learnt to rely on kerosene lamps and candles for lighting. Faults in the power-supply systems have, as usual, scarcely received the prompt attention of the engineers of the National Electric Power Authority (NEPA).

Provision for drainage and for the removal of solid and liquid wastes is very inadequate. Each interviewer after questioning households also undertook a systematic assessment of each house and its surrounds in regard to environmental quality. These assessments showed that almost three-fifths of the sample have house frontages that are dirty. The presence of human and/or animal waste around dwellings is not widespread in Olaleye. However, in Iponri, almost 40 per cent of the houses studied have evidence of human or animal waste in their surroundings. Over a quarter of all houses had what the interviewers described as a foul smell arising from open drains, human waste, dead animals and overflowing garbage dumps. This is not surprising as most gutters and drains were blocked and not cleaned, and there is no systematic form of public waste disposal. In Olaleye, about 96 per cent of the drains are blocked with rubbish and not cleaned at all. In Iponri, 82 per cent of the drains are recorded as blocked, while about 96 per cent are recorded as not clean. Garbage disposal facilities within the vicinity of dwelling exist for 70 per cent of Olaleye while in Iponri these exist in 59 per cent of the cases.

In conclusion, there are serious deficiencies in virtually all forms of basic infrastructure and services: water, facilities for cooking, washing and personal hygiene, sanitation and drainage. These findings were confirmed in a survey carried out by Lagos State's Ministry of Economic Planning and Land Matters, which compared deficiencies in infrastructure and services, and in the environment in 42 different low-income settlements.[31] Olaleye-Iponri was one of the worst of these, being characterized as unplanned, constantly flooded, with poor and sub-standard housing, an unlandscaped site, a socio-economically deprived population and lacking basic services, facilities and infrastructure. The fieldwork and the survey also showed that the settlement was poorly served by roads both access and internal roads. Provision for the collection of solid wastes was very inadequate.

Health Problems

Our research made no provisions for epidemiological and laboratory studies – the funding available did not allow their inclusion. Such studies could have substantially enriched the findings. The emphasis here is on examining certain features: the prevalence of diseases and ailments, the evidence of mortality as provided by respondents, the perception and definition of health needs and health-related deficiencies or obstacles in the settlement's physical and social environment.

In terms of health-care provision, Olaleye-Iponri is located within the jurisdiction of the Lagos Mainland Local Government. Local government authorities, when questioned, could not produce information on the total number of health institutions and facilities (both public and private) located within the jurisdiction. The only information they had was on health facilities provided by the government. These are as follows: one teaching hospital, the Lagos University Teaching Hospital, owned by the federal government; two health centres located at Ebute-Metta and Suralere, and owned by the state government; and, five family health-care centres, located at Ebute-Metta, Abule-Abe, Suralere, Badiya and Ijora Oloye. In addition, there are seven treatment centres for primary school children and three health clinics, located at Makoko, Iwaya and Moshalashi.

The local authorities claimed to employ only 119 nurses and midwives and two doctors at the time of interview (December 1985). This was for an area with an officially estimated population of about 800,000 people, with an average annual attendance of 3,000 patients at the maternal services and between 25–30,000 at the child welfare clinics. The school treatment service also averaged an annual attendance of 18,000.

Local authority personnel suggested that the main causes of infant and child mortality were diarrhoea, chest infections, measles, tetanus, malaria and malnutrition. The main causes of adult mortality were pneumonia, hypertension, malaria and road traffic accidents. Asked to identify the main problems affecting health care delivery in the Local Government area, officials noted, in order of priority: i) inadequate funding; ii) shortage of trained health personnel; *and* iii) inadequate provision of health-support materials such as drugs and equipment. The most common health problems in the area were identified by officials as consisting mainly of: i) those deriving from poor environmental sanitation – in particular, there is a high occurrence of malaria attacks, as a result of bad drainage and flooding; ii) overcrowding and inadequate housing – particularly with regards to sizes of rooms, ventilation and lighting; *and* iii) inadequate supply of potable water.

Olaleye-Iponri residents were questioned about their perceptions of illnesses, ailments and causes of death. The questions sought to find out their perceptions of the most common illness or ailment in their household, the illnesses or ailments for which respondents and/or members of their households have sought treatment in the six months before the survey, the illness and ailments that respondents believed have led to the death of people in the community in the six months preceding the survey, and the sex and age of those who died.

Table 3.4: Respondents' identification of the most common illness in their household

Ailments	*Olaleye*	*(percentages)*	*Iponri*
Colds	1.4		1.8
Malaria	70.9		89.0
Bronchitis/Pneumonia	3.7		–
Measles	15.6		9.1
Chicken pox	–		–
Dysentery/Diarrhoea	5.4		–
Coughs	2.4		–
Others	0.6		–
Number	295		110

The vast majority of respondents identify malaria as the most common ailment in their households with measles next in importance. Perhaps surprisingly, dysentery and diarrhoea account for only 5.4 per cent of the Olaleye cases and do not feature at all in Iponri. However, the pattern identified supports the fact that environmental factors are a strong determinant of the pattern of prevalence of disease.

The fact that diarrhoea and dysentery do not figure prominently might reflect the way the question was posed, as the question concerning ailments suffered in the past six months produces a different pattern of responses. When asked if members of their households have sought treatment of any form for any ailment in the past six months, only one-quarter of the sample in both cases provided a negative reply. For both Olaleye and Iponri, in three-quarters of the sample either the respondents or other members of their households have experienced illnesses warranting some treatment (see Table 3.5).

Malaria is still the most common illness, followed by measles. After measles comes dysentery and diarrhoea, which more than one-tenth of the sample in both Olaleye and Iponri identify as the third most common illness. Other ailments include "coughs" (which are a manifestation of other ailments), colds, chicken pox, back pain and rheumatism.

What is interesting, apart from the differences in the pattern of response between the more general question and the one that is period-specific, is that the ailments identified as having occurred in the past six months are mainly related to a deprived urban environment and deficient sanitary conditions. Malaria has been noted as having a strong relationship with the standard of environmental sanitation, particularly the presence of stagnant water in which the vector mosquitoes may breed. Measles, dysentery and diarrhoea also have strong associations with poor quality, overcrowded housing and poor sanitation.

Table 3.5: Respondents' identification of illnesses suffered by themselves and their households in the previous six months

Ailments	*Olaleye*	*(percentages)*	*Iponri*
Colds	1.0		–
Malaria	50.3		43.5
Bronchitis/Pneumonia	5.2		–
Measles	18.8		8.7
Chicken pox	3.7		33.3
Dysentery/Diarrhoea	13.6		11.6
Coughs	4.7		2.9
Others	2.6		–
Number	191		69

Respondents were also asked if they could recall specific cases of illnesses/ailments which resulted in death in the past six months. They were asked to provide the age and sex of the victims. The response rate for this question is quite low. This could be because not too many deaths have occurred within the six months or because respondents are not keen to discuss the subject of death.

Of the 21 cases of death that respondents could recall, 10 (47.6 per cent) are adduced to measles – all the victims were children. Clearly this is an avoidable killer that, with public education and the necessary action, can be prevented. Malaria comes next, accounting for seven deaths (one-third of all the cases) with diarrhoea/dysentery identified as the cause of the remaining two deaths. Again – like measles – malaria, dysentery and diarrhoea are causes of death that possess close linkages with lower socio-economic status, poor and deficient environments, and housing. Of the seven cases identified for malaria, five are adults and two are children. The two cases of dysentery and diarrhoea were both children. Thus children are the greatest victims, accounting for two-thirds of all the mortality cases that respondents could recall. It should be noted that respondents do not mention deaths caused by traffic accidents, fire and such other mishaps. Informants pointed out that traffic accidents within the settlements are minimal as the roads are often impassable by motor vehicles. They confirm that, although fire outbreaks were regular, they have not caused deaths in the past six months or recent years. They admit that regular domestic accidents do occur with children such as accidents with boiling water and hot cooked substances. But these have not directly caused deaths as far as they could remember. Other accidents that have caused death include drowning in a well by a toddler and death from head injuries sustained from tree-climbing by one of the young members of the settlement.

How residents cope with their health problems

The interviews included questions to gauge respondents' awareness of the health facilities and provisions in their communities. A general question sought to find out whether respondents were aware of any health-care provisions (no matter which one) in their community. We found a very high level of awareness of some form of health provisions. No less than four out of every five respondents are aware of some provision. The next set of questions were directed at pinpointing the health facilities of which residents were aware. Asked whether they were aware of any government-owned health facility in the settlement, we found an overwhelming negative response. No respondents in Iponri are aware of any, while 96 per cent of those in Olaleye hold this view. The small proportion of Olaleye respondents who answered in the affirmative might have been referring to the Desalu health centre which serves the Apapa Road and Oko-Oba communities, and which is not too far from Olaleye Village.

As to the existence of private medical provisions either very close by or within the community, responses simply confirm the actual state of things. Only about 14 per cent of the Iponri respondents and some 45 per cent of the Olaleye subjects answer in the affirmative. There are no private medical clinics located inside the settlement. There are one or two nursing homes and a few nurses who provide services such as maternity services, first-aid and administering drugs for a fee. More interestingly, Olaleye Village which shares a boundary with Apapa road via the railway line is closer to this other community which contains not only a public health centre but several private clinics. At the time of survey, two such private clinics were distinctly identifiable only a few metres away from the settlement across the railway line. Again this might account for the larger proportion of affirmative responses from Olaleye Village.

Box 3.5 Adebayo and Moni's family.

Adebayo is 58 years-old and a wood-plank merchant; Moni is 42 and works for the government. They have five children ranging in ages from 31 to 16 years. Some are working while the two youngest are in secondary school. Adebayo is the landlord of the 12 room-house.

The family lives in two rooms and has been in the settlement for 24 years. The building itself is made up of the products of Adebayo's trade – wood plank and zinc sheets. They have a well and fetch drinking water from the public tap. They have one bathroom and one toilet, which they share with the other households. There is no designated kitchen.

The children when they were young were susceptible to malaria, colds, cuts and sores, and ring worm. The adults suffer from fever and rheumatism. They treat themselves either with herbs or with products purchased from the chemist. They go to the hospital whenever things get serious. Four of their children have died: they claim that two of the deaths were caused by convulsions (probably malaria) but they do not know the cause of the other two. The main health hazards in the community are poor toilet facilities, bad roads, no water and no bins for garbage.

On the awareness of other forms or means of providing health, we found that respondents show greater knowledge of the presence of these in their settlement. For instance, over three-quarters of the Olaleye respondents and more than half of those in Iponri are aware of private pharmacists and patent-medicine stores in their settlement. Their role in low-income communities in Nigeria is important. Although some shop owners and attendants might be unqualified, they often provide the first or initial level of consultation and advice on ailments. They recommend and prescribe cures and drugs and advise on their potency and particular suitability for specific diseases. As such, they provide a significant point of contact in health matters, even if their lack of professional knowledge and the absence of a set of professional ethics may make their services dangerous. They are seen by some as being more useful and reliable than traditional medical practitioners or "native doctors".

Most respondents are aware of the existence and availability of native doctors. As for their complement, spiritual healers (found mainly in spiritual churches in Nigeria), a lesser number of respondents are aware of their services: about 46 per cent in Olaleye and two-thirds of the Iponri sample.

This information on awareness demonstrates the residents' lack of access to formal public health institutions, provisions and facilities. Their awareness is far more of private provisions, and in most cases, informal and/or customary private provisions. This point is further confirmed by the fact that an overwhelming proportion of the respondents are in no way aware of any recent attempts at mass immunization in their settlement. About nine out of every ten respondents are not aware of any such attempts. This information is of particular interest if it is realized that the survey was carried out between June 1984 and January 1985, at the heart of the Government and United Nations Childrens' Fund (UNICEF) campaign supporting the Expanded Programme on Immunization. This programme obviously had not penetrated this particular low-income settlement at the time of study. Further probing on awareness of how long ago any immunization programme had occurred yielded interesting answers. To the few who could answer this question, about 72 per cent of those from Olaleye claimed that such had occurred more than a year ago. In fact, most of these respondents claimed over three years ago. As for Iponri, 80 per cent of those who answered claimed that such a campaign last took place over five years ago.

The health profiles in Boxes 3.1 to 3.5 provide some insight into the needs of residents. It is interesting that these residents, apart from asking for health centres, focus their health needs mainly around better provision of basic services and infrastructures closely related to shelter. They ask for good water, better toilets and bathrooms, better drainage and roads, waste disposal facilities, and the control of flooding. They also advocate better conditions for environmental sanitation.

When asked to identify the main problems of the settlement, 86 per cent in Olaleye and 78 per cent in Iponri point to inadequate and poor infrastructures and services as the most pressing problems of the community. For them this means mainly roads, waste disposal facilities, toilets, drainage and flood controls. No respondents identified politics as a problem. Economic hardship as a settlement problem is mentioned by only one per cent of the respondents in Iponri and four per cent in Olaleye.

Asked what happens during the rainy season, over nine out of every ten respondents identify flooding as a problem. Most of them advocate immediate government measures to include sand-filling of the swamps, dredging the canal behind the settlement and building better drains and roads. The floods during the rains not only constitute health hazards (they increase vulnerability to all forms of ailments); they also impede movement to places of livelihood and disrupt social and economic interactions that normally take place in the streets or in the open air.

The inhabitants of Olaleye-Iponri do possess some elementary knowledge of what their health conditions and needs are. They know their prevalent ailments and diseases, and although they cannot always specify the causes, they are aware of the basic improvements that should be made. The survey and family profiles suggest that the main health problems in Olaleye-Iponri as presented by the people are environmentally-related problems. The diseases – malaria, measles, dysentery and diarrhoea – all have a strong relationship with the degree of environmental and social deprivation. On mortality, the information from the profiles presents more concrete evidence about the extent of infant and child mortality in various households. At least six of the ten households for which profiles were done have suffered one or more infant or child dying. Again the importance of basic health knowledge and services in preventing some of these deaths cannot be underestimated. A lot of the deaths that respondents claim occur from convulsions, malaria, dysentery, diarrhoea and cholera are preventable in the light of current medical knowledge and health technology.

The greatest awareness of medical services is of the presence of pharmacists and chemists in the settlement. The profiles confirm that they are often used as the first line of defence in cases of illness, accidents and other ailments. This suggests perhaps the most important lesson that public authorities need to learn in the provision of health care. That is: it must be accessible, available, close-by and have minimal overheads. The people in low-income settlements know this for themselves but clearly public institutions are further behind. This final point raises the question of public response and initiatives, and community efforts as they pertain to health and habitat issues.

Chapter Four

Housing and Health in Three Squatter Settlements in Allahabad, India

H. N. Misra

Introduction – the development of Allahabad City

The City of Allahabad lies almost at the centre of the densely-populated north Indian plains, which are among the most densely-settled parts of India and also among the most economically backward and least urbanized regions in the country. Allahabad's site is on the confluence of two of India's most important rivers, the Ganga (Ganges) and the Yamuna (Jumna), so that these rivers bound the city to its north, east and south. In 1981, the city had 642,000 inhabitants and was the fifth largest city in the State of Uttar Pradesh, India's most populous state, which itself had 111 million inhabitants. The contemporary city owes its origin to a fort built at the order of the Mughal emperor Akbar in 1583, and this fort remains one of the landmarks in Allahabad today. Under Akbar's rule, the city also became one of the 15 provincial headquarters through which Mughal rule was administered. The Ganga and the Yamuna Rivers were widely used as transport arteries; the Yamuna also runs past Delhi (India's current capital) and Agra (founded by Akbar as his capital).

Under British rule, Allahabad was also an important administrative centre. In 1858 it became the headquarters of a new administrative division (the Province of Oudh) and then capital of the North-Western Provinces, later called the United Provinces, when Oudh and Agra provinces were joined. In 1950, the United Provinces were renamed Uttar Pradesh (literally "northern province"). Although Lucknow became the State capital around 1930, Allahabad still retains some state-wide functions. For instance, Uttar Pradesh's High Court remains in Allahabad.

Allahabad is also a district headquarters and the setting up and expansion of administrative offices, courts, police, post office, a government printing press, hospitals and dispensaries were important for its development in this period. Allahabad was also an important centre for the army and for education; the University of Allahabad was founded in 1887 and is one of India's oldest universities. The city has one of the main railway stations on the line linking India's capital, Delhi, with its largest city, Calcutta. Population growth was particularly rapid between 1853 and 1872; as figures in Table 4.1 show, its population almost doubled in these two decades.

During the twentieth century, Allahabad's importance within India and within Uttar Pradesh has declined. Lucknow, a large industrial centre with over one million inhabitants some 200 kilometres to the northwest, is the state capital. Kanpur, also some 200 kilometres away and close to Lucknow, developed as one of India's main industrial centres and had 1.7 million inhabitants in 1981. Varanasi, 124 kilometres to the east of Allahabad, and Agra, 328 kilometres to the west, also had populations exceeding that of Allahabad in 1981.

Table 4.1: The growth in Allahabad's population

Date	*Population*
1853	72,093
1872	143,693
1881	160,118
1901	172,032
1921	157,697
1941	260,633
1961	430,730
1981	642,420

As Table 4.1 shows, the city's population declined between 1901 and 1921 largely as a result of epidemics, especially bubonic plague. Although Allahabad has attracted some industry, the basis for the city's economy derives from administrative, religious and educational activities. In 1981, 68 per cent of the workforce were working in the service sector. The city retains an important religious function since the confluence of the two rivers has long been regarded as a sacred site. Every year, a large religious festival takes place on land just by the confluence and attracts hundreds of thousands of pilgrims.

Some of the main formative influences on the city's physical development can still be seen in the city plan. The oldest parts of the city are close to the fort built under Akbar's rule and these remain the most densely populated parts of the city (see Map 4.1). Here is located the central business district and the main market; the streets are narrow and are often congested. The lack of a plan to guide this early city development is evident when compared to the area known as the Civil Lines, to the north west of the old city, which was laid out in 1858 and developed by the British colonial administration as their city. Here the road network is carefully planned and most of the land devoted to western style residential sub-divisions with bungalows located in large lots. A report in 1868 pointed to the fact that all the roads in this area, inhabited by the European community, were surfaced, with good provision for drainage, unlike much of the city proper.[1] The cantonments – barracks for the army – also show up on the contemporary city plan and these too have a colonial origin. So too does the area around the railway stations where railway colonies grew; originally, these stations were located outside the built up areas.

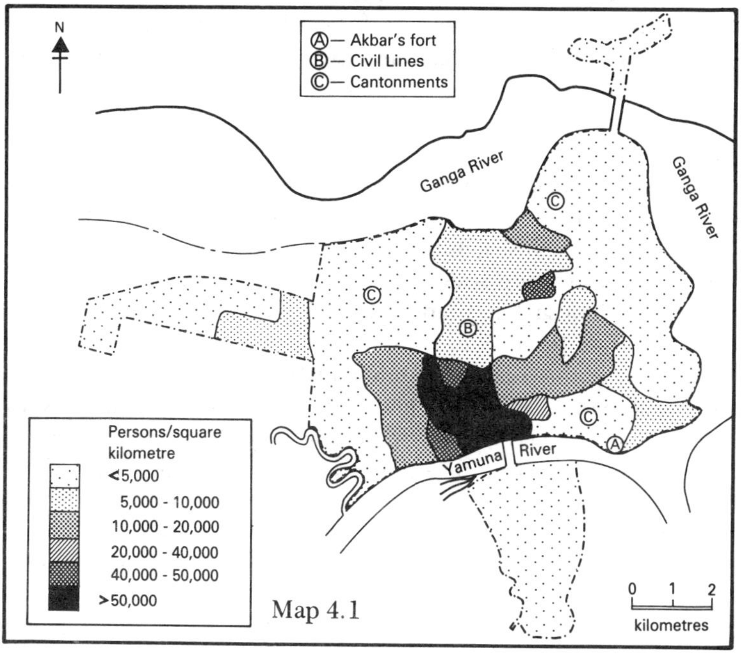

Map 4.1

The area encompassed by city boundaries has grown from 27.2 square kilometres in 1818 to 41.6 in 1901 and 70 in 1951. By

1971, there were 27 wards but in this year, the city boundaries were increased to encompass 82 square kilometres with the city later coming to be divided into 40 wards. The city's expansion has to take place towards the west – since rivers limit its physical growth in other directions – and to the north and south on the other side of the rivers, along roads leading out of the city. This physical expansion has meant the incorporation of many villages into the city. For instance, some 65 villages were incorporated into the area under the jurisdiction of Allahabad Municipal Corporation between 1957 and 1960.

Over two-fifths of the city's households live in one-room flats, houses or shacks. The municipal corporation and the city's development authority recently identified 45 slums within the city each with populations of between 1,000 and 4,000. Most of the lower income groups live in illegal settlements. These first grew on sites subject to flooding or marshy lands, since these were the vacant land-sites best located in terms of access to city jobs and where, because of the flooding or waterlogging, the people stood a better chance of not being evicted. In 1981, an estimated 188,000 people were living in illegal settlements. Typically, these settlements have little or no infrastructure and services in the way of paved roads, piped water, provision for the removal of household and human wastes, schools and health-care centres. The sites are unhealthy and, at least for part of the year, waterlogged. A high proportion of all these settlements are close to the river banks and subject to flooding. The housing is overcrowded – most of it being one-room or at best two-room structures.

One reason for the scale of these illegal developments on land ill-suited to housing is simply the lack of better sites; the city is hemmed in on three sides by rivers and one-fifth of the city lands belong to the three army cantonments located around the central area. A second reason is the low income of so many of Allahabad's inhabitants; as noted earlier, Allahabad is in the middle of one of the poorest but most densely-populated parts of India and many individuals or households in the city are people who could not make a living in the surrounding rural areas. In-migration has contributed a lot to the city's population growth and historically, Allahabad has had a highly-imbalanced sex ratio: for the censuses between 1941 and 1981, there has always been less than 800 females per 1,000 males. Many migrants are male agricultural labourers from "backward" or "scheduled" castes[2] or from the local tribal population; in the 1981 census, 15 per cent of the city's population were from scheduled castes.

A third reason is the failure of the urban authorities to intervene in the land market to guarantee lower-income groups cheap, legal house plots despite the fact that much of the land in the city is under public ownership. Although public authorities have been relatively tolerant of squatters who build their shelters on public land, they have not used public land to increase the supply of affordable, legal, serviced plots for lower-income groups. In addition, obtaining official approval for a building or for a sub-division is both difficult and time consuming.

Land tenure within the city is complicated by the fact that much of it is still held under a system imposed by the British for agricultural land. Within the 82 square kilometre boundaries, 39.4 per cent of the land is "estate" land – land the British confiscated from landowners who fought against them in 1857.[3] A further 8.6 per cent is *nazul* land – land which was originally unclaimed and then taken by the Colonial government and given to people for cultivation, although no written title to the land was given to the cultivator. Virtually all other land is held freehold (28.6 per cent of the total) or is part of the cantonments (22.3 per cent). Many low income settlements have grown up on *nazul* or government estate land. In both, public authorities have the power to transfer tenure to the inhabitants. Only rarely have they done so.

Some government action was undertaken in Allahabad to improve health conditions in the last few decades of the nineteenth century, including the construction of some public latrines and an attempt to close down deep-pit latrines, since these helped to contaminate the water drawn from nearby wells. In 1891, a piped water system began operation, although with restricted coverage and with inadequate or no provision for the removal of waste water. Growing drainage problems prompted the design of a drainage system and work on this began in 1913. By 1917, a water works began operation with some water-borne sullage and sewage disposal collected and pumped across the Yamuna for use in irrigating land.[4] A more interventionist municipal government dates from 1909 when an Improvement Trust was set up, under whose direction many new roads were constructed. Despite its original goal to provide healthy housing for the displaced population, the new model townships ended up in middle-class hands. Further work was undertaken after the 1920s when Town Planning Improvement Trusts were set up in many of India's more important urban centres after a recommendation of the Plague Commission. As in so many other nations, mounting health problems provided an important stimulus towards city government. An Improvement Trust was established in Allahabad in 1921 and this sought to acquire land from Kastkars (land tillers who did not own the land) and landlords but with little success. In 1960, the Trust became a Municipal Corporation. In 1974, the Allahabad Development Authority was set up to execute a masterplan, but it has not proved successful.

During the 1970s, the city government tried to acquire land for low-income housing. With powers provided by the federal government's Urban Land (Ceiling and Regulation) Act of 1976, a ceiling was set on individual's undeveloped land holdings of 1,500 square metres. A total of 660,000 square metres was declared surplus (held above the limit) out of a total land area of 106 square kilometres.[5] But less than half of this has been handed over to the magistrate by the authorities and very little of this land has been used to provide lower income groups with housing sites. Meanwhile, there is a large illegal land market which despite its illegality, still prices land sites beyond the reach of most lower-income households.

The development of Chheetpur

Chheetpur is a small settlement with some 500 inhabitants in 108 households, located close to the railway line in the southern part of the city. The site is less than one hectare and is subject to flooding almost every year during the rainy season. It is well located within the city, with a market just across a railway line to the south and the Indian Hume Pipe factory just to the north. A brick road connects it to a major road linking the Civil Lines to the Sangham (the site where the rivers converge).

The longer term residents of Chheetpur were forced off two other sites nearby. On the first of these sites, a settlement was formed largely by unskilled, landless rural people who migrated to Allahabad and built mud huts on vacant government land close to the site of the present Swaroop Rani Hospital. They were evicted when the Civil Lines area was developed by the colonial government in the second half of the nineteenth century. Some of those evicted built huts on land, very close to the current site, which belonged to the Trust which manages the K.P. College. They were forcefully evicted from here too and around 18 families moved away from the area to other low income settlements while five families came to the present site. This site also belonged to the Trust but some of these people were employed by the Trust as peons or security staff and they were allowed to stay, after agreeing to pay a nominal rent. When they moved to the new site it was forested, with serious water-logging, and ever since settling here the inhabitants have tried to raise its level. Gradually, the settlement grew. Friends and kin came to join the original families, in part responding to demand for labour by the Indian Hume Pipe Company. Other families derived incomes from work as masons, labourers and rickshawpullers. Some newcomers built their own huts while others rented rooms in existing dwellings. The K.P. Trust sought to prevent this growth in the settlement's population; some new huts were removed while others were set on fire by students from the K.P. College on the instructions of the Management Trust. In recent years, such actions to discourage the settlement's physical growth have become common. In March 1984, seven newly-built huts were burnt down. The inhabitants have refused to pay rent to the Trust and the Trust has filed a suit of eviction against some of the households. This has been pending since 1974.

Chheetpur's inhabitants have organized to fight eviction. A Harijan and Backward Development Committee, was constituted in 1980. Another local organization, the Chheetpur Development Committee, was constituted in 1983 at the initiative of the Sanjay Vichar Manch (a political party named after the late Sanjay Gandhi). This committee, however, is no longer in existence.

Although there are high-caste Hindus and Muslims among the inhabitants, 95 per cent are from the backward and scheduled castes. Table 4.2 shows the occupational structure of the working population which constitutes some 45 per cent of the total population and includes a substantial proportion of women and many children. Nearly three-fifths of the working population work as labourers for daily wages while 16 per cent work in some government or semi-public institution (for instance the railway, the municipal corporation or an educational institution). Vegetable vending, rickshaw pulling and work as masons constitute the other most important sources of income. Perhaps not surprisingly, the few upper-caste workers all have jobs in government. Most of the scheduled caste earn a living by selling vegetables; 29 per cent of the workers from this caste run small, illegal vegetable shops by the side of the road. Some are semi-permanent structures, others temporary wooden structures and others four-wheel carts designed to carry vegetables or seasonal fruits.

Table 4.2: Employment in the three squatter settlements

Occupation	*Percentage of working population engaged in*			
	Chheetpur	*Kydganj*		*Lowther Road*
		(Male)	*(Female)*	
Labourers (daily wages)	59	–	–	26
Government or semi-govt.	16	–	–	7
Rickshaw pullers	5	6	–	46
Vegetable vending	5	–	–	–
Masons	4	–	–	–
Tea stall	3	–	–	1
Betel/bidi stall	1	–	–	1
Basket makers	–	81	100	–
Junk collectors	–	11	–	7
Cycle repair	–	–	–	9
Others	7	2	–	3
Total	100	100	100	100

Chheetpur, like the wider city of Allahabad, has a highly-unbalanced sex ratio; in 1984 there were 281 males to 211 females. Women and children of backward and scheduled caste households are important secondary-income earners. Several women sell vegetables from door to door while others work as maids in nearby middle-or-upper-income families' houses. The number of dependents per household is higher among Muslim and high-caste households since women are not expected to work outside the house. Household incomes are typically below $300 a year, and below $200 a year for 56 of the 108 households. Only two households have incomes of more than $400 a year.

Most households are *de facto* owner occupiers although 23 are tenants (see Table 4.3 for details). Of these, two pay no rent because the original household has moved away or died. Six pay rents of between $1 and $2 per month for a small room; these have been living in the settlement for around ten years. Rent levels are higher for more recent arrivals; tenant households who moved in very recently pay more than $5 per month for a room while those who moved in earlier but within the last six years pay between $2 and $4. Among the 23 tenant households, seven pay to absentee landlords who only visit the settlement to collect rent.

Table 4.3: Land and house tenure

Kinds of house or land tenure	*Percentage of households in* *Chheetpur*	*Kydganj*	*Lowther Road*
De facto owner occupation (squatting)	79	100	59
Renting land from legal owner	–	–	41
Renting house without payment to de facto owners	2	–	–
Renting shelter with payment to de facto owners	19	–	–
Total	100	100	100

Two-fifths of the households live in one room with another 44 per cent living in two rooms. Half of all households have less than two square metres per person while 88 of the 108 households have less than four square metres per person. Mud, bamboo, wood, tiles and grasses are the most common building materials since they are easily available and relatively cheap. Tiles are made by the inhabitants themselves; so too are most of the bricks which are sun-baked. Most shelters (70 out of 108) are made with mud walls and tiles with another 28 with brick walls and tiles. Just ten have brick walls and cement. None of the houses meet official building norms or codes since the inhabitants see little possibility of their tenure being legalized.

Up to 1972, the community's main source of water was a well. This supply was frequently contaminated. In 1972, one public standpipe was set up with another provided in 1976. These remain the main source of water and large queues build up around each standpipe, especially early in the morning and evening. These two standpipes are where most people wash their clothes. Lack of facilities for drainage have led to stagnant pools there which serve as breeding grounds for mosquitoes. But the whole site suffers from waterlogging. A sewer connection to the settlement has been proposed but never implemented. A public latrine remains half constructed, after strong objections by some households to its location. Excreta is usually disposed of in the open and children often defecate in and around the settlement. No house has a latrine, nor indeed provision for separate kitchens or bathrooms. Problems of hygiene are compounded by the fact that goats, pigs and hens are kept by many households and in such an over-crowded settlement, it is impossible to keep these separate from humans.

Until 1978, no electricity was provided. Most households finished their daily tasks during daylight, including cooking and eating, although some used kerosene lamps. In 1978 the municipal authorities set up one electric pole, while another was recently set up. Many inhabitants have taken illegal connections off these poles. School provision is inadequate; there is no good primary school nearby and the only nursery schools are private and beyond the price of the inhabitants. Only 30 per cent of the inhabitants are literate.

Health-care services are available closeby at the Swaroop Rani Hospital but the inhabitants rarely go there since they usually have to wait for several hours before receiving treatment. Although in theory this hospital should provide free medical treatment, it is not uncommon for doctors to advise patients to come to their private clinics if they want proper treatment and these are expensive. There is also a children's hospital in a wing of a medical college some three kilometres away but several families told of poor treatment there. Chheetpur's inhabitants feel doctors do not pay attention to their needs because of their low socio-economic status. A few families have used a private doctor; although costly, this doctor is trusted by these families. A social/religious organization sends a doctor to Chheetpur every Sunday and he distributes homeopathic medicines free of charge. Most births are delivered in the houses, usually supervised by *chamains*, traditional mid-wives with no training. Tetanus is one of the main causes of infant deaths and infection usually takes place during delivery.

The development of Kydganj

This settlement, with 237 inhabitants in 1984, is near the Yamuna River (see Map 4.2). A small road runs through the settlement which is built on land belonging to the federal government's Defence Department since it is legally part of the cantonment area. The settlement was begun in 1978 on what had previously been vacant land by people whose shelters had been destroyed when the Yamuna River broke its banks. Hundreds of people who lived close to the Yamuna Bridge were made homeless.

The inhabitants are almost all from a scheduled tribe known as Dharkar; this tribal name is of a community which traditionally

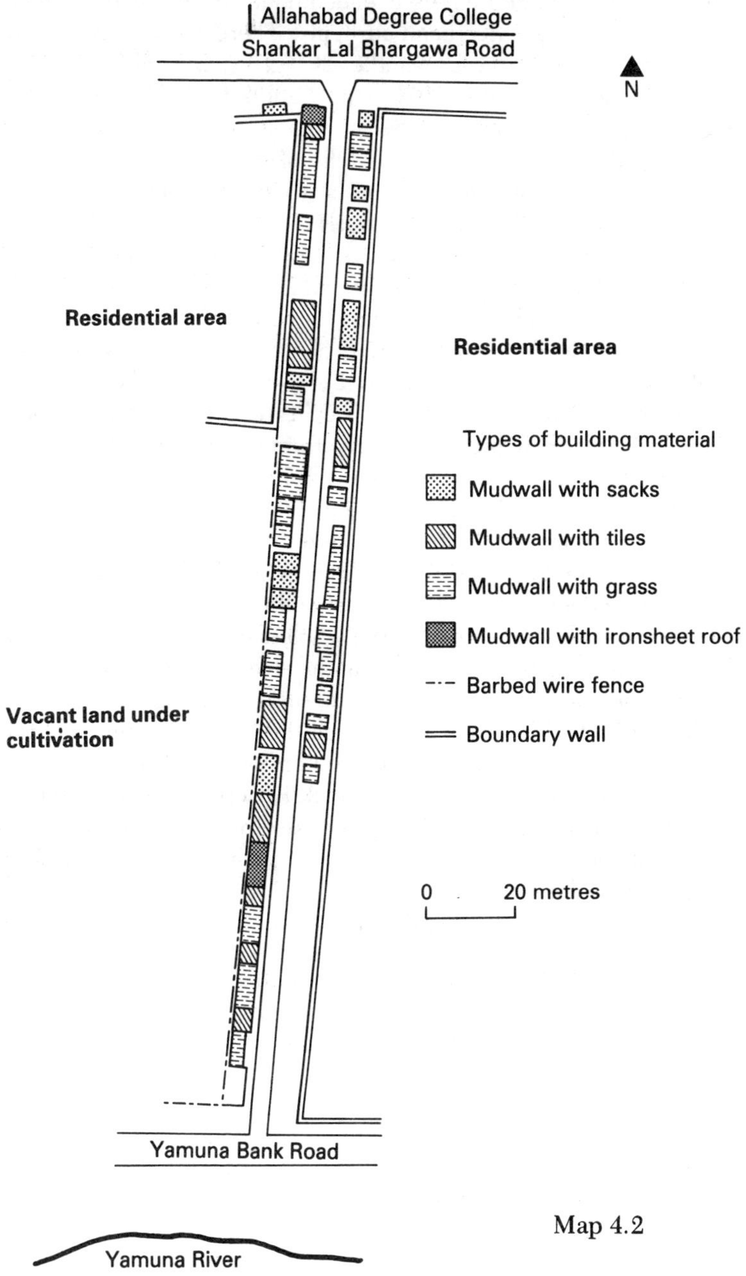
Allahabad Degree College
Shankar Lal Bhargawa Road
N
Residential area
Residential area
Types of building material
Mudwall with sacks
Mudwall with tiles
Mudwall with grass
Mudwall with ironsheet roof
Barbed wire fence
Boundary wall
Vacant land under cultivation
0 20 metres
Yamuna Bank Road
Yamuna River

Map 4.2

depended on bamboo for its livelihood and many inhabitants still make baskets and other bamboo items. There are no Muslims or people from backward castes in the settlement, and only one household from another caste. Older inhabitants tell of the Dharkar's migration from Madhya Pradesh, the state to the south of Uttar Pradesh. One, in his seventies, tells of the growing shortage of bamboo and of oppressive landlords who forced many to migrate to Allahabad some 30 years previously.

Two days after the flood had destroyed their homes some 21 families had settled at Kydganj, while within a week another 15–20 families had joined them. Initially, all slept out in the open but gradually, over a period of two months, some families built rudimentary shelters made out of sacks, tiles, broken pieces of wood and brick and other materials collected from around the city. The site is relatively high and so free from the threat of floods.

There are 56 households within the 237 inhabitants and a sex ratio of 897 females to 1,000 males. The inhabitants have few interactions with other groups within the city. Basket making is the main source of livelihood for 44 of the 56 households with seven relying on scrap collection and four on rickshaw or cart pulling. There are 52 men and 34 women basket-makers, and the wholesale market for bamboo is less than one kilometre away, along the riverbank. One household, the only one not of the Dharkar caste, makes a living as a wholesale junk dealer. This household has much the highest income and this averages around $500 a year. Most other households earn between $240 to $480 per annum. Among the 237 people, 215 are illiterate, including all members of the upper-caste household which helps explain its occupation and its isolation within this settlement from other households of the same caste.

All the inhabitants built the houses they live in; there are no tenants. The inhabitants feel insecure, especially since on several occasions, local residents and people from the Defence Department have threatened them. Most structures are made of canvas, sacks, mud, rags and tiles and all but five of the houses have one room. Floor space per person is under three square metres in 41 of the houses and under one square metre in 12 of them. Seven households live in canvas and sack dwellings while 33 have one-room mud-wall houses with thatched roofs. The cost of materials for more than half the houses is estimated at less than $20.

There is no provision for water supply on the site. There is a public tap some 350 metres away; water collection is usually done with buckets loaded onto rickshaws or bicycles or hand carried. Sometimes, water direct from the Yamuna River is used. There is no provision for drainage or for the removal of household or human wastes. There is no electricity supply and most households are too poor to afford kerosene lamps. Cooking is done using cowdung or garbage as fuel. The nearest hospitals and dispensaries are nearly two kilometres distance but Kydganj's inhabitants have similar problems to the inhabitants of Chheetpur in obtaining treatment. The inhabitants are not on the voting list and do not seem to have organized to bring pressure to bear either on elected politicians or on government officials. The inhabitants are also not entitled to a ration card which would give them access to cheap foodgrains, sugar, cloth, kerosene, soap and other basic essentials from "fairprice shops". While all citizens are entitled to such cards, these are issued after application has been made to a district magistrate and these are issued only to people with an "authentic address" and the illegal occupation of a land-site does not qualify.

Health problems are compounded by the difficulty in obtaining water and in the inability to safeguard water stored in the house. Pigs are kept as important supplements to food supply and income but keeping pigs in close proximity to humans adds to health problems.

The development of Lowther Road

This settlement is close to Chheetpur, some 800 metres to its west, and just north of a railway line (see Map 4.3). In 1985, it had 310 inhabitants within 80 households. The settlement's name comes from that of the road just to its west. It covers nearly two hectares of low-lying land owned by the Railway Board and a nearby Degree College Trust. The location is good for employment opportunities: nearby are four coal stores, three fuel-wood stores, three motor workshops, two sawmills, an enterprise which rents rickshaws and two warehouses for storing paper to be used for making pulp. Bus and railway stations are close-by and the Chowk Market in the business district is less than a kilometre distance.

The site becomes waterlogged or muddy after rain although a small drain towards the west helps remove some of the rainwater. The residential part covers only 20 per cent of the total area so 310 people live on a site of less than half a hectare. Around 40 per cent of the site is covered by the commercial and industrial enterprises mentioned earlier with the other 40 per cent remaining vacant.

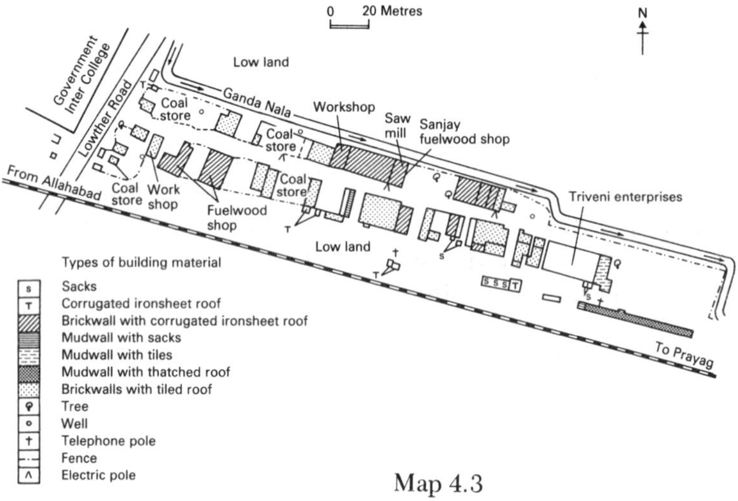

Map 4.3

Of the 81 households, 32 migrated from Madhya Pradesh State, with 16 from Bihar and 14 from districts to the north of Allahabad, within Uttar Pradesh. The remaining 19 are from the city of Allahabad. The site was vacant 25 years ago and was used as a garbage dump before nine households came and built small huts. These households had been forced to move off a site close-by when the state government decided to build a medical college there in 1961. In the 1960s and 1970s, the population grew slowly, but in the 1980s, its growth has been more rapid. In 1985, over three-fifths of the households had joined the settlement since 1979, including 20 tribal households from Madhya Pradesh who had entered the settlement after 1982.

These tribal households originally to Allahabad came as labourers hired by local contractors; the land they occupy belongs to the Railway Board. They decided to stay in Allahabad since they have no property in their area of origin and the land they occupy in the settlement is free; the Railway Board has not taken any action against such illegal occupation. The Trust which owns the rest of the site is concerned about the illegal occupation of the other households and has tried to evict the inhabitants.

The commercial and industrial activities grew along with the residential areas; many households first came as sub-tenants of these enterprises and have built huts beside them. These households pay nothing to the Trust which owns the land but pay the owners of these enterprises. These owners have also brought pressure to bear on the Trust not to evict their workers. Many of the enterprises are relatively new; for instance, since 1980, tea-pan shops (shops serving tea and a popular cheap snack comprising of betel nuts and spices wrapped in betel-leaf), retail stores, coal and fuel-wood stores have developed and a shed has been constructed for buffaloes; the milk they produce is sold outside the settlement but the dung is used for cooking fuel.

As in Chheetpur, most households are from backward or scheduled castes and tribes – 64 households in all. Twelve households are Muslim and seven upper caste. The sex ratio is seven females to every ten males. Table 4.2 shows the occupational structure of the households with rickshaw or cart-pulling being the most common job, followed by labouring – much of it in the enterprises mentioned earlier. The settlement's location close to bus and railway stations and a major market helps explain the predominance of rickshaw pullers. The owner of the rickshaw hire enterprise makes a good living while his brother earns a living running a rickshaw repair shop some 500 metres away from the settlement. Six households earn a living collecting junk or garbage. Just three households derive their income from working for government agencies and three of these are upper-caste households. Three households, including two of the upper caste households, have opened small-scale general stores within their huts, while another has opened a small temporary wooden structure as a tea-pan shop. Of the 150 people who work, 42 are women and most are from backward or scheduled caste households. Some of the women work as labourers outside the community in construction activities while others sort and pack different kinds of paper cuttings in the two paper warehouses. A few women work as maids for wealthy households nearby.

Most households' incomes are less than $400 a year while for 13 households, they are less than $240 a year. Backward and scheduled caste families dominate the lower-income groups while upper-caste households tend to be among the best-off households.

The households whose fathers own the rickshaw hire and the rickshaw repair enterprises are among the only four households whose annual income exceeds $720. Two-thirds of the households are reported to be illiterate although most of the Muslim and upper-caste households have one or more literate members.

Of the 81 shelters, 67 are one-room units. Twenty-three are made of canvas and sacks, 26 of mud walls and thatch or tiles and 23 of brick walls and tiles (see Table 4.4). There are nine buildings made of brick, with corrugated iron roofs;

Table 4.4: Materials used for housing units

		Percentage of housing units in	
House type	*Chheetpur*	*Kydganj*	*Lowther Road*
Canvas huts or shacks	0	13	9
Mud walls with thatch or tiles for roof	65	87	32
Brick walls and tiled roof	26	–	28
Brick walls and cement or iron roof	9	–	11
Total	100	100	100

most of the bricks were collected as scrap with mud used to hold them together. These include four which house commercial or industrial enterprises. For more than half of all households, internal floorspace per person is less than two square metres while in 22 households it is less than one square metre.

Land and house tenure is complicated. Thirty-three of the households pay rent to the Trust on whose land they have built their dwellings. The monthly rent is between $2 and $4 with the terms of tenancy renewed by the Trust every five years. The other 48 households pay nothing to the landowners; 15 are on Railway Board land while the rest are on Trust land but refuse to pay rent since they claim to be tenants of the owners of the commercial and industrial enterprises there. These owners encouraged their workforce to squat and have helped protect them against the Trust. But this is to their advantage for they do not pay their employees minimum wages.

The main source of water is an open well which is close to an open drain. The high water table helps ensure that the well becomes contaminated during the rains. This one well provides water for washing, cooking, bathing and laundry, as well as providing for the needs of the enterprises on the site. One of the inhabitants works as a peon in the chemistry laboratory of the neighbouring college and has managed to obtain some potassium permanganate to treat the well water. But the cost of adequate supplies of the chemical are too high. Three households installed their own handpumps in 1983 but one no longer works. With no proper drainage system, water-logging is a perpetual problem. The one open drain often becomes clogged with garbage.

A few households have electricity provided by the owners of industrial units who have set up three electric poles; users have to pay. Three households have illegal connections from one of the motor workshops. Many people use kerosene lamps for light but their use is limited, given the high cost of kerosene. As in Kydganj, the fact that the inhabitants do not have legal tenure means that they do not receive ration-cards. At a government run "fairprice shop" kerosene is two-thirds the open market price but this can only be obtained with a ration-card. No health care services are provided in Lowther Road and the inhabitants have problems comparable to those of the Chheetpur inhabitants in obtaining medical treatment.

Health and nutrition

In Chheetpur, where research on health was concentrated, information about mortality and health were gathered from three sources: a questionnaire to all the settlement's inhabitants; clinical tests to identify anaemia (blood tests), intestinal worms (stool tests), jaundice (urine tests) and TB (X-rays) for 150 people (around 30 per cent of the population with all age groups represented); and informal talks with selected inhabitants and local informants. The questionnaire included questions designed to identify the number of children who had died between 1970 and 1984 and the causes of death. A dietary survey was compiled through a series of interviews. In Lowther Road and Kydganj, a questionnaire was used to identify the number of persons who had died – and the cause of death – in the period 1979–84, with 20 families selected for detailed enquiry into the number of children born, the number that had died and the causes of death.

In Chheetpur, the main health problems at the time of the survey (1984) were malaria, injuries and infections arising from accidents and burns, diarrhoea/dysentery, jaundice, intestinal worms and scabies. Anaemia was common, especially among women. There were eight cases of malaria, five of hydrocele (swelling of the scrotum, a side effect of filariasis transmitted in urban India by a mosquito which breeds in blocked drains or stagnant, polluted water), ten of conjunctivitis and seven of TB. Every winter, there is an outbreak of scabies, a highly contagious skin disease. At the time of the survey, 60 per cent of the population had scabies. Mumps and whooping cough are common every winter and measles common in the summer; every season, around 20–30 children become infected and measles is one of the main causes of child death (see Table 4.5).

Table 4.5: Causes of infant and child death

Causes of death	*Chheetpur (entire pop'n 1970–84)*	*Kydganj*	*Lowther Road*
		(sample of 20 households 1979–84)	
Premature delivery	11		
Tetanus, accidents and burns	33	4	
Diphtheria	4		
Measles	7	2	
Malaria	35	4	2
Diarrhoea, dysentery or cholera	29		
Jaundice	20	4	
Chickenpox	–		6
Not known	4		8
Total number of infant and child deaths	143	14	16

In stool tests for around 30 per cent of Chheetpur's population, 50 per cent had worm infections with the incidence being higher in the case of children (55 per cent) compared to adults (45 per cent). The dietary survey revealed that most of the population had an average intake of less than 1,500 calories a day. Among the 126 females over 15 years of age, including seven who were pregnant, all but 12 (including all those pregnant) had average daily intakes of below 1,500 calories, with 24 of them having intakes below 1,000 calories. Among 159 males over 15 years of age, 101 had average daily intakes below 1,500 calories. Among infants and children up to the age of four, 93 per cent of females and 87 per cent of males had average daily intakes of less than 750 calories although the optimum intake should be of the order of 1,000; the average daily intake of around half the children is less than 500 calories.

In Chheetpur, 143 children's deaths were recorded from household interviews in the period 1970–84. The most commonly identified causes of death were malaria (35); tetanus, accidents and burn injuries (33); diarrhoea, dysentery or cholera (29); jaundice (20); premature delivery (11); and measles or chickenpox (7). Of these 143 deaths, 73 died as infants (that is, before their first birthday) with tetanus, diarrhoea and dysentery, malaria or premature delivery stated as the reasons in most instances.

In Kydganj, a total of 42 persons had died in the five-year period, an average of close to one per household. Of these, 15 were attributed to jaundice, diarrhoea or dysentery; eight to malaria; eight to TB or anaemia; six to "fever"; and three to pneumonia. Of the 35 children born to 20 families in the five-year period between 1979 and 1984, 14 had died, including seven before their second birthday. The causes identified were tetanus (4); jaundice, diarrhoea or dysentery (4); malaria, sickness or "fever" (4); and measles (2).

In Lowther Road, a total of 55 persons were reported to have died in the period 1979–84. The causes of death according to local records, medical professionals and information from the families suggest that 13 died from malaria, nine from jaundice, diarrhoea or dysentery; eight from measles; and six from pneumonia, with five as a result of post-natal or delivery deaths. Others are not easy to attribute to any specific cause – for instance, six persons died of "unknown fever" while the death of five persons was associated either with TB or anaemia.

Among the 20 families selected for detailed enquiry, a total of 37 babies had been born over a five-year period and 16 had died, seven of them before their second birthday. Chickenpox was reported as the cause of six of these deaths with malaria accounting for two; the rest were attributed to an "unknown fever".

Some tentative conclusions

Without more detailed and sophisticated research, it is impossible to be precise about the causes of the health problems. Indeed, a large number of factors which affect any person's health always inhibits precise diagnoses as to causes of ill-health. But clearly, inadequate provision of water and the fact that each of the sources is open to contamination (even standpipe water may be contaminated as intermittent water supply, low pressure and leaks in water pipes can mean contaminated water is sucked into the water-supply system) is an important factor in the high incidence of diarrhoea and dysentery. No doubt this is also linked to the lack of provision for the hygienic disposal of household and human wastes and to the very low incomes (and thus inadequate food intake) of most inhabitants. The fact that half of a sample of 30 per cent of the residents in Chheetpur had intestinal worms must also relate to insufficient supplies of clean water and inadequate provision for sanitation. The high incidence of anaemia is probably connected to the large numbers of people with intestinal worms. The high incidence of scabies results from lack of washing and bathing which is due largely to inadequate water supplies that make washing and bathing difficult in cramped space with no drainage and little possibility of privacy. The incidence of malaria is linked to the fact that malarial mosquitoes are known to breed in stagnant pools in and around the settlements. The high incidence of infant and child deaths attributed to tetanus, accidents and burns has obvious links both with over-crowded conditions, the use of open fires for cooking, the inadequate provision of infant and child health care, and the total lack of emergency life-saving services.

In-depth interviews with 13 households reinforced this impression of very high infant and child mortality. The two worst affected were one in Chheetpur and one in Kydganj. In the former, both husband and wife were in their forties. They had had 12 children, but only four had survived. Their youngest daughter of seven was found to have jaundice and serious worm infestation, and was suffering from malaria at the time of the interview. In the latter, the husband was about 35, the wife 32. All five of their children, born in the last eight years, had died at birth or very soon afterwards. A daughter lived until the age of three but then died of diarrhoea.

Chapter Five

WATER SUPPLY AND THE URBAN POOR

Sandy Cairncross

The undue emphasis on water quality

In 1975, it was estimated that only 74 per cent of the Third World's urban population had access to a safe water supply. Ten years later, in 1985, half way through the International Water Decade, the number of people served had increased by more than 300 million, an increase of over 70 per cent. However, the towns and cities of the Third World had grown so rapidly that 25 per cent of their population still lacked adequate access to safe water. In fact, 100 million more people were unserved in 1985 than in 1975.[1]

Those not served are obliged to use water from streams and other surface sources, which in urban areas are often little more than open sewers, or to purchase water from insanitary vendors. It is little wonder that their children suffer frequently, often fatally, from diarrhoeal diseases, which worldwide kill a child every 20 seconds. In other words, since you started reading this chapter, a child in a city in the Third World has died from diarrhoea, which could very probably have been prevented by a better water supply.

It is well known that contaminated drinking water can cause water-borne epidemics of these diseases. However, it is by no means the only hazard, and probably not even the greatest of the health risks to which the urban poor are exposed by shortcomings of the water supplies in most Third World nations. There is good reason to believe that difficulty in obtaining enough water is at least as prejudicial to their health as water contamination, if not more so, for two reasons. First, the lack of sufficient water to maintain adequate hygiene can promote transmission of any of the diseases which are potentially water-borne, and several more besides. Second, the high price which the urban poor have to pay for water diminishes the amount they have to spend on food, and so undermines their often precarious nutritional status. Unfortunately, few of the engineers and planners responsible for urban water supply are aware of this, or understand its important consequences for policy. This chapter seeks to correct the picture.

There are three main reasons which can account for the emphasis usually placed on the risk of water-borne disease, to the neglect of disease due to water scarcity. The first is historical. John Snow's demonstrations of water-borne transmission of cholera in nineteenth-century London stand among the first triumphs of the science of epidemiology, and European water engineers still shudder at the memory of the famous water-borne epidemics which their networks of piping helped to spread: the typhoid epidemic of 1937 in Croydon, UK, for instance, or that in Zermatt, Switzerland, in 1963. Most water engineers practising in the Third World have been trained in Europe or North America or at least with the textbooks of Europe and North America, and their professional attitudes have been formed in a context in which these traumatic experiences figure large.

The second possible reason is that water-borne disease can attack everyone in the community, rich and poor alike, whereas water scarcity is not a serious problem for the middle classes and the elite. A contaminated water supply is likely to lead to a sudden surge of cases of disease, and so to a major public outcry. Politicians, journalists and the engineer are equally at risk, and therefore equally aware of the need to prevent that risk. By contrast, disease and hardship due to water scarcity afflict only the poorest in the community. The impact is not a sudden and dramatic epidemic, but dispersed and inconspicuous individual cases. The engineer whose house has running water may not even know how many people in his or her city have to queue or pay for water, or how long they have to queue, or how much they have to pay.

Third, the responsibility for water quality lies clearly with those who supply the water. When water-borne transmission of disease is suspected, the first to be questioned – and even, sometimes, arrested – are the operators of the water supply. It is not so clear who is responsible when a poor family does not have enough water for its needs, and it is easier to blame the victims. They should have installed a house connection, one might argue, or bought a bigger bucket, and spent less on alcohol, tobacco or televisions.

The importance of water quantity

In the last two decades, however, an increasing amount of evidence has accumulated for the importance of access to water in adequate quantities as a means of improving health. Over the last 30 years, there have been more than 70 studies of the health impact of water supplies. A review of these studies[2] found that in most of the cases where water supply improvements were shown to have brought about a reduction in diarrhoeal disease, these improvements had included an improvement in access to water in quantity. The review concluded that water quantity appears to be more important than water quality as a means to control diarrhoeal disease in contaminated environments.

This conclusion does not refer to the occasional epidemics of typhoid, cholera and other enteric infections which attract public notice and are sometimes water-borne, but rather to the endemic diarrhoeal disease which continually afflicts low-income communities, particularly small children, and is a major cause of child mortality in the Third World (see Box 5.1).

In addition to increased water availability having an impact on diarrhoeal diseases, it has also been found to play a role in the control of trachoma, an eye infection causing widespread blindness in the Third World,[3] and it probably helps to control infectious skin diseases and infections carried by body lice.

Box 5.1: Endemic vs. epidemic

A graphic illustration of the difference between a water-borne epidemic, and water-washed endemic disease, is provided by a study of a typhoid epidemic in the town of Kosti in the Sudan. The epidemic curve is shown in Figure 5.1. The epidemic was found to have been water-borne, due to an interruption in the disinfection of the town's water supply from July 1 – 19, 1976. On 20 July, a Ministry of Health team identified the cause of the epidemic, disinfection was immediately restored and the water quality was meticulously monitored thereafter. However, the graph shows that typhoid had been endemic in the town before the incident, and typhoid cases continued to be reported long after the restoration of disinfection and the expiry of the 10-day incubation period for the disease.

Box 5.1: (continued)

These additional cases were clearly not water-borne, and must therefore have arisen from contamination of items such as food, hands or utensils. Transmission of disease by routes such as these is most likely where not enough water is available in the home for hygiene purposes. The number of cases in the epidemic was large, but a far greater number of endemic, hygiene-related cases must have occurred in the town during previous and subsequent years.

Source: Elzubier, A.G., *An Outbreak of Typhoid Fever in Kosti Town, Sudan*, DTPH dissertation, University of London (1977).

Distance and demand

If an increase in the quantity of water used in the home can bring about significant health improvements, how can this be promoted? The most obvious measure is to provide water as close as possible to the home. In this context, it is remarkable how few people have studied the way in which the distance to the water source affects a household's water consumption, as the distance water must be carried and the water consumption per capita are both fundamental design parameters of any water distribution system. Nevertheless, some half a dozen studies of the question have been carried out in various countries in Africa and Asia, and their results fit a common pattern (Figure 5.2).

As the water source is brought closer to individual homes, it has been found that the average household's consumption tends to increase. This is a result one would expect, but what most of us would not expect is that at a certain threshold distance a plateau is reached; bringing the water source closer than this does not produce an increase in consumption until it is less than one hundred metres from the home. The exact magnitude of the threshold distance has varied a little between studies, from "about a mile" in East Africa[4] to some 400 metres in Sri Lanka.[5] At the other end of the plateau, water consumption increases slightly when the source is less than one hundred metres away, and then shoots up by a factor of two or three when water is available in the home or on the individual family's plot.

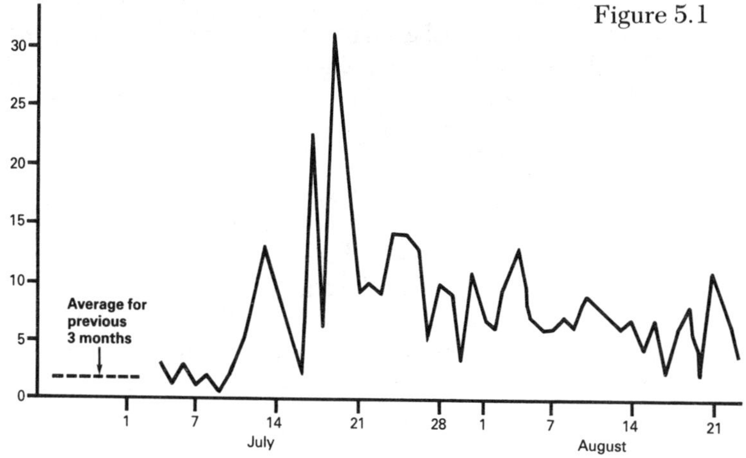

Figure 5.1

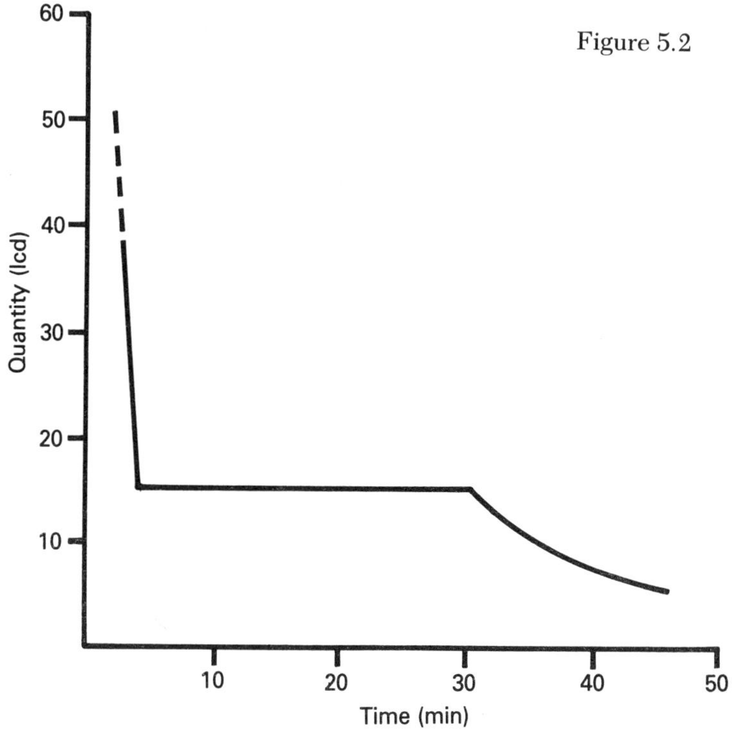

Figure 5.2

When the only cost of water is the cost in time spent collecting it, this finding has important policy implications for the water engineer who seeks to bring about a health benefit. First, priority should go towards serving those whose existing water sources are more than, say, 1 kilometre from their homes. Those whose water sources are further away than the threshold distance are most likely to increase their consumption if water is provided at a well, borehole or standpipe closer to their homes. They will also benefit most from the savings in time and effort which stem from a more convenient source of water, and so be most willing to pay for it. If, on the other hand, everyone has a water source within the threshold distance of their home, it may be necessary to provide individual connections, at least at the level of a tap in each person's yard, if a significant health benefit is to be obtained.

Cost

However, distance is not usually the only consideration among low-income urban communities. The urban poor not only have to fetch water, but frequently they have to pay for it. They usually pay by the bucket, and they are often charged an exorbitant price by the owner or operator of the well, tap or tanker truck, or by the vendor with their yoke or donkey-cart who comes calling door-to-door. White and others[6] found that those buying water from kiosks in Nairobi's Mathare Valley were paying ten times as much per litre as the wealthier citizens with private connections. Adrianzen and Graham found in Lima, Peru, that the price of water bought from tanker trucks was 16 times the metered rate.[7] Indeed, as they commented, it is expensive to be poor.

The practice of water vending is very common in the Third World. In a brief survey, Zaroff and Okun found it to be prevalent in rural and urban areas throughout Asia, Africa and South America, and to serve an average of 40 per cent of the households in the 12 low-income communities which they studied in detail.[8] In half of these communities, the cost of water amounted to one-fifth or more of the income of a typical household. Briscoe has estimated that water vendors serve 20 to 30 per cent of the urban population of the Third World.[9]

Moreover, it has been estimated that money paid to water vendors often accounts for a large share of the total income from vendors often accounts for a large share of the total income from the sale of water.[10] In one of the few detailed field studies of water vending, Whittington and others found that the total sum paid to water vendors in a Kenyan community amounted to twice the revenue paid to the water supply agency.[11] The existence of this thriving informal market in water is evidence of a demand unsatisfied by the official government (or private sector) water agencies. It is also evidence of the money value which even the poorest are ready to give to the time they would have to spend carrying water if they did not buy from vendors. It is an indication of how much they would be willing to pay for an adequate conventional water supply, were it to be made available to them.

Problems of the formal sector

Most Third World water engineers are unaware of the scale of water vending in the area which falls under the jurisdiction of their agency. They would also be shocked to learn of the price at which the vendors resell the water, since most vendors obtain their water supplies from the public water mains system. Meanwhile, the engineers struggle to overcome the almost intractable problems presented by the piped water-supply systems which they manage.

The first, and most apparent, of these is that the system's capacity generally falls far short of the demand. As a result, roughly half the urban water supplies in the Third World operate intermittently, sometimes providing water for only one or two hours each day. Those who can afford private connections can usually install their own storage tanks, so the poorest suffer most from the impact of the shortfall. The prospect of obtaining sufficient funds to provide a constant water supply is generally remote. In many urban water supply improvement schemes, such as the $480 million Bombay water-supply project,[12] it is assumed at the design stage that the water supply will continue to be intermittent.

Intermittent water supplies encourage vandalism, if only through the frustration of those trying to obtain water. Conversely, vandalised taps make it more difficult to provide a constant water supply. In the case of the Bombay project, the large number of *chawls* or one-room tenements in which all the taps were stolen was the principal reason for keeping the supply intermittent. It is not only among the poor that water shortage provokes anti-social behaviour. When pressure is low, many consumers with private connections pump water directly from the mains to their storage tanks, whether or not this is illegal. This further reduces the pressure in the distribution system, and can even cause negative pressures.

One of the reasons for the shortfall in capacity of many a city's water supply is the high rate of leakage from the distribution system. Typically, 30 per cent of the water treated and pumped into the water supply of a tropical town, and commonly as much as 60 per cent, is lost in this way.[13] It may result from incompetent pipe-laying, from exposure of mains pipes due to soil erosion, from construction of houses over mains due to poor physical planning, or from sheer age of the system. Leaky distribution mains present an additional hazard with intermittent supplies or where there are low pressures, as pollution from drains and sewers may enter through the leaks when the pressure drops. Repair of leaking mains is made more difficult by the lack of accurate records showing pipe locations.

The leakage is frequently exacerbated by the numerous unauthorized connections to the water mains made by private individuals. They are often improvised out of inappropriate materials such as old motor tyres and wire. They may result from high water charges, from delays and corruption in the allocation of water connections, or from a refusal to provide connections to squatters. The resulting erosion of the water agency's revenue makes it hard to lower the charges, the leakage from incompetent connections diverts the agency's resources (so making it difficult to shorten the delays) and attempts to police the illegal connections frequently result in increased corruption.

Finally, the unauthorized connections are only one among various factors contributing to the large proportion of water which is supplied but not paid for. Other causes include broken water meters, defaulting by consumers, and exemptions for government installations. Even when water is paid for, the invoiced tariffs are often barely sufficient to cover the cost of operating the water supply, let alone to finance the new investment needed to increase its capacity. The problems which beset most urban water supplies in the Third World are thus interrelated, exacerbating one another in a vicious circle.

A number of solutions to these problems have been proposed.

Policy-makers have sometimes put their faith a little too enthusiastically in some of the simpler ones. The main ones are discussed in turn.

Privatization

The popularity of this panacea in the industrialized countries has spread to the major aid agencies, which are now advocating it to their clients in the Third World. It has been argued that the private sector can provide and charge for water supplies in the Third World with greater efficiency and with less political interference than public bodies, without undue prejudice to equity.[14]

However, it is important to distinguish between privatization and efficient cost recovery. If users pay the full cost of the water they consume, it does of course make it easier to persuade private companies to manage the supply. However, management by the private sector does not necessarily guarantee full cost recovery. The advocates of privatization have not successfully answered the question of what happens in the event of bankruptcy of a private water company; no government would allow the water supply of a major city to be simply abandoned in such a case. A company operating the supply can therefore use the threat of bankruptcy, abandonment or sale to an asset-stripper to extract a subsidy from the government or municipality, particularly in a small, underdeveloped economy where there are few competitors able to take over the running of a large system at short notice.

On the other hand, private enterprises are not necessarily free from the bureaucratic and political interference which can prevent a public body from charging water prices adequate to recover costs. Governments do not limit their control of prices to public sector goods, and there are important political reasons why it would be hard to persuade them to do so. Water-price riots are not unknown in the Third World.

Nor is a private company certain to provide better coverage of the population, by seizing the commercial opportunity afforded by the unmet needs of the poor. In those large tropical towns where no public water supplies exist, there is hardly a queue of private firms eager to build one. The lack of convenient standpipes in many squatter settlements or illegal subdivisions is not always due to a lack of entrepreneurial initiative on the part of the public water supply agency, but is often a consequence of government policy not to provide infrastructure in "illegal", unplanned squatter areas. In such cases, a private water company cannot necessarily be certain of obtaining the necessary wayleaves from the legal owners of the land to lay its pipes.

Finally, it is not at all certain that any gains in efficiency will be passed on to the consumer, as this requires firm government regulation. If there are limits to the British Government's power to control the recently privatized telephone service, the task is much more daunting in what are usually highly stratified Third World societies, where the owners of private companies are likely to have far greater political influence than a mass of poor, over-charged water consumers. Perhaps a closer British parallel is nineteenth-century London, where it took 50 years for the private water companies to fulfill the simple obligation of the Waterworks Clauses Act 1847, that they should provide a 24-hour supply, seven days a week. The threat of government intervention means little to the prominent political figures who control Nairobi's hugely profitable privately-operated water kiosks, when they in turn can control the government.

Metering

The explicit policy of the major agencies funding most large urban water-supply schemes is to encourage water utilities "to introduce tariffs based on the incremental costs of service, with a view to encouraging economically efficient use".[15] Payment by metered volume, it is argued, will help to prevent waste. It is also advocated as a means to facilitate the use of a progressive tariff system, whereby those using larger than average amounts of water, usually for luxury purposes such as watering lawns or washing cars, are required to pay more than the basic rate for their water. The additional revenue can be used to subsidise a cheap "lifeline" tariff for the smallest consumers, or the supply of water free of charge from public standpipes. The additional revenue needed for this is not very great, because "the poorest 40 per cent of households would normally account for only some 6–10 per cent of water consumption in a city with a fully developed system in a developing country".[16]

The reality of metering, however, is less auspicious. For example a study of the metering system in Lahore by the World Bank concluded that of 7,500 meters, only 3,500 were working. The authors added that

> meters are frequently stolen or tampered with, often with the connivance of meter readers; honest mistakes are also made in meter readings (particularly for dial-type meters)... repair facilities are inadequate; there are difficulties in getting spare parts; consumer complaints are numerous; and the average length of life of a meter is only about five years.[17]

The problems of meters are particularly acute with intermittent supplies. When the pressure is off, water is drained from the mains pipes as the lowest taps are opened, so that the pipes are filled with air. When the flow of water is re-established, the rush of trapped air through the meter of the first consumer to open a tap causes it to spin, and an incorrect, sometimes very high, consumption figure is recorded.[18] If the meter is not sabotaged by the irate consumer confronted by a correspondingly high water bill (more than proportionately high, if a progressive tariff is in force), it is likely to be damaged by the physical shock when the first water coming down the pipe hits it at high speed.

In practice, the cost of repairing and replacing water meters can amount to a sizeable part of an urban water agency's recurrent budget, and in countries which do not manufacture their own meters it is largely a foreign exchange cost. In one African country recently, the cost of replacement meters regularly used up half the water agency's foreign exchange allowance; there was a small local capacity to manufacture meters using imported mechanisms, but even this was not enough.

Little is known of the degree to which water consumption is reduced by metering under the conditions of Third World countries. When meters were introduced in Rangoon, Burma, in 1965–66, a saving in water use of about 30 per cent was achieved.[19] Fifteen years later, 90 per cent of these were not functioning properly,[20] but even were they to have survived, the investment might not have been justified. The Lahore study mentioned above concluded that on average, metering would have to reduce water consumption by 80 per cent or more to be worthwhile.

Nor is metering an essential prerequisite for the introduction of progressive tariffs. Several countries have used criteria based on plot size, house size or rateable value as a basis for water rates. Tariff systems such as these can ensure with reasonable equity that consumers pay in proportion to their resources, which usually increase in slightly greater proportion to their water consumption as one goes up the socio-economic scale. They are recognized as equitable by most consumers at all levels, and are easier to administer than metered tariffs.

Water demand management

If meters are a wasteful way of preventing waste, what more efficient methods are there? Some of the most wasteful uses of water, such as the watering of lawns and washing of cars, occur out of doors. If meters are not installed, it is still possible to charge for them, using a system of hosepipe licences such as that which has worked for many years in the United Kingdom.

Another approach is to control leakages from the distribution system. Reducing the leakage rate from 60 per cent (a figure common in Third World nations) to the 12 per cent typical of systems in Europe and the USA, would more than double the amount of water available for use. It may not be feasible in practice to achieve such a dramatic reduction in full, but significant improvements can be made even with a modest effort, as roughly 80 per cent of the losses typically occur at only 20 per cent of the leaks.[21] The example of Sao Paulo, Brazil, where the proportion of unaccounted-for water has been reduced by about 50 per cent over ten years, shows what can be done even in a large and sprawling metropolis.[22]

Other measures include the use of water-saving fittings, particularly low-volume flush toilets. The flushing of toilets accounts for about one-third of the water use of a typical household with a private connection, and is more than the total amount of water used by a typical family served by a standpipe. The large volume of 10–20 litres used to flush a conventional cistern-flush toilet is unnecessary for efficient operation. By efficient design of the toilet bowl, it can be reduced to about 3–6 litres per flush, as has been shown by the widespread introduction of more efficient cisterns and flushing pans in Scandinavia. The introduction of such fittings can be assured by building regulations and by-laws, and by government house-building policy. Any such measures which produce economies in water use would bring similar benefits to waste disposal, because less water used is less water to be disposed of.

Other solutions

In general the popularity of other approaches to improving access to water by the poor tends to decrease in proportion to the degree of creativity they demand from the engineers and administrators responsible for the sector. One which is relatively simple to implement and whose popularity is well justified, is to provide yard taps, an intermediate level of service between the standpipe and the full house connection. Families served by hand pumps or public standpipes typically use about 20 litres per capita per day (l.c.d.) while those with house connections use some 100 l.c.d., rising to over 200 l.c.d. in the wealthier low-density housing areas with extensive gardens.[23] Provision of a single tap in the yard of each household generally causes consumption to increase from standpipe level by a factor of two or three, to some 60 l.c.d. There is reason to believe this is sufficient to achieve most of the health benefits associated with increased water availability, as well as most of the savings in time which a convenient water supply can bestow (see Box 5.2 for more details on relative costs).

Box 5.2: The cost of conventional water supplies

The cost of building urban water supplies varies widely, depending largely on the availability of water resources. For instance, in monsoon-drenched South-East Asia, a water supply with house connections costs only $60 per capita, whereas in the arid Middle East it is likely to cost five times as much. A typical figure for a Third World nation would be $120 per person served.

One cheaper alternative to water piped into each house is public standposts from where those living close-by collect water. Public standposts cost roughly half as much to build as house connections, say $60 per head. The difference is not due primarily to savings in the cost of distribution pipes, as the distribution system normally accounts for only one-third of the total cost of a water supply. Rather, the lower cost of standpost supplies is due to the fact that those who use them consume much less water than households with private connections, so that they put less demand on the water abstraction, treatment, pumping and storage capacity of the system. Households with taps in the yard of their homes use roughly half as much as

Box 5.2: (continued)

those with house connections, so that the cost for them is nearer to the lower figure – say $80 per capita.

In order to combine the construction costs with the annual operating costs of a system (typically about $0.35 per cubic metre of water supplied), it must be converted to an equivalent annual amortization cost, as in the table below.

Typical costs of urban water supply (in US$ per capita)

Level of service	*Typical construction cost*	*Equivalent annual amount*[1]	*Typical water consumption*[2]	*Annual operating cost*[3]	*Total annual cost*
Public standpost	60	8.88	20	2.55	11.55
Yard tap	80	11.84	60	7.66	19.50
Private connection	120	17.76	150	19.16	36.92

1. Converted on the basis of amortization over 10 years at 10 per cent interest.
2. In litres per person per day.
3. Calculated on the basis of $0.35 per cubic metre.

Source: Data from WHO (1987), see note 1.

Single-tap yard connections can be installed more cheaply than laying on piped water to a series of taps and fittings in each house. Small pipes of 12 millimetres diameter will suffice, and water demand is not as great as with full piped water so that there is less pressure on treatment, pumping and storage capacity. In neighbourhoods where a distribution main already runs down every street, the additional cost of pipes for yard connections need not be great.[24]

Where the nearest main is some distance away, the principle of a progressive tariff can be extended to the charges made for house connections. The first person in an area to apply for a private connection, generally one of the better-off residents, is charged the full cost of laying a pipe to their house which is large enough to serve all the houses near it. Then, when poorer neighbours apply, a pipe has already been laid down their street and they need only pay for a small branch from it.

There is also room for creativity in the engineering design of distribution pipes. Water distribution networks are often designed to the demanding criteria originally developed in the industrialized countries. Recently, computer-aided design and cost estimation of these networks has made it possible to calculate quickly the cost savings which result from a change in these criteria for a specific town. In the Philippines, for instance, it was found that a reduction in the minimum pipe size from the diameter normally specified could reduce the cost of the network by 45 per cent.[25]

In many tropical cities, however, the existing treatment plant, pumping mains and storage capacity are already heavily overloaded so that there is little benefit in extending the distribution network until the overall capacity of the whole system can be increased. Until then, a variety of local solutions are possible. One option is to install a series of small independent networks of water points, each served by a local source such as a spring, well or borehole. These networks can be designed in such a way that they can be connected into the city's overall system, and house connections offered to those who wish them, when the main system's capacity allows.

For the engineer willing to countenance the unorthodox, yet more options are worth study. These include grants to householders towards the cost of guttering and rainwater tanks, on the grounds of their reduced consumption from the city supply. Alternatively, local wells in poor urban neighbourhoods may provide water of good quality if a few basic precepts are observed in their construction. They will normally cost less per person served than an extension to the main city water supply, and certainly be easier to install. They will also have the virtue of being under the community's control.

Support to vendors

A still more unorthodox solution, though one which has been advocated by some eminent and thoughtful engineers[26] is to provide assistance to water vendors with a view to rendering their service more efficient. It might appear that the water vending systems of the informal sector involving transport by truck, by animals or on people's backs, are hopelessly inefficient by comparison with formal water supply systems using pipelines. However, the fact remains that, for all their efficiency, the formal systems still fail to serve a quarter of the population of a typical tropical city, and the shortfall in service is largely made up by vendors.

Compared to further funding for formal water supply construction, an intervention to increase the number and efficiency of these vendors might produce a more rapid and replicable improvement in the standard of service provided to their clientele. Since this clientele consists mainly of the urban poor, they would be the ultimate beneficiaries. The intervention could thus be an effective form of aid to the poorest. However, the engineering, financial, economic and social aspects of vending systems have hardly been studied at all.[27] They must first be examined in order to judge the feasibility or the most suitable means of providing support for them.

An example of the potential fruits of such study is provided by recent research in Khartoum, Sudan.[28] Communities paying vastly different prices for water were compared, but the price was found to have no measurable impact on water consumption. This was a remarkable result, as the average household in the community paying the highest price was spending more than half its income on water. Even more startling was the finding that household income had a similarly negligible effect on water consumption, as is shown in Figure 5.3. Since households at all income levels purchased the same amount of water, they all spent the same amount. Thus, the poorer the household, the greater the proportion of its income this represented. Since most households spent almost all the remainder on food, the poorest households were clearly having to sacrifice most of their expenditure on diet in order to meet their need for water.

A consequence of such inelastic market conditions is that even a slight constraint on the supply side – that is, on the availability of water – should lead to a much greater increase in price. This was found to be the case in one of the study areas, where the closure of only one out of several boreholes in the vicinity was accompanied by a fourfold increase in the water price. The same logic also implies the converse; that is, a slight improvement in water availability, such as an increase in the number of boreholes or the number of vendors, should lead to a major drop in price.

In Khartoum, some 300,000 people depend on the services of about 6,000 vendors. Poor households often pay many times more per litre than richer households. This has serious consequences, especially for their children (see Box 5.3). But an important constraint on cheaper water is the limited number of vendors which in turn is linked to the lack of credit to allow the purchase of a donkey and cart. In order to finance a new donkey and cart for each of them every five years, or to increase the number of vendors by 20 per cent each year, a revolving fund of $900,000 would be sufficient. Since the price of water is typically $2.25 or more per cubic metre, and the average consumption of vendors' clients is over 25 litres per capita per day, the water vending market in Khartoum is worth at least $6.2 million annually. Thus, if the revolving fund were to cause a 20 per cent reduction in the price of water, it would quickly pay for itself by permitting an annual saving of some $1.2 million from the budgets of the poorest households in the city.

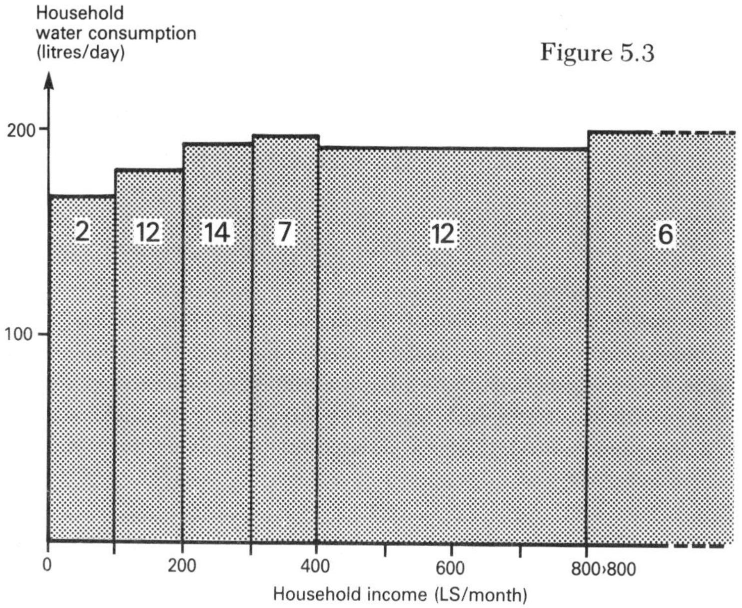

Box 5.3: What is water worth?

Consider two families of five in Khartoum. One uses 500 litres/day from its private tap and pays water bills of $2.60 per month. The

Box 5.3: (continued)

other, poorer, family has no private connection and is obliged to depend on a vendor who sells water door-to-door from a donkey cart. He charges $0.90 for each drum of 200 litres, and they use 120 litres/day, so that water costs them $16 per month.

If a limited amount, delivered erratically and unhygienically by a vendor, is worth $16 a month, the real value to the first family of unlimited quantities of water piped into the home must be far more than it really pays.

Even the poorer family would probably be prepared to pay more. Vendors in some parts of Khartoum charge twice as much, but the price does not seem to affect consumption, as can be seen from the figures below, for two areas in the city.

Area	*Price per drum*	*Consumption (litres per day)*	*Average monthly income*	*% of income spent on water*
Meiyo	$0.45	24	$93	11
Karton Kassala	$1.40	27	$118	35

Apart from water, most of the income of a typical family in these areas is spent on food. Payments for water come out of the food budget, exacerbating the prevalence of malnutrition and so contributing to the high levels of child mortality. So the cost of water is high indeed; there are children who literally pay for it with their lives.

Chapter Six

LOW COST SANITATION

Gehan Sinnatamby

Who needs sanitation?

More than two billion people – that is approximately 60 per cent of all those who live in the Third World – have no sanitary means to dispose of human wastes. An even greater number lack adequate means to dispose of their other waste-water, known as sullage. At present, little over half of the Third World's urban population have access to adequate sanitation, even where adequate sanitation is defined in the most modest terms possible and based on government estimates. Only one rural dweller in six has any sanitation facility (see Table 6.1)

Table 6.1: Sanitation coverage by region in 1985 (per cent)

Region	*Urban*	*Rural*
Africa	73	25
Americas	79	27
South-East Asia	33	10
Europe	92	69
Eastern Mediterranean	68	9
Western Pacific	94	66
Average	65	18
Average (excluding Europe)	59	16

Source: World Health Organization, *The International Drinking Water Supply and Sanitation Decade – Review of Mid-Decade Progress* (Geneva, 1987).

In most Third World cities, between 30 and 60 per cent of the population live in informal or illegal settlements (see Table 6.2); in these settlements, the proportion served by sanitation facilities is typically no better than that in rural areas. In many cases they are in fact much worse. Amongst the slum dwellers of Sao Paulo, for example, only two per cent have any form of sanitation[1] as compared to 41 per cent in rural Brazil. However, the consequences of a deficiency in sanitation facilities for health and the environment differ dramatically between rural and urban communities.

Table 6.2: Estimates of the percentage of city populations in informal settlements in 1980

City, Country	*Per cent urban population in informal settlements*	*Per cent urban population without sanitation*
Luanda, Angola	70	71
Bogota, Colombia	59	45
Ankara, Turkey	51	24
Lusaka, Zambia	45	66
Tunis, Tunisia	50	30
Manila, Philippines	40	35
Mexico City, Mexico	40	30
Karachi, Pakistan	37	51
Caracas, Venezuela	34	30
Nairobi, Kenya	33	35
Lima, Peru	33	33
Sao Paulo, Brazil	32	22

Source: United Nations Centre for Human Settlements, *Global Report on Human Settlements* (Oxford University Press, 1987) and World Health Organization, *The International Drinking Water Supply and Sanitation Decade – Review of Mid-decade Progress* (Geneva, 1987)

Among the urban poor who dwell in densely-populated areas, there is a strongly felt need for sanitation. This arises from the need for privacy and the need to spend less on waste disposal. The urban poor often pay large sums to private individuals for services such as nightsoil collection and emptying of pit latrines. All indications are that the demand for urban sanitation will increase.

Benefits of improved sanitation

As noted in Chapter 1, an increasing volume of literature suggests that the health problems that result from – among other factors – the lack of sanitation facilities are greater among the urban poor living in overcrowded, cheap rental accommodation or informal or illegal settlements than they are either in the rest of the urban areas or in rural areas. In Manila, for example, diarrhoea among the urban poor was observed to be twice as common as in the rest of the city.[2] The infant mortality rate in the old city (slum area) of Kabul, Afghanistan was observed to be 1.5 times that for the rest of the city.[3] In Port au

Prince, Haiti, mortality rates among slum infants were observed to be three times that of rural infants.[4] Likewise, in Villa El Salvador, a low-income settlement developed by squatters on the outskirts of Lima, Peru, the observed infant mortality rate was twice the city average.[5]

A variety of intestinal parasites is usually present in poor urban populations, with roundworms and whipworm often observed at higher levels than in corresponding rural populations. In Dakar, Senegal, one-third of the peri-urban dwellers tested for roundworms were found to be positive, compared to less than one percent of the rural population tested.[6] In Singapore, the prevalence of hookworm, roundworm and whipworm among squatters was more than double that found among flat-dwellers.[7] Chapters 2 and 4 also mention the high proportion of the population in San Martin and the squatter settlements in Allahabad which were suffering from intestinal worms.

Likewise, the accumulation of waste-water as a result of the limited available soil area to absorb waste-waters in densely-settled urban areas has led to increased transmission of filariasis in many cities.

While the fundamental reason for undertaking sanitation is to promote health, the extent to which sanitation can influence health varies considerably, depending on other factors such as personal hygiene and levels of water supply. Some understanding of the potential impact that sanitation – alone or as part of a comprehensive package – could have on the health of a community is essential in devising a suitable programme to address the specific health problems of a community. The classification of excreta-related diseases, their modes of transmission and the potential impact that sanitation and complementary interventions can have on improving health are well documented in Kalbermatten and others (1982), Feachem and others (1983) and Cairncross and Feachem (1983).[8]

While it is intuitively believed that improved provision for sanitation will reduce the spread of diseases and result in a number of social, environmental and other benefits, it has proved very difficult to demonstrate this causal relationship in practice (see Box 6.1). The inability to pin-point and quantify most benefits from sanitation interventions is one reason why these have not received the attention they deserve. A detailed discussion of the problems and methods of measuring the impact of water and sanitation facility provision is given in UNCHS (1987).[9]

Improved sanitation can also improve the quality of the environment and thus the quality of life. The desire for privacy when defecating is also important, especially among women. Having access to toilets that could also be used at night was perceived by women in Nepal to be a primary benefit; it is common for women to eat little or nothing at night to avoid the necessity to go to the toilet. Such benefits are usually secondary to the benefits to health, and equally difficult to assess (see Box 6.2).

Direct economic benefits usually override all other considerations and sanitation tends to be ranked below other needs such as improved water supply or drainage, as in some low-income settlements of Brazil and Haiti, and more basic needs such as food.

Box 6.1: Health effects of improved sanitation

In India alone, it is estimated that some 73 million work days are lost every year due to excreta-related infections and that the lost production is worth around US$600 million per year.[10] Likewise in an estimate of the cost of *Ascaris* (roundworm) infection to Kenya it was concluded that the largest single component was the estimated reduction in food absorption and utilization of those infected; this loss was assessed to be of the order of US$4.4 million each year, compared to US$0.7 million for all other costs such as treatment, health care, and transport to health care facilities.[11]

Despite many problems of measuring health improvements, it is possible to compile an overall picture of the effect of improved sanitation – and its relative merits in relation to improving the quality and quantity of water made available – based on a single, but important, health problem: diarrhoeal disease in young children. As noted in earlier chapters, about five million children under five in the Third World die each year from diarrhoea and related causes. The results of a recent literature review by the World Health Organization show a clear reduction in disease following the provision of sanitation facilities. The same study also noted that the reductions in the death rates were even greater. The changes necessary for an effect on health are most likely to occur where there is a real demand for sanitation, such as in high-density urban areas. (Box 6.1 continues on p. 131.)

Typical effects of improved water supply and sanitation conditions on diarrhoeal morbidity

Condition	*Median reduction in diarrhoeal morbidity (per cent)*
Improved water-quality	16
Improved water availability	25
Improved water quality and availability	37
Improved excreta disposal	22

Source: Esrey, S.A. *et al.*, "Interventions for the control of diarrhoeal diseases among young children: improving water supply and excreta disposal facilities", *Bulletin of the World Health Organization* (Geneva, 1985), vol. 63, no. 4.

Box 6.2: Reasons for constructing latrines in Nepal

In surveys conducted in five urban centres in Nepal to determine the reasons why people built toilets outside a special government subsidized programme to introduce low-cost pour-flush latrines, the following responses were recorded:

Principal reasons for constructing latrines	*Percentage respondents*
Increased prestige	8
Increased comfort/privacy	10
Increased comfort/privacy/prestige	25
Improved health	28
Other	29

Source: UNCHS (Habitat), *Sociocultural Perspective on Sanitation in Nepal: A Survey Report* (Nairobi, 1986).

Types of excreta disposal-systems

The conventional, water-borne sewerage system is by far the most convenient sanitation system for the user. However, it is very expensive and may cost seven to ten times as much as a simple, but equally hygienic, latrine. Starting in the mid-1970s, international agencies and national governments made a concerted effort to identify alternative (low-cost) sanitation technologies that could be adequately applied in rural and low- to medium-density urban settlements. These technologies were of limited applicability in a high proportion of low-income urban areas where population densities were high.

National agencies in countries such as India, Zimbabwe and Vietnam have made major developments in applying low-cost technologies. Despite these efforts, the rate of provision of urban sanitation in the three main Third World regions was barely sufficient to keep pace with the increase in urban population over ten years. Sanitation for high-density low-income settlements presents the single most important challenge to those concerned with environmental health in the Third World in the 1990s (see Table 6.3).

Table 6.3: Percentage urban sanitation coverage

Region	*1975*	*1980*	*1985*
Africa	75	54	73
Latin-America	80	56	79
South-East Asia	31	31	33

Source: World Health Organisation, *The International Drinking Water Supply and Sanitation Decade – Review of Mid-decade Progress* (Geneva, 1987)

There are over 20 different excreta disposal-systems which offer differing degrees of user convenience, protection against the spread of diseases and water demand for their operation.[12] Some of the most promising options for use in the Third World are described here. It is not the intention of this chapter to provide detailed information on each option, but rather to describe them, to give examples of their use, to point to their advantages and disadvantages and to indicate where more details may be obtained.

Ventilated Improved Pit (VIP) latrines

The pit latrine is still by far the most common sanitation system in the Third World, particularly in rural areas, mainly because it is the cheapest and simplest to operate. It can cope with the discharge into it of bulky anal cleaning materials (few rural dwellers use or could afford toilet paper) and does not need water for its operation. In its most basic form, a pit latrine has three components: an excavated pit, a covering platform and a superstructure. Unfortunately, in its basic form, the pit latrine can produce offensive odours and give rise to fly and mosquito nuisance; the pit can collapse, and the platform can lead to the transmission of hookworm if it cannot be adequately cleaned. Most of the objections to the use and acceptance of pit latrines have largely been overcome with the development of the Ventilated Improved Pit (VIP) latrine.

In VIP latrines, the pits are provided with a masonry collar lining around the upper part of the pit to prevent collapse (see Figure 6.1).

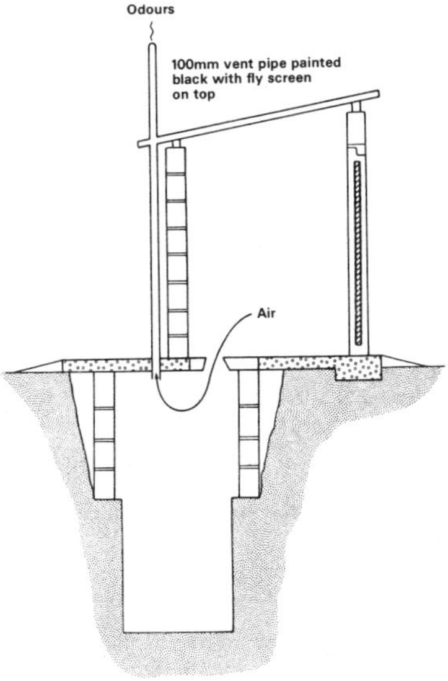

Figure 6.1

This is particularly important in loose soils or where the pit is full of water. The lining permits the seepage of fluid into the surrounding ground. The improved latrine also has a concrete squatting slab (or a seat) to prevent the soiling of the floor and permit its easy cleaning. The squatting slab may be reinforced with steel, or cast in a domed or conical shape to remove the necessity of using reinforcement.

The single most important feature of VIP latrines is the ventilation pipe. The action of wind blowing past the top of the pipe draws air from the pit through the pipe and causes a downdraught of air through the drop hole. This circulation of air removes odours coming from the faecal matter in the pit. The vent pipe is covered with a gauze screen that prevents flies from entering the pit and traps any newly emergent adult flies. The vent pipe is made large enough to let light into the pit, and if the superstructure is sufficiently dark, the adult flies that enter the pit through the drop-hole of the squatting plate to lay their eggs, and others hatched in the pit, will try to escape up the vent pipe and will be trapped. Controlled studies in Zimbabwe have shown that the provision of a screened vent pipe dramatically reduces the number of flies emerging from the latrine. Design considerations and other details of VIP latrines are given in Kalbermatten and others (1982) and Mara (1984).[13]

While most pit latrines are sufficiently deep to avoid the need to empty them for several years, digging such a deep pit might prove expensive under certain conditions – such as in rocky ground. Here, it is often cheaper to build twin-pit VIP latrines. In this version, one pit is used for at least a year until it is full, when the second pit is put into use. When the second pit is full, the first pit is emptied and used again. The advantage of leaving material in the pit for a year before removal is that by then it is an inoffensive humus, which will be effectively free from disease organisms. The removal of the material can therefore be undertaken with ease. Details of this form of pit latrine are given in van Nostrand and Wilson (1983) and Carrol (1980).[14]

In conclusion, the principal advantages of VIP latrines are its:

- extremely low cost;
- ease of construction and maintenance;
- possible use of all types of anal cleansing materials;
- minimal water requirement for successful operation;
- low level of municipal involvement for operation; *and*
- potential to be upgraded.

The main disadvantages are that they are not suitable for high density settlements (over 300 persons/hectare), and when full, the pits require emptying. They also do not solve the problem of households' waste-water from food preparation and washing (known as sullage): households usually require separate provision for disposing of this. Box 6.3 gives examples of pit latrine programmes in Mozambique, Ghana and Malawi.

Box 6.3: Pit latrine programmes in Mozambique, Ghana and Malawi

MOZAMBIQUE: After several years of research, the Mozambican government developed five types of pit-latrine with modifications to suit ground conditions. The latrines were widely promoted in urban areas through the centralized production and sale of non-reinforced domed pit slabs. These slabs were produced on a commercial basis and sold for US$ 14 per 1.5-metre diameter slab and US$ 10 per 1.2-metre slab. Production costs were approximately half this. Cooperative workshops for producing the slabs were set up, distributed throughout the settlements. Since transport was by two-wheel hand carts, a distance between workshops of two kilometres was considered to be the maximum. Training in slab production, accounting and the use of hand puppets for advertising was provided for the production crew. More than 25,000 slabs have been sold and latrines installed, benefiting some 125,000 people.

GHANA: Under a pilot-scale programme, in-house bucket latrines were converted to in-house twin-pit VIP latrines. Initially, the external parts of the pits were excavated and lined with open-jointed brickwork. The pits were then extended 45 – 60 centimetres inside the house, passing below the foundation wall; timber was used to support the foundation during this excavation. The pit lining was then completed, the reinforced cover slab placed in position and the old bucket latrine access doors bricked up.

MALAWI: The Ministry of Local Government through the various local authorities is promoting improved sanitation through the use of pit latrines. The Ministry has focused on their use in the urban low-cost housing areas since the needs and problems of poor sanitation are greatest in these settlements. The local authorities have created a number of Sanitation Centres within these settlements to promote the improvement of existing latrines and the construction of new ones. The new latrines contain the following improvements on the traditional latrines.

- Hygiene and child security have been improved.
- Fly nuisance has been controlled by use of a tight-fitting cover.
- The useful life of the latrine has been extended to over 20 years by increasing the pit volume to one cubic metre per user.

Box 6.3: (continued)

The key element of the programme is the production and sale of a small prefabricated concrete platform (60 by 60 by 5 centimetres) which includes an elevated foot-rest, a key-hole-shaped drop hole which makes the latrine safe for use by small children, and a tight-fitting lid. The sanitation platform only costs US$ 2, and is light enough (32 kilos) to be readily transported. The Sanitation Centres also sell screened vent-pipes and materials for constructing improved latrines, and train local contractors and other personnel in their construction. The Centres also serve to inform and demonstrate the technology to the public. The Sanitation Centre concept has proved to be a success and over 1,000 traditional latrines have been converted in under six months.

SOURCES: See note 15.

Pour-flush latrines

Pour-flush latrines consist of a squatting pan for excreta deposition with a steeply-sloped base and a syphon, or water-seal trap, attached underneath to provide a water seal of 2–3 centimetres (see Figure 6.2).

The pan is connected to one of two sealed leachpits and is flushed manually with a small quantity of water (usually 2–3 litres) after use. The excreta are carried through a connecting pipe or drain into one of the pits. The water seal ensures that there are no problems with flies or odours and since the pit is offset by up to ten metres, it is not only easier to empty but also requires a less sophisticated toilet superstructure. The use of a water seal also permits the toilets to be located at any level within a house or building. Pour-flush toilets are widely used in Asian countries where anal cleansing with water is traditional.

In Latin America, pedestal toilet seats are used instead of the squat-pan and while these have been essentially of the cistern flush type, they are often flushed manually, especially in low-income settlements. Cistern-flush toilet bowls require large volumes of water to flush, usually 8–20 litres. More recently, a number of purpose-made low-volume pedestal toilet seats have been developed that require only 3–5 litres to flush, either manually or automatically.[16] Such low water requirements are a considerable advantage for households who have to collect and carry their water supplies. The low water requirement of the pour-flush latrine makes it suitable for use in settlements where the inhabitants are presently served either with communal standpipes or with taps provided within the yard of their house and have yet to receive multi-tap, in-house piped water supplies.

Figure 6.2

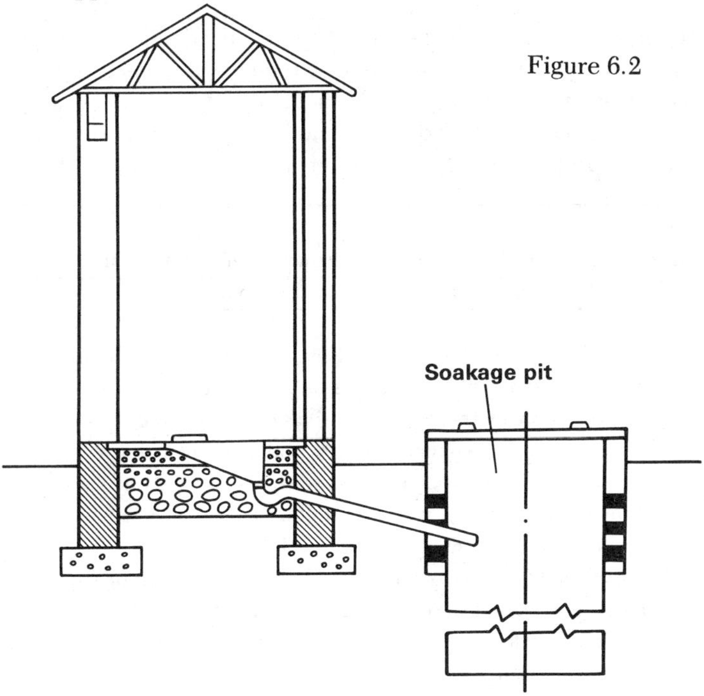

It is usually better for pour-flush latrines to have two leachpits, so these can be used alternately, as in the twin-pit VIP latrines, since this permits the safe removal (manually if necessary) of inoffensive humus after the waste has been stored for over one year. Usually, each pit is designed to last at least three years before it becomes full. A junction chamber is provided to permit the diversion of the waste-waters from one pit to the next when the first becomes full. If emptying is to be done mechanically, one pit can prove adequate. The pits are lined with open brickwork to facilitate the seeping of flush waters into the surrounding soil.

The pour-flush latrine has the following advantages:

- –no odour or insect problems;
- –the possibility of locating the latrine within the house and in multi-storey buildings;
- –little or no involvement of sanitation agencies needed for the proper operation of this system; *and*
- –the potential to be upgraded through connection to small diameter sewers (as will be described in a later section).

They have the disadvantage that they are unsuitable where bulky anal cleansing materials are used. Although only small quantities of water are required to operate them, a reliable water supply is still needed. Design considerations and other details of this form of sanitation are given by Roy and others (1984) and Mara (1986).[17]

Box 6.4: Pour-flush latrine programmes in India, Indonesia, Pakistan, Nepal, Brazil and Colombia

INDIA: The Indian Government has launched a programme to provide low-cost pour-flush latrines on a large scale in urban areas. As a matter of policy the government has decided that urban centres with a population less than 100,000 will have pour-flush latrines only, instead of conventional piped sewerage. As part of its efforts to eliminate the degrading and unsanitary job of scavengers (whose job it is to empty bucket latrines), in 1979 the government undertook a study of the feasibility of widespread use of latrines in urban areas in 21 states and unions. Some 40,000 latrines were built as part of a demonstration effort. The technology was refined and cheaper pans and water-seal units were developed. Many states such as Gujarat, Tamil Nadu, Kerala, Madhya Pradesh and Uttar Pradesh have borrowed from the World Bank Group's International Development Association to finance the low-cost sanitation programmes. Together these projects have channelled US$70 million to the construction of pour-flush latrines.

The institutional models through which each state seeks to extend the use of these latrines vary. In Kerala, for example, the local authorities within each urban centre have overall responsibility and supply the pan and water-seal while the beneficiaries (in whose shelter the latrine is being built) hire local trained masons to construct the latrine. The local authority provides funds direct to

Box 6.4: (continued)

the beneficiaries, who pay for the components and labour and repay the loan in monthly instalments over five years. In Tamil Nadu, the State Water and Drainage Board is responsible for promoting and constructing the latrines. Once a household's application for a pour-flush latrine is approved, the Board's engineering branch takes bids and awards the work of installing them to private contractors. The cost is recovered through property taxes. The state of Gujarat uses a mix of the two institutional approaches but the beneficiaries are expected to put the money up front. Most states provide some form of subsidy which usually amounts to approximately 50 per cent but in exceptional cases of need this can go up to 100 per cent. The cost of each latrine, including the superstructure, is between US$150 and US$200.

In the state of Bihar, the conversion of bucket latrines to pour-flush latrines has been undertaken since 1974, through a partnership between local governments and a non-profit voluntary social organization, Shulabh International. To date some 200,000 bucket latrines have been converted to pour-flush latrines. The NGO has a staff of over 2,500 workers who receive monthly wages which are marginally better than government salaries. It has an annual turnover of work of approximately US$15 million. The main source of income is through nominal overheads (between 10 and 20 per cent) charged for implementing large conversion contracts. Households who want their latrine converted approach the municipality or local authority and, after agreements are signed, the NGO is given the money to construct the latrine. Half the cost is covered by a central government loan and the other half recovered through property taxes. Without the superstructure, the latrine costs a maximum of US$115. The NGO also provides free maintenance up to the time of the first desludging (or emptying) operation. The NGO therefore acts as a turn-key contractor and the overheads have proved adequate to sustain and expand its operations. In another case outside New Delhi, an NGO known as Asha Sadan has set up a revolving fund and lends to households to construct their own latrines to required specifications. Full cost recovery has been achieved from low-income families with a monthly repayment of between 50 and 100 rupees

Box 6.4: (continued)

(US$ 4.5.– 9).

INDONESIA: Many housing schemes in Indonesia have, for many years, been provided with pour-flush latrines. One such settlement is the Klander housing scheme, constructed in 1976 in a suburb of the capital, Jakarta. The average gross density of the settlement is 335 persons per hectare. Initially each house was provided with a pour-flush toilet and a single 0.8 metre diameter leachpit, 2 metres deep, lined with traditional woven bamboo. Household sullage was discharged into stormwater ditches. An evaluation done seven years later found that the people approved of the technology but felt that the pits were too small. Over 70 per cent of households had increased the capacity of the pits from the original volume, using burnt brick lining to prolong their life and reduce the frequency with which they had to be emptied. The cost of the expanded pit was US$100, compared to US$50 for the original (smaller) pits. The householders themselves paid for the subsequent improvements. The cost of this form of sanitation, although not tackling the problem of sullage disposal, was observed to be a quarter of the cost of conventional waterborne sewerage.

The settlement was serviced by municipal desludging tankers. After five years of use, it was observed that only 17 per cent of the enlarged pits required emptying compared to 50 per cent of small pits. Once the small pits were emptied, it proved necessary to repeat the operation annually as they rapidly filled up with liquid due to the clogging of the natural soil surface. This was not the case with the larger pits. The leaching pits are located to the front of the plot in the newer developments to provide easier access for the desludging tankers.

PAKISTAN: The pour-flush latrine is being increasingly used in the Sind and Punjab provinces of Pakistan to upgrade sanitation in squatter settlements. Baldia, for example, is a large squatter settlement on the periphery of Karachi with over 200,000 residents. Water is supplied through standpipes by the Karachi Municipal Council. A majority of the population was served with bucket latrines while a small proportion had traditional pour-flush and single leachpit systems. These pits were constructed of locally

Box 6.4: (continued)

available sandstone and were located in the streets. Traditional pits with their small capacity had to be emptied frequently. This proved expensive since the cost of doing so was between US$20 and US$30. The passage of vehicles over the pit covers also led to frequent failure. In a bid to overcome these shortcomings and to promote the wider use of more hygienic sanitation systems than the bucket latrines, efforts were made by UNICEF to encourage the construction of pour-flush latrines with twin alternating pits within the household plots.

Initially some 10 latrines were offered free of charge to families who agreed to construct them within their plots. This encouraged others to opt for this form of sanitation. As the project team became accepted, and community workers were able to orient and inform families, especially the women in the families, it proved possible to get people to build their own twin leachpit pour-flush latrine solely by providing the basic materials for their construction. The cost of the latrines was further reduced by negotiating acceptable construction rates with local masons.

Soon, as many as ten latrines were being constructed each week. The project role changed to being the purchaser and supplier of building materials, obtained at wholesale rates, and training the community to construct the latrines themselves. The poorest families were identified by the project team together with local community leaders and given priority. The community, viewing the project as a springboard for other development work, gave the project team an office within the settlement and prepared their own sanitation information and publicity materials. The cost of the latrines excluding the superstructure averaged US$75. Since no provision was made for the disposal of waste water (sullage), it also proved necessary for the Municipal Corporation to construct stormwater drains so that the unsurfaced roads were not made impassable by standing water.

NEPAL: At the beginning of 1981, only 19 per cent of urban and hardly any of the rural population had access to any form of sanitation. In a bid to promote the use of hygienic toilets, the

Box 6.4: (continued)

government launched a programme to construct pour-flush latrines in eight towns. A subsidy in the form of a pour-flush pan, waterseal, cement and steel was provided to beneficiaries selected by locally elected leaders. Masons were trained to construct the latrines and government technicians checked the quality of construction and ensured these conformed to standard designs. A total of some 2,000 latrines were constructed by 1986. The response to the programme has been positive in all towns and applications for the toilets reached a point where the administrators refused to continue maintaining a waiting list.

BRAZIL AND COLOMBIA: Leachpits are widely used in various parts of Latin America in both urban and rural areas. The principal difference from their form in Asia is that the pits are used in conjunction with standard cistern-flush toilets and only a single large capacity pit is used instead of two. Most coastal cities of Brazil north of Rio de Janeiro use this form of sanitation in areas with no sewers. For the past two decades, all new housing schemes in the cities of Natal and Fortaleza have been provided with this form of sanitation. Both toilet wastewaters and sullage are discharged into the pits and the system has operated for many years without any problems due to the very favourable soil conditions in these cities.

In Colombia, leachpits have been used with a low volume (three litre) manual flush pedestal toilet. More recently, similar improved pedestal toilet bowls have been developed in Brazil and are produced by two commercial manufacturers. Both can be upgraded, when in-house plumbing becomes available, through connection to a low-volume discharge, overhead cistern. Since the digestion of wastes proceeds more rapidly and completely under wet conditions, the pits only need desludging every 3–5 years. Most municipalities in Latin American cities offer a desludging service with tankers for both leachpits and septic tanks. The capital cost of these cistern-flush and leachpit systems, excluding the superstructure, averages between US$150 and US$250. They provide for the disposal of sullage as well as excreta.

Source: See note 18.

Septic tanks

The septic tank is a watertight settling tank to which wastes are carried by water flushing down a short length of pipe. Solids settle on the bottom of the tank where they are digested anaerobically while the effluent overflows to a soakaway, drainfield or sewer system. Septic tank and soakaway systems are very common in Third World cities in low-density, middle and high-income areas not served by sewers. Since population densities in these areas are typically less than 100 persons per hectare, there is sufficient space within each house plot to dispose of the effluents. It has been suggested that a tank with three compartments could be used in somewhat higher density areas (with some 200 persons per hectare).[19] Here, the first two compartments would be used in series for the processing of wastes from the toilet which then overflows to a third chamber which also receives sullage.

The use of septic tanks in the Third World has been restricted by their high cost. A cheaper alternative is the use of communal septic tanks serving two or more houses. There is ample scope for locating and designing communal tanks with sub-surface irrigation within designated green areas of new low-income housing schemes. Alternatively, a whole settlement could be planned with a series of communal septic tanks connected to a network of small-bore sewers (see below). The per capita investment cost of septic tanks decreases with the increase in the number of persons served, as illustrated by the case of Karachi (see Figure 6.3).

Similar cost relationships were also observed in Northeast Brazil.[20] Any reduction in unit tank cost may, however, be offset by the increase in the length of pipework connecting the houses to the common tank.

Septic tanks and soakaways were developed for use in isolated and remote buildings in Europe and North America and so their design has been based on standards inherited from these countries, essentially for conditions of temperate climate and individual household usage. Under such conditions, these tanks require considerable per capita capacity and function essentially as settling tanks. But in the tropics, they function more as biological reactors and should be designed as such. The design of communal septic tanks also differs considerably from that of individual household septic tanks. A comprehensive design method that allows for tropical conditions and communal usage is given in Mara and Sinnatamby (1986).[21]

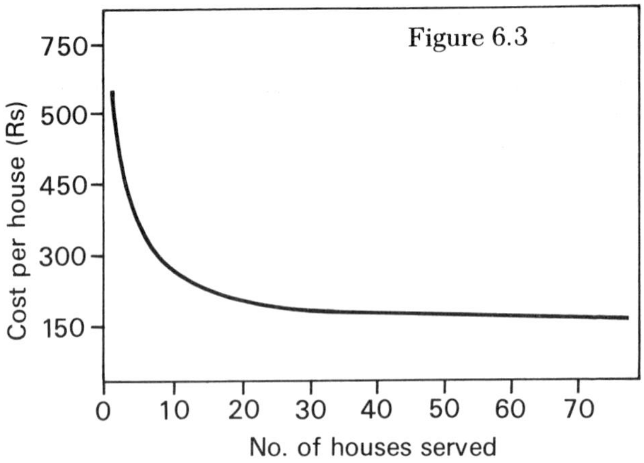

Small-bore sewers

Sanitation systems using on-site leachpits or soakaways can all be upgraded by connecting them to a small-bore sewer system so that their partially treated effluents are removed for treatment and disposal off-site. Such upgrading may be warranted when the level of water consumption increases, as a result of an increased or improved water supply. More often, it is the result of an improved level of service such as the provision of water taps to each house's yard, to replace communal standpipes. New sanitation systems may also be designed using small bore sewers. In such cases, it is common to construct a septic tank for each premise, from which the effluent is discharged into a sewer.

Since the effluent conveyed in small-bore sewers has already passed through one of these interceptor tanks, it is free of gross solids, grit and grease. Consequently, lower water flow velocities are required to prevent solid deposition within them. As a result, smaller diameter pipes (50 millimetres and upward) may be laid at flatter gradients or slopes than required for conventional sewers. This means savings in both pipe costs and the cost of excavation. The interceptor tanks settle and degrade the solids and in so doing, relieve the off-site treatment plant of between 40 and 60 per cent of its treatment requirements. This allows further cost savings because of the construction of a smaller treatment plant. Some of these savings will be offset by the need for regular removal of the accumulated sludge from the interceptor tanks. Detailed information regarding the design and operation of small diameter sewer systems is given in Otis and Mara (1985).[22]

Although the evidence appears to be somewhat conflicting, the construction of a new small-bore sewer system including both the network of pipes and the interceptor tanks is often only marginally cheaper than installing conventional sewerage. An exception to this is the Orangi Pilot Project, Karachi (see Box 6.5). The economic merits of the system arise chiefly when it is considered as a means of upgrading existing on-site systems, or intended for use in areas with unfavourable ground conditions such as high ground water tables or rocky ground.

Box 6.5: Small-bore sewers in Orangi, Karachi.

Orangi is a large unauthorized settlement on the outskirts of Karachi, Pakistan. Apart from the provision of water (supplied through standpipes) there are few other urban services in this settlement of over a million people. Over the last decade a non-governmental organization known as the Orangi Pilot Project (OPP) has been organizing and assisting the local communities to help themselves. Part of this has been the construction of small-bore sewers, which was organized and implemented with no support from the municipal authorities. This has proved OPP staff's original suggestion that a cheap but effective sanitation system could be installed and paid for, if local residents were fully involved.

To initiate the process, social motivators hold meetings with those living in 10–15 adjacent houses each side of a lane to explain the sanitation programme and the technology proposed. A single lane is considered the basic social unit and each lane is asked to elect its own lane managers. OPP technical staff then conduct land surveys and prepare plans and cost estimates and present these to the lane managers. The lane managers then collect the money from the residents, call meetings to sort out social problems, receive various tools from OPP to undertake the work and make arrangements to hire OPP-recommended masons and plumbers to carry out the work. OPP helps supervise construction.

Each house is provided with a single chamber septic tank which receives all domestic wastewater before it is discharged to the sewer.

Box 6.5: (continued)

Although strictly speaking this receiving sewer is not a small-bore sewer but a common 100-milimetre diameter concrete pipe, it nonetheless represents the cheapest locally available small-diameter pipe. The size of the septic tank is often not determined by any technical criteria but by what the user can afford. The effluents are discharged into the nearest watercourse.

During the last ten years the project has managed to service 458 of a total of 3,050 lanes in the project area. An additional 742 have built their own sewers as a ripple effect of the project. The average cost of the small bore sewer system is no more than $66 per house. This is estimated to be a quarter of what it would have cost the city authorities to provide the same service. OPP capital and administrative inputs to achieve this coverage have been no more than one-tenth of the capital inputs of the community. OPP has also developed a health programme working through women's groups, also at the level of the lane, with advice provided on hygiene, nutrition, disease prevention, family planning and kitchen gardens, an income generating programme which provides credit and advice to small businesses and a project to help upgrade the schools in Orangi.

SOURCE: Arif Hasan, "Community groups and non-government organizations in the urban field in Pakistan", *Environment and Urbanization*, vol. 2, no. 1, April 1990, pp. 74–86 and Trudy Harpham, Tim Lusty and Patrick Vaughan (eds), *In the Shadow of the City* (Oxford University Press, 1988).

Shallow sewers

Except for the small-bore sewers, all the sanitation technologies so far discussed are primarily applicable in low- to medium-density settlements. In high-density settlements, such as many consolidated squatter settlements or densely developed illegal (or legal) sub-divisions, these on-site systems are sometimes appropriate, but they often require too much space. There is also the problem of disposing of sullage. Small-bore sewerage is a possibility, although it is not always low in cost; it is also often difficult to get the desludging equipment close enough to empty the interceptor tanks. Meanwhile, conventional sewerage is too expensive.

The shallow sewer system has emerged as a result of adapting the design standards of conventional sewerage (which are very conservative – see Box 6.6) to suit the physical conditions of urban low-income settlements and taking advantage of recent advances in sewer design and operation. Shallow sewers are designed to accept all household wastewaters – excreta, toilet flush water and sullage – in their fresh state, for off-site treatment and disposal. Sullage is usually passed through a grit and grease trap before it is discharged into the sewers. The sewer network consists of small-diameter (100 – millimetres upwards) pipes laid to flat gradients (1 in 167) away from paths or roads with heavy imposed loads (such as road vehicles). They are usually laid in backyards and narrow back alleys.

Box 6.6: Conventional sewer design too conservative

Sewers are designed to be laid at a gradient which ensures that peak flows carry away any solids deposited during periods of low flow. These self-cleansing velocities do occur, at least once a day, in large downstream sewers, but not in the small diameter individual house connections and street laterals where the flow is intermittent. Solids are shifted along these pipes by the flushing action of sequential waves of waste-water: as the solids deposit on the pipe invert, the subsequent waste-water flow backs up until the pressure is sufficient to move the solids along the pipe.

Unable to model this process, engineers resorted to rules of thumb which have become more conservative over the years. This has added unnecessarily to sewerage costs. For example:

- Minimum diameters for street laterals and house connections are sometimes as large as 200 mm, yet there is little justification for a minimum diameter of more than 100 mm – in fact smaller diameter pipes have better solids transport properties.
- A minimum gradient of 1 in 70 is often set for a minimum of 20 houses connected to a 100 mm street lateral, where this diameter pipe is permitted. Yet in Brazil, a gradient of 1 in 167 has been successfully used for many years, for up to 60 houses connected to a 100 mm diameter pipe.
- The minimum velocity of flow considered essential for self-flushing is often specified to be as high as one metre per second. In practice, sewers do not function on the basis of self-cleansing velocities, and

Box 6.6: (continued)

any velocity greater than 0.3 metres per second is sufficient to transport inert materials.

- A maximum velocity of flow between four and six metres per second is often specified to avoid sewer pipe wear. Studies have shown, however, that such sewer wear through pipe erosion is negligible.

Field investigations in the UK have demonstrated that sewer blockages are principally caused by poor workmanship, infrequent usage and extraneous matter gaining access to the pipe. No correlation was found between blockages and gradients. In fact more blockages were found in pipes set at the recommended gradients (1 in 30–70) rather than on flatter ones, and sewers laid as flat as 1 in 1,200 were observed to function well for many decades.

Shallow sewer design seeks to maximize the frequency of discharges to increase the efficiency with which solids are transported in small diameter pipes. It avoids the use of long pipelines serving few houses. Conventional UK practice dictates that each house be separately connected to the street lateral, and this sometimes necessitates very long house connections. More recently, up to four houses have been allowed to use a common connection. If 20 houses were permitted to use a common connection, cost savings of up to a third could be achieved. Higher numbers, as promoted by the shallow sewer concept, would achieve even greater economies.

Source: Sinnatamby, G., *et al.*, "Shallow systems offer hope to slums", *World Water*, January–February 1986.

Typical layouts for shallow sewers are shown in Figure 6.4. These allow shorter overall pipe lengths because not every street requires a sewer but only those which contain emerging block sewers. The sewers are laid in shallow trenches (typically 0.3-metre pipe cover to soffit) with small inspection chambers to facilitate house connections and provide access for maintenance. The shallow depths of the sewers emerging from the blocks are maintained, as far as possible, by locating them along footpaths immediately adjacent to property boundaries. Where street crossings are inevitable, suitably designed concrete collars around the pipe can serve as

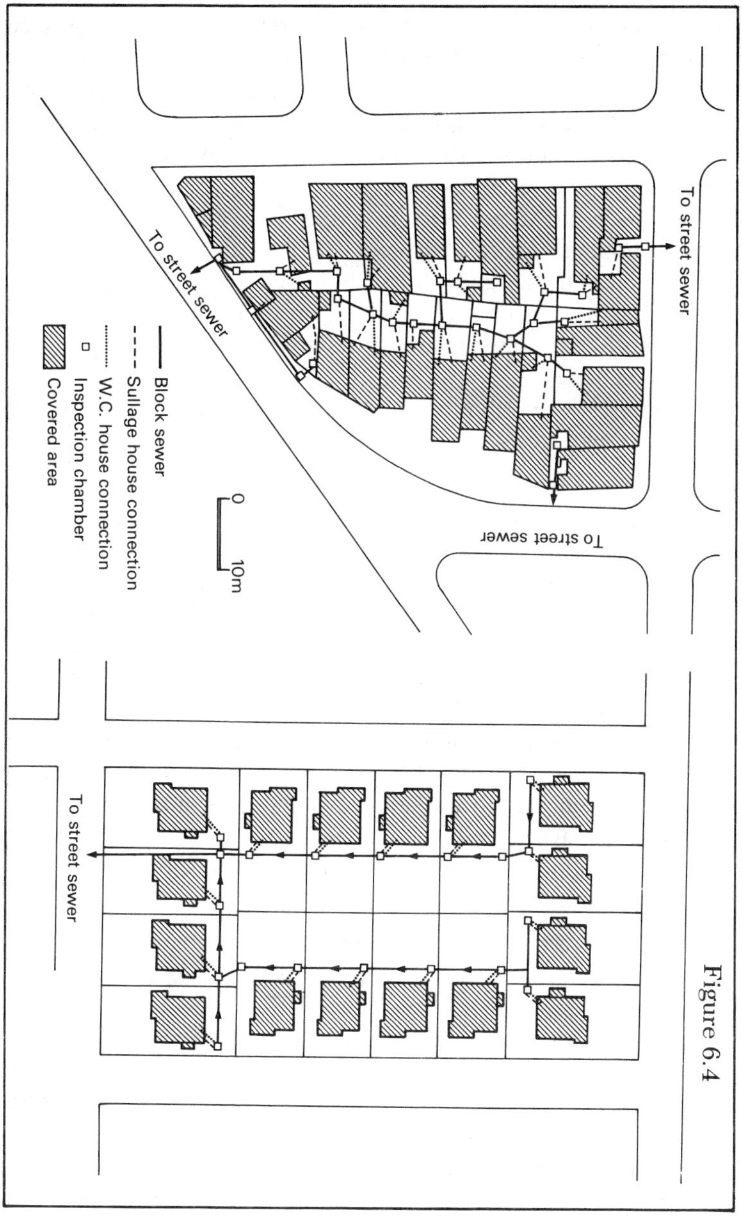
To street sewer
To street sewer
To street sewer
To street sewer
0
10m
Block sewer
Sullage house connection
W.C. house connection
Inspection chamber
Covered area

Figure 6.4

protection. Shallow sewers do not rely on large quantities of flushing water for their trouble-free operation: instead, they rely on the high frequency with which waste-waters pass through them. Densely-populated areas offer ample scope for such operation. Consequently, shallow sewers have been introduced in areas where the per capita water consumption does not exceed 27 litres and where supply is through standpipes.

The success of shallow sewerage depends on attaining a high rate of connection; essentially all houses in a block should be connected. This is ensured by designing the system such that it is affordable and by undertaking consultative planning involving the community in the whole process, from planning through construction, to operation and maintenance.

Collecting waste-waters in the manner described above has the following advantages:

- reduced water requirement – it may be used with low-volume flushing pans and seats in areas supplied with only a standpipe level of service;
- reduced overall length of pipework – in an efficient layout, a reduction of the order of 50 per cent is possible over conventional layouts;
- reduced excavation cost through reduced length and depth of pipework;
- reduced material cost through the use of small pipe diameters and simple inspection chambers;
- reduced maintenance through frequent sewer flushing ensured by the pipe layout; *and*
- high connection rates, since block and street sewers are constructed concurrently.

Box 6.7: Shallow sewer systems in Brazil, Pakistan and Sri Lanka

BRAZIL: Shallow sewerage was first used in Brazil in the city of Natal by the sanitation research unit of the State Water and Sewerage Company (CAERN). This unit was evaluating sanitation alternatives for two low-income squatter settlements, Rocas and Santos Reis, which had a total population of 15,000, two-thirds of which were living below the poverty line. The average population

Box 6.7: (continued)

density was 350 persons per hectare, and almost all households had at least a water tap in their yard and a pour-flush ceramic toilet bowl. The community wanted sewers, a common aspiration among urban dwellers, but conventional sewerage was far too expensive and beyond their means. By modifying the conventional sewer design and discussing it with the community, the CAERN unit came up with the idea of shallow sewerage as being the only way in which the aspirations of the community could be made compatible with what they could afford. The community collaborated fully with CAERN and a pilot scheme was built to demonstrate and test the technology. House-to-house visits and surveys were made and community meetings held to obtain community support for the system.

Each household agreed to the construction of common house connections in their backyard, and to take responsibility for maintaining the length of sewer laid on their property; a simple inspection box was built at each connection for this purpose. CAERN was responsible only for the maintenance of the very reduced length of street sewers. An unprecedented connection rate of 97 per cent was achieved in the year of construction. The system has operated satisfactorily for over eight years. Total capital costs in both settlements were $325 per household, and full cost recovery is being achieved by a surcharge on the water bill of only 40 per cent (the surcharge for conventional sewerage is 100 per cent on a much higher water bill and this still falls short of full cost recovery – most households in Rocas and Santos Reis are unmetered and pay only the minimum tariff). Shallow sewerage has been installed in dozens of site and service schemes at much reduced capital costs, (between $120 and $180 per household) and in other upgrading projects in the state, and other parts of Brazil.

PAKISTAN: Shallow sewers were introduced to Pakistan in 1984. Chisty Nagar, a low-income Bihari community on the outskirts of Karachi, was selected for a demonstration project. The population density was 193 persons per hectare and most households obtained an intermittent supply of water from standpipes. Water consumption was low; only 27 litres per person per day. Shallow sewers

Box 6.7: (continued)

designed as in Brazil, received the waste-water from manually-flushed squat pans and also all household sullage; a grit and grease trap was used to act as a focus for sullage discharge and as a preventive maintenance device. Despite the low flows, the system has functioned well for nearly five years, showing that despite the relaxation in standards, properly designed and constructed sewers do not need vast quantities of water for trouble-free operation. The investment cost per household was incredibly low – a mere $45, which covered the squat pan, grit and grease trap, house connection, street lateral, collector main and primary treatment.

SRI LANKA: Shallow sewers have been built in Colombo in two urban settlements as part of the government's Million Houses Programme. Population densities in these settlements exceed 500 persons per hectare and shallow sewers proved to be the most economic and technically appropriate alternative. Water was supplied to both communities through communal standpipes. The total capital cost of the shallow sewer system including a wet sanitation core for each house (a squat pan, grit and grease trap, ground level water tank, house connection and street lateral) was no more than $60. In comparison to earlier upgraded slums which were provided with more costly communal bathing facilities or which used on-site pour-flush toilets built through individual household initiatives, a distinct preference was expressed by the communities for the shallow sewer system that removes both sullage and toilet waste-waters.

Source: Sinnatamby, G. *et. al.*, "Shallow systems offer hope to slums", *World Water*, January–February 1986; Sinnatamby, G., "Shallow sewer system – a low-cost sanitation option", *Developing World Water*, (Hong Kong: Grosvenor Press International, 1987); and Sinnatamby, G. S., *Summary Report on Mission to Sri Lanka)*, report to UNCHS/NHDA, *(Colombo, 1986).*

The shallow sewer system is both technically and economically best applied under the following conditions:

- *High population density*: shallow sewer systems, like all pipe networks, demonstrate marked reductions in unit household costs as the density of settlement increases, and become more economical than on-site sanitation systems at a given density. In Natal, for example, this transition density occurred at 160 persons per hectare (see Figure 6.5);

- *Adverse ground conditions*: shallow sewers are often feasible even under adverse ground conditions such as shallow rock, high groundwater table and low soil permeability; *and*
- *High water consumption*: since shallow sewer systems dispose of both toilet waste-waters and sullage, they may be readily applied in areas where water usage is extensive.

Detailed information regarding the design, operation and maintenance of shallow sewer systems, including relevant case studies are given in UNCHS (1986).[23]

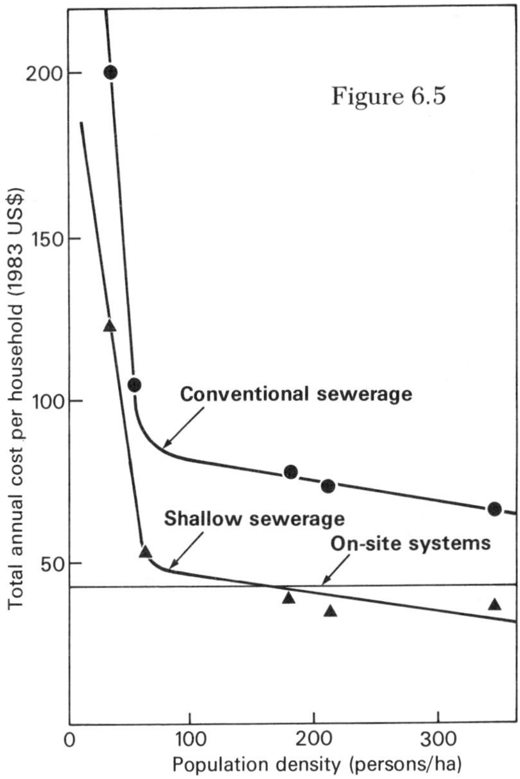

Figure 6.5

Factors affecting the choice of sanitation system

The main factors which affect the choice of sanitation system are:

water usage and sullage disposal; the density of the settlement; ground conditions; social factors; and system costs.

In terms of water usage and the disposal of sullage, all the sanitation technologies discussed above do require modest quantities of water for trouble-free operation and are usually compatible with water systems where supply is through communal standpipes. But not all systems can cope with large water usage without complementary investments in some form of sullage-disposal facility. Standpipes are sometimes recommended in urban low-income settlements so that water usage may be made compatible with on-site sanitation systems which make no allowance for the disposal of sullage. This invariably falls short of community aspirations. Communal standpipes are therefore rarely maintained and hold little prospect for recovering capital and operating costs, except for a few cases of water vending through kiosks. Most residents in illegal or informal settlements seek to obtain the quantities of water they require either by making illegal connections to street mains (as they did in San Martin, described in Chapter 2) or by building large storage tanks on their premises which they fill by connecting them to the standpipe through a hosepipe.

There is also ample evidence that water piped into each house or at least to a tap in each building's yard provides substantial health benefits. As described in Chapter 5, this will usually lead to water consumption of 60 litres per person per day or more.

Box 6.8: Baldia squatter settlement revisited

Baldia, a squatter settlement on the periphery of Karachi has a very successful low-cost sanitation programme based on the provision of pour-flush twin pit toilets (see Box 6.4), but a closer evaluation of this settlement reveals serious problems in sullage disposal. Although water to the settlement is provided only through standpipes, the fact that no provision was made for sullage disposal, meant that sullage was discharged to the streets. As the streets were not surfaced, many became inaccessible to pedestrians and soon the residents were obliged to seek the Karachi Municipal Council's (KMC) assistance in installing open drains. The settlement was therefore provided with open drains although the topography in the area slopes sufficiently to ensure natural drainage, and rainfall

Box 6.8: (continued)

in this semi-arid region is concentrated in a period of two weeks in any single year.

With the advent of the open drains, most people now found a convenient place to discharge not only their sullage, but in many cases also their toilet waste-waters. Those who had any form of vault or septic tank discharged the contents of these into the drains to eliminate the need to have them emptied which could cost US$20 to US$30 a time. Even those who had constructed pour-flush latrines under the sanitation programme and were not conversant with their proper mode of operation soon overflowed the pits into the nearest open drain. The drains also became receptacles of household refuse as there was no regular refuse collection service. Consequently the drains, which were not designed to facilitate dry weather flow, soon became the focus of complaints from residents. These complaints were founded not only on the odour from the drains and public health nuisance they presented but also on the physical danger to children, some of whom had fallen into them. The fact that most drains were also located at the front of the houses only served to reinforce the complaints. In the final analysis, adding the cost of the complementary investments in open drains to the original cost of providing sanitation to the settlement, the twin pit pour flush latrines proved to be much more expensive than they seemed. There were also the additional public health risks posed by the drains.

Settlement density is also an important factor in the choice of a sanitation system. On-site systems such a VIP latrines require adequate space within each house plot both for their construction and to allow for the infiltration of all waste-waters discharged into them. Such space becomes difficult to find as the density of settlements increases. The cost per house plot of providing on-site sanitation facilities such as VIP latrines remains constant irrespective of the settlement's population density. By contrast, all sewer networks demonstrate reductions in the cost per plot serviced as the density of settlement increases (see Figure 6.5), and become cheaper than on-site sanitation facilities at a given population density.

Adverse ground conditions can increase the costs of certain sanitation options and make others technically unfeasible. For instance, under adverse conditions such as shallow rock, high groundwater table or low soil permeability, sanitation systems that rely on the ability of soil to absorb waste-waters and require some form of excavation can prove technically unfeasible or too expensive. Under such conditions there is always scope for ingenuity in design such as raising latrines above ground level and laying pipes at shallow depths.

Social factors should also influence sanitation system choices. Some sanitation systems may prove unfeasible if they are incompatible with social customs. For example, low-volume pour flush toilets might become blocked if used in communities that use bulky anal-cleansing materials. Other social factors that merit consideration in planning sanitation systems are given in Kalbermatten and others (1982) and Cairncross and Feachem (1983).[24]

A variety of factors affect the cost of any given sanitation system and many are specific to each site. For each project site, the capital cost of all technically and socially feasible alternatives should be determined to guide system choice. The final choice of the most appropriate design and technology must lie with local residents and their community organizations, taking due account of their ability and willingness to pay. Table 6.4 gives the typical range of capital costs for various sanitation alternatives, excluding the cost of latrine superstructures.

Table 6.4: Typical range of capital costs per household of alternative sanitation systems (1990 prices)

Type of system	*US$*
Twin pit pour-flush latrines	75 – 150
Ventilated improved pit latrine	68 – 175
Shallow sewerage	100 – 325
Small-bore sewerage	150 – 500
Conventional septic tanks	200 – 600
Conventional sewerage	600 – 1,200

Capital costs alone cannot provide a meaningful basis for determining the cost of a system since some systems are more expensive than others to operate and maintain. What must be determined are the total discounted capital, operation and maintenance costs for each household. Then the charge that must be levied for the service can be determined and also it can be established which households can afford to pay this amount. Where the monthly cost of providing sanitation exceeds five per cent of the family income, it might be deemed unaffordable. Most low-cost sanitation alternatives come within this limit even for the poorest of communities, especially urban communities.

Nevertheless, most low-cost sanitation programmes are still heavily subsidized – often in excess of 50 per cent. Consequently the provision of low-cost sanitation facilities is fast becoming associated with grants, a trend that requires prompt modification. There would appear to be little justification for continuing this practice in future, considering that the cost of the systems decribed in this chapter represent a sixth to an eighth of the costs of conventional sewerage. One of the strongest arguments in favour of the promotion of alternative technologies, at the start of the 1980s, was the fact that the reduced construction costs would eliminate the need for subsidy and enable the establishment of self-sustaining programmes for wide scale replication. To greatly increase the number of urban inhabitants adequately served with sanitation systems, there is a need to find ways in which low-cost technologies can be marketed without subsidy and in response to true demand. A prerequisite to achieving this is the promotion of sanitation systems that people want and are prepared to pay for, and which are affordable – that is, which satisfy effective demand.

Chapter Seven

Surface Water Drainage in Urban Areas

Sandy Cairncross and E. A. R. Ouano

The problem

Many low-income communities in urban areas of the Third World consider stormwater drainage to be their most urgent need as far as urban infrastructure is concerned. This is partly because their houses are often built on unsuitable land. As noted in Chapter 2, they often have no alternatives. In areas sufficiently close to the city centre or other concentrations of job opportunities for the journey to work to be affordable, both housing prices and the price of land on which housing can be built tend to be beyond their means. The only land which they can afford, or on which the owners will allow them to stay as squatters, is land which is unsuitable for other purposes. This is often on steep hillsides subject to erosion and landslides, or low-lying, marshy land often subject to flooding.

Most of the Third World's major cities are seaports, located on coasts. Many are on the estuaries of rivers which served as commercial arteries for the transport of goods to and from the hinterland. The flat estuarine terrain and soft, often impermeable alluvial soils make drainage difficult, and the coastal regions of the world are where the highest average rainfall is found.

Even in the arid areas where average rainfall is low, tropical rainfall when it comes is more intense than in temperate climates, and the lack of vegetation and of adequate drainage means that torrents of water can arise in minutes, causing damage to homes and property which may take years to repair. Not only is rainwater a problem. Leaking water-mains, waste-water from washing and bathing, and the sewage from overflowing septic tanks and blocked sewers constitute a health hazard and can damage buildings and cause flooding if an adequate drainage system does not exist.

The lack of drainage is especially serious where the ground is steeply sloping or very flat. In settlements built on very steep sites, as in parts of Rio de Janeiro, Luanda or Hong Kong, stormwater flows fast and violently, damaging buildings, eroding the land and sometimes causing landslides. Soil eroded from a hillside is usually deposited at the foot of the slope; soil eroded in a single rainstorm has been known to bury houses completely in this way. In other cases the land is flat; in cities such as Jakarta, Manila, Bangkok, Calcutta, Colombo, Dar es Salaam, Lagos, Recife and Guayaquil, many neighbourhoods are flooded at least once or twice a year, and people have to learn to cope with water inside their dwelling. Sometimes people build homes on stilts and connect their houses by elevated pathways; in Guayaquil, for instance, hundreds of thousands of people live on homes built on stilts over the tidal flood plain.[1] However, their construction is rickety, and it is easy to lose one's balance and fall into the muddy, polluted water underneath. In the houses on stilts in Guayaquil, many children have died by drowning or suffocation in mud, as a result of falling from the walkways which connect the housing.

Health consequences

Deaths due to drowning in floods or burial beneath landslides or collapsing homes are perhaps the most dramatic signs of the suffering which drainage can help to alleviate. Less noticeable to an outsider, but of greater impact on the residents' lives, is the steady toll of disease, disability and death caused by standing water in a poor community.

First in public health importance are the many faeco-oral infections transmitted by consumption of contaminated food and drink. The micro-organisms which cause them are found in the excreta of infected people or animals, and surface water becomes contaminated with them from sources such as blocked sewers and overflowing septic tanks, and often from defecation in the open by livestock and by people who have no toilet. This contaminated surface water can then infect people in many ways. It can contaminate their hands, their utensils, or their drinking water supply (see Figure 7.1).

Children are particularly exposed to infection when playing or bathing in the water.

The faeco-oral diseases include well-known water-related diseases with a high mortality rate such as cholera and typhoid fever, but

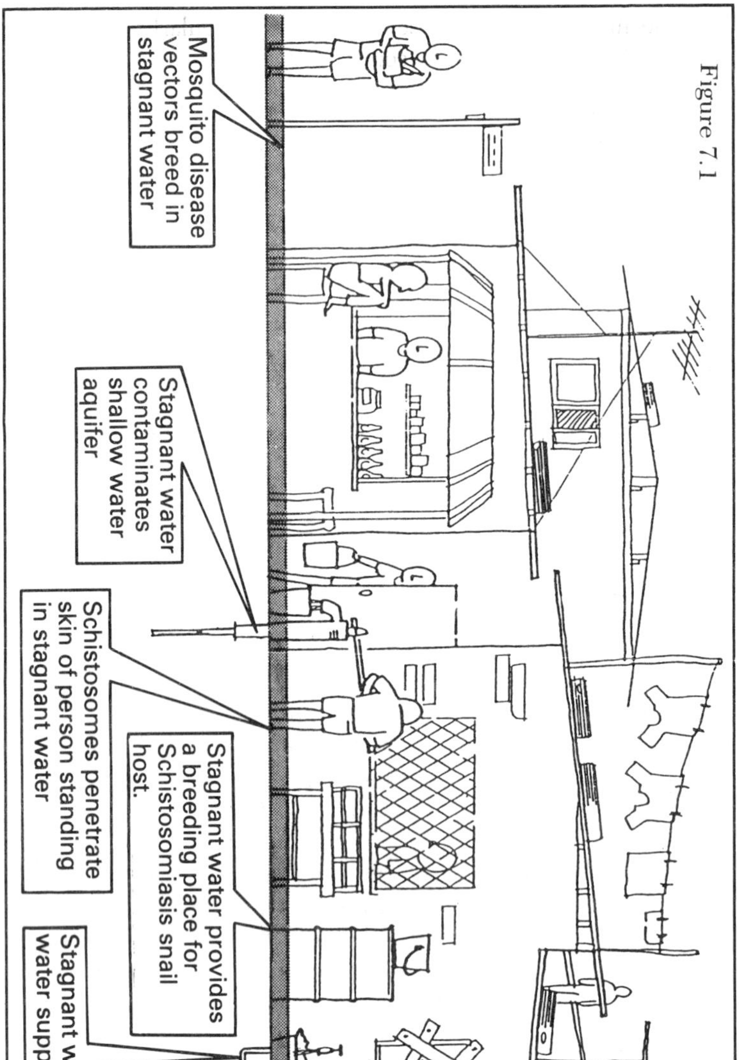
Mosquito disease vectors breed in stagnant water
Stagnant water contaminates shallow water aquifer
Schistosomes penetrate skin of person standing in stagnant water
Stagnant water provides a breeding place for Schistosomiasis snail host.
Stagnant water contaminates water supply
People urinate and defecate into water due to difficulty building latrines

Figure 7.1

also the many diarrhoeal diseases which particularly affect young children in the Third World, contributing to malnutrition and often killing more children than any other cause. Important measures to control them are improved water supply and sanitation, but these are almost impossible to install in areas subject to frequent flooding.

In those countries where schistosomiasis (bilharzia) is endemic, poorly-drained urban areas present ample opportunities for transmission of the disease (see Figure 7.1). Contamination of standing water with the faeces of infected persons (or, for one species of the disease, their urine) enables the schistosomes, the microscopic parasites which cause this infection, to reach the small aquatic snails in whose bodies they multiply. From every infected snail, thousands of parasites emerge each day and swim in the water. Local residents become infected when they enter the water and the parasites penetrate their skin.

Schistosomiasis may sometimes be thought of as a rural disease, but it is often no less prevalent in urban areas where drainage is lacking. Some of the species of the snail-host thrive and breed rapidly in the heavily-polluted stagnant water which often accumulates there. Moreover, a single infected person in an urban area can cause sufficient contamination to infect very large numbers of the people living in his crowded neighbourhood, because even a small number of snails, once infected, can produce many thousands of schistosomes over a year or so.

Another important group of diseases related to poor drainage is transmitted by mosquitoes. Different diseases are transmitted by different species of mosquito, and each chooses different bodies of water in which to breed. Some prefer water which is heavily polluted, others prefer it clean; some breed in flooded areas, some in the drains themselves if they are blocked by rubbish or vegetation or are laid to an uneven level so that there is standing water in them.

Malaria is the best known of the mosquito-borne infections, and is transmitted by the *Anopheles* species, many of which bite animals as well as humans. Transmission can be particularly intense in urban areas where there are relatively few animals to divert the vector species of mosquitoes from human-blood meals. Anopheline mosquitoes do not usually breed in heavily-polluted water, but can multiply in swamps, pools, puddles, and also in streams and stormwater canals in which there is standing water.

Anopheline mosquitoes breeding in poorly-drained low-income areas can transmit malaria to adjacent wealthy parts of town. A particular danger of malaria transmission in a city is the large amount of population movement to and from it, which increases the risk of the importation of new and possibly drug-resistant strains of the disease.

Another family of mosquitoes, the *Aedes* species, can transmit several viruses, such as dengue and yellow fever, in urban epidemics. In recent years, a more virulent form of dengue has been observed, known as dengue haemorrhagic fever (DHF). Both DHF and yellow fever are often fatal. *Aedes* mosquitoes are well known to breed in clear water, for instance in domestic storage vessels; but they have also been found to multiply in swampy and flooded areas, and in open drains and stormwater canals.

Finally, there is the particularly urban problem of Bancroftian filariasis, which causes the irreversible swelling of the legs known as elephantiasis, as well as other disabling symptoms. Although transmitted in rural areas by *Anopheles* species, which appear to be the original vectors of the disease, it seems to have adapted to transmission in urban areas by the *Culex pipiens* species group, which generally multiply in heavily-polluted bodies of water. Transmission of the disease is a relatively inefficient process, so that many years of exposure to intense night-time mosquito biting are needed for the average case to develop. Nevertheless, more than 80 million people in the Third World are infected. In many countries, such as India, it is especially prevalent in urban areas. Filariasis transmission by *Culex pipiens* mosquitoes is now common in Asia, is occurring in cities on the east coast of Africa and South America, and may soon emerge in the large poorly-drained urban areas of West Africa where both the disease and the vector mosquito already exist.

Drainage construction is an effective mosquito control measure. It requires a one-time capital investment, followed by recurrent costs for maintenance, which may be minimal in cash terms, if a good level of community participation can be obtained. In many cases, the initial investment costs less than one year's supply of insecticide. The difference will become more prominent in time, with the continued spread of insecticide resistance, and the consequent need for more expensive compounds. In fact, drainage construction can help to slow down the induction of insecticide resistance by reducing the amount of pesticide used. The use of insecticides for public health purposes usually carries little environmental risk, but drainage construction is, by definition, an environmental improvement. Contrary to chemical-control programmes, environmental modifications such as drainage construction are much less affected during periods of political, social or economic instability.

Urban planning implications

The urban poor may often build on land with drainage problems, but good urban physical planning can help to avoid making those problems worse. One of the simplest planning measures is to set out regular plots before house building starts in an area, leaving space for well-aligned roads. Adequate road width and alignment will make it much easier to build drains when they are needed later. Site-and-service schemes are expensive and take a long time to plan and implement, but such a "site only" scheme should be within the means of any municipality. Once the overall layout of a neighbourhood has been planned, residents (or future residents) can be shown how to set out individual rectangular plots with nothing more sophisticated than a tape measure, or even a piece of string with knots at regular intervals. A 3-4-5 triangle is used to mark the first right angle. Some degree of discipline over house building is necessary, to ensure that plot boundaries are observed, to prevent houses from obstructing existing drainage paths, or from occupying land needed for future drainage works. The residents themselves are in the best position to enforce this.

The development of residential areas can increase drainage problems in other ways. As vegetation is removed, the capacity of the ground to retain water and resist erosion is reduced. The increasing area covered with roofs and road surfaces diminishes the area of ground into which water can infiltrate, leaving a greater volume of water to be removed by drainage. Low-lying areas subject to flooding play a role in storing the water from sudden rainstorms until it can drain away gradually; when these are filled in for housing, this may cause flooding in other areas.

Roads must be built above the flood level, and the embankments this requires can obstruct natural lines of drainage, or can channel water alongside them causing erosion. In some cases, as in parts of Bangkok, roads have been built by filling in existing channels, causing serious flooding. Where the natural drainage channels are not filled in or obstructed by buildings, they often become blocked by domestic refuse.

On the other hand, drainage improvements in one area are closely interrelated with drainage problems elsewhere, and are best planned in the context of the city as a whole, or at least of a whole catchment area. Better drainage in one neighbourhood means that surface water flows away faster, imposing a greater burden on the capacity of the system downstream. At the same time, drainage improvements at a local level may be of little use if water still backs up because this downstream capacity is insufficient. This has been a serious problem in Jakarta, where improved local drains were often submerged by water held back by constrictions in the city's major canals.

Of course, it is possible for a community to make local improvements, even without the support of the city planning authorities, but at least some consideration should be given to the body of water into which a new drainage system will discharge. Whether this is a main sewer, river, lake or sea, the maximum level to which it floods will normally set the minimum level for the drainage system. The discharge of drainage water also affects the quality of the "receiving water" into which it flows, especially when sewage or septic tank effluent is released into the drains. In Bangalore, for example, the discharge of sewage into several dams in the city led to intense breeding of mosquitoes until measures were taken to breach or bypass them.

The need for collaboration

Drainage improvements are not only a job for a drainage engineer. They involve several professions and need the co-operation of several sectors if they are to succeed. Drainage is of great concern to town planners, and if some houses have to be relocated to make room for new drains, architects and builders may also be involved. Drains are usually built beside roads, and the roads department will have an interest because good drainage is essential to protect the road surface.

Maintenance of the drainage system depends on an efficient solid-waste collection service, because without one the drains will soon fill with rubbish. Moreover, the street cleaning and solid-waste collection service will often be the most suitable municipal department to clean the drains regularly, as it will have the necessary vehicles to remove the solid materials such as silt, vegetation and refuse which will accumulate in them. The health department will be concerned to ensure that the cleaning is done well and regularly, and that the drains are not built in such a way as to make this difficult or to promote disease transmission. This in turn involves several specialities, such as medical entomology.

The community has a key role to play in this. Whether or not local residents participate in construction, their co-operation is needed in obtaining the necessary land. Some people may have to sacrifice part of their premises, or agree to relocate their houses, to make room for the new drains. Whether or not the community takes responsibility for maintaining the system, a responsible attitude on their part will be a great help towards its upkeep, reducing the amount of rubbish thrown into the drains, and damage done to them by vehicles, building work or vandalism. A single unco-operative resident who blocks the water flow, or neglects to clean his or her section of the drainage line, can harm the interests of the whole community. Proper drainage therefore calls for the close co-operation of the community and their leaders, and also of those who work with the community, such as educators and health workers.

A co-operative attitude, however, is not enough. Effective collaboration between municipal departments, which also involves the community, has institutional implications.

At the level of local government, the most fundamental consideration is that some department at least must have the primary responsibility for urban drainage. In many cities there is no clear definition of who is responsible for cleaning and maintaining the drainage system (including the natural drainage system) and in some it is not even clear who is to build it, or which national government department is to finance major drainage works. An example of the absurd situations which can arise in such cases is for one department to clean rubbish from the drains, the solid-waste collection service to refuse to collect it from where it is dumped on the adjoining roads, and for the roads department to sweep it back into the drains again!

Ideally, the regular cleaning of urban drains should be the job of the street cleaning and solid-waste collection service. However, other sectors will usually be responsible for drainage construction and repairs, so that several sectors are inevitably involved. Some arrangement for regular liaison meetings should therefore be set up, and a single department should be responsible for convening them. The health department should be represented.

Some institutional arrangements are also needed in the community, to mobilize and co-ordinate the community's contribution and to ensure that it is not undermined by the anti-social behaviour of a minority. If possible it is best to build on existing community institutions, although these may already be fully occupied with other day-to-day tasks. In many cases, a useful initial step will be to form a drainage committee to organize the community's contribution to planning, implementation and maintenance of drainage improvements.

Developing a drainage programme

A typical neighbourhood drainage improvement programme passes through four principal phases:

- initiation
- planning
- construction
- maintenance

The first two of these are fundamental, as they determine all that follows.

Initiation of a programme may arise from the community's own identification of the need for better drainage, possibly after a particularly serious flood or as a result of drainage improvements in other neighbourhoods. In many cases, however, it is catalysed by some external agency such as the municipality, a political party or a non-governmental organization, or a concerned individual such as a teacher or health worker. This phase involves identification of the need for drainage, formation of a consensus regarding the scope of the problem and the desired solution, and establishment of the drainage committee, at least on an interim basis. Where the initiative comes from outside, it is also likely to include a certain amount of work in the community to develop awareness of the problem and mobilize support for a drainage programme.

Planning is the most important phase of all, as it involves the most fundamental decisions. The more decisions that can be taken in the planning stage, the better it is for the future of the programme. The most basic decision for the community is whether to implement the drainage programme on a formal basis through the local authorities, or to attempt a "do-it-yourself" project on their own. Formal drainage projects tend to be expensive, so that the first task of the drainage committee is to lobby and persuade the local authority to agree to support the programme, unless of course the authority itself initiated the scheme. The authority will usually have to obtain finance from some other agency, which is likely to require a feasibility study and design by a consulting engineer before a contractor is given the job of building the new drainage system. All this takes time – typically 3 – 10 years – and the community may prefer to carry out some "do-it-yourself" interim measures themselves, while they wait (Figure 7.2).

Whichever approach is followed, it is important to define not only the layout and design of the new drainage system but also the community's role in the construction and maintenance phases, and how its contribution is to be organized.

For more information on the other two phases, – construction and maintenance – the reader should refer to the longer and more comprehensive report on which this chapter is based.[2]

Figure 7.2

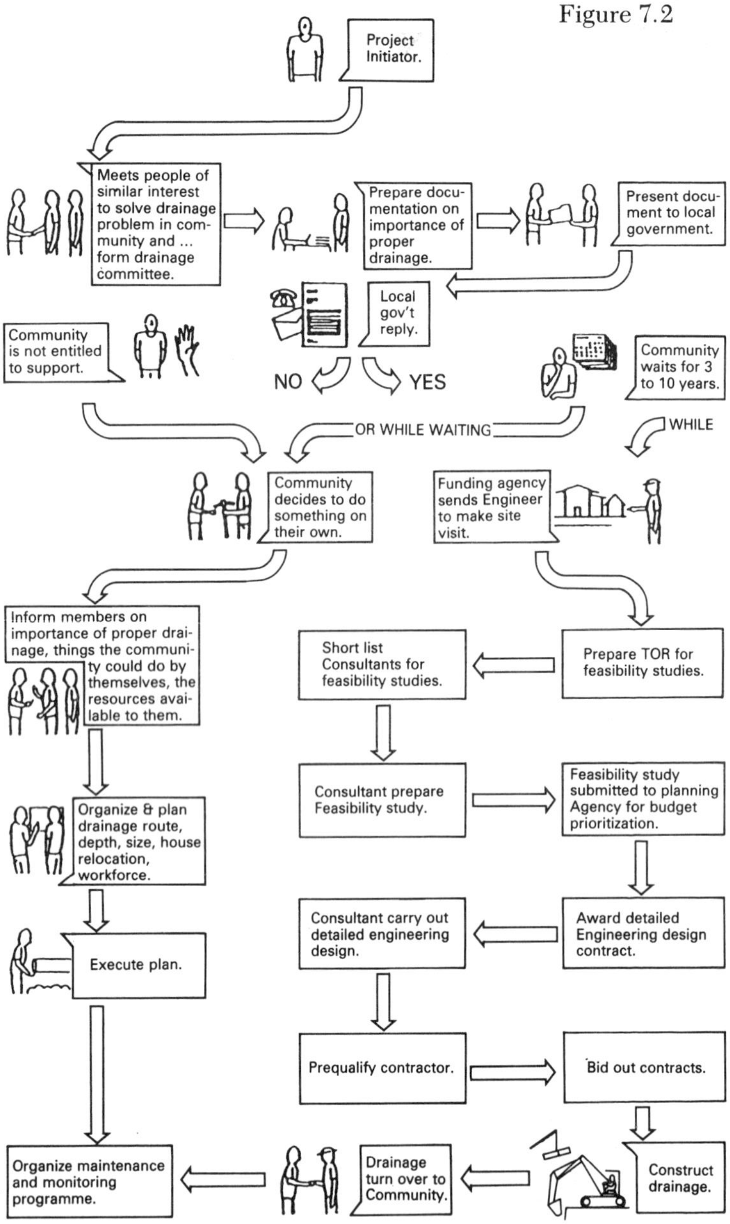
Project Initiator.
Meets people of similar interest to solve drainage problem in community and ... form drainage committee.
Prepare documentation on importance of proper drainage.
Present document to local government.
Local gov't reply.
NO
YES
Community is not entitled to support.
Community waits for 3 to 10 years.
OR WHILE WAITING
WHILE
Community decides to do something on their own.
Funding agency sends Engineer to make site visit.
Inform members on importance of proper drainage, things the community could do by themselves, the resources available to them.
Short list Consultants for feasibility studies.
Prepare TOR for feasibility studies.
Organize & plan drainage route, depth, size, house relocation, workforce.
Consultant prepare Feasibility study.
Feasibility study submitted to planning Agency for budget prioritization.
Execute plan.
Consultant carry out detailed engineering design.
Award detailed Engineering design contract.
Prequalify contractor.
Bid out contracts.
Organize maintenance and monitoring programme.
Drainage turn over to Community.
Construct drainage.

Chapter Eight

The Collection and Management of Household Garbage

Stenio de Coura Cuentro and Dji Malla Gadji

Introduction

Chapter 1 noted the poor performance of most government services in collecting and disposing of household wastes. An estimated 30 – 50 per cent of solid wastes generated within urban centres is left uncollected,[1] although in some cities the proportion is higher.

The resulting problems are obvious when wastes are dumped on streets, the spaces between houses, open land, drainage ditches and rivers, streams and lakes. Piles of garbage are scattered by scavengers or animals and serve as food or breeding grounds for disease vectors – primarily flies and rats.[2] Dangers to health arise both from pathogens in the refuse itself and from disease vectors which breed or feed there. Uncollected refuse often clogs drainage channels which then become stagnant pools and may overflow; if the drainage channels are carrying liquid wastes which include excreta (which is commonly the case in poorer settlement) this means further extensive site contamination. Uncollected garbage is thus a serious health-hazard for all inhabitants, perhaps most especially for children who play on streets or open ground contaminated with refuse. It is also a fire hazard.[3]

Poorer households usually suffer most.[4] It is overwhelmingly the poorer areas of a city which have no service to collect garbage – or very inadequate levels of service provision. Most low-income households' problems are further compounded by a lack of space within their homes to store garbage, or the space and means to have dog- and rat-proof dustbins outside their homes.

Part of the reason for inadequate service to poor households is that they throw away less wastes which can be profitably reclaimed by the staff collecting the garbage, or the scavengers or recycling businesses with which the staff deal. Private companies often operate profitable garbage-collection services, as long as they collect only from richer neighbourhoods where service charges can be higher and where the value of reclaimed or recycled materials is much higher.

Another reason for this inadequate service is the fact that so many live in settlements regarded as illegal by the public authorities, so that there is no recognition of their right to public services. But even if the local authorities do recognize the right of those in illegal settlements to a service, there are major obstacles to providing that service. Garbage collection is usually the responsibility of the local municipal government; but most poorer households are in the poorest municipalities, which have the least resources with which to pay for public services. If there is no system through which some of the revenue generated by richer city districts are transferred to help pay for services in poorer city districts, garbage-collection services (and all other services which rely on local revenues) will be particularly deficient in poorer districts. The collection and disposal of solid wastes is expensive and often consumes as much as 20 – 40 per cent of a municipal authority's total budget.[5]

There is the additional problem that poorer areas of a city are often more expensive to service. As previous chapters have noted, many poor settlements develop on terrain – for instance, on steep hills of flood plains – to which access by motor vehicles is difficult. Many houses are built close together with access to them only by pathways. As such, conventional garbage-collection trucks cannot get close to them. Meanwhile, most engineers associated with solid wastes still see the solution to the problem as an increased use of large, sophisticated collection trucks and solid-waste treatment plants whose cost is far beyond the means of local governments. Even if the funds were found, these would still be useless for people living on inaccessible sites.

The many poor families who make a living out of garbage also suffer from the ambiguous or hostile attitudes of local authorities to their work. Most major cities have thousands of households dependent on incomes generated by reclaiming material – for instance glass, plastics, metal goods, paper, rags – from household garbage for resale.[6] Some make a living through collecting wastes by going from door to door in residential areas. More pick their way through garbage once it is collected or when it is unloaded at the official city dump. In many cities, there are also hundreds of businesses ranging from some large formal enterprises to small, informal, family-based firms who manufacture a range of goods out of reclaimed materials.[7] All these people may be judged by public authorities to be a nuisance and their work to contribute to public health problems. Of course, these people face special risks to their health in their daily handling of refuse. Many settlements have developed on or next to refuse dumps, housing those who make a living from garbage picking.[8]

There is a need to reconcile a more effective system to remove garbage (especially in poorer communities) with limited municipal budgets. The poorer, more distant, more inaccessible settlements whose inhabitants have the least capacity to pay are usually those in most need of better services. There is also the need to address the health problems faced by those who make a living out of garbage.

There have been important changes among certain professionals in attitudes to waste management in recent years. One is the recognition of the need to develop local solutions which match local needs and possibilities; this usually implies solutions very different from those taught to engineers whose training is overwhelmingly based on Western models and precedents.[9] Conditions vary so much from city to city in (among other factors) the scale and type of refuse generation, the type of vehicles needed to get to each building in different settlements, local possibilities for recycling or reclaiming part of the refuse, local traffic conditions, the availability for land sites for city dumps and the resources at the disposal of local authorities for the collection and management of garbage disposal. A second change, linked to this, is the recognition that different kinds of refuse-collection vehicle are needed for different settlements. Carts which are pushed or carried manually, or modified tricycles or animal-pulled carts, are often the most appropriate means for serving many low-income areas. A third change is the recognition that district or neighbourhood-level garbage-collection schemes devised and managed in collaboration with the residents are often the cheapest and most effective solution. This is especially the case when the reclamation of materials and the recycling of part of the waste (for instance composting) is involved. This leads not only to additional employment but also to significant cost-savings since a reduction in the volume of waste needing to be collected and transported to a waste dump means a reduction in one of the major costs in a garbage collection and management service. A fourth change in attitude is the recognition that scavengers, rag pickers and recycling businesses can be made an important component within garbage management systems but that they need a supportive framework – perhaps most especially in the provision of services to address their health problems. In many nations, it is largely women and children who reclaim materials from garbage so such health programmes must address their particular needs.[10]

A final change in attitude among these professionals is the recognition of the connections between garbage collection and other improvements in infrastructure and services. For instance, paving roads to and within peripheral settlements can reduce garbage-collection costs while, in turn, improved garbage-collection ensures that drainage systems work better and so lessens water pollution.

The first case study presented here, written by Stenio Cuentro, illustrates how these changes in attitude led to the development of new approaches to garbage collection and management in Recife, Brazil.

The second, by Dji Malla Gadgi, is a case study of an innovative community-based project to improve refuse collection in N'Djamena, Chad. As in other chapters, the case studies are not models for replication in other cities but examples of how and in what way new and appropriate solutions were sought in a particular context.

The development of low-cost garbage collection and disposal in Recife, Northeast Brazil

Greater Recife grew from 554,000 inhabitants in 1940 to over 2.3 million in 1980. It is made up of twelve municipalities, of which Recife (with 1.3 million inhabitants), Olinda (330,000 inhabitants) and Paulista (242,000 inhabitants) are the most populous.

With the possible exception of electricity, there are serious deficiencies in the supply of most public services and utilities in Greater Recife. Garbage collection may rate as one of the most inadequate. The deficiencies stem largely from the fact that municipalities have been unable to cope properly with the rapid growth of population. Each of the 12 municipalities which make up Greater Recife is in charge of street cleaning and waste collection and disposal services, within its boundaries. Each of them face increasingly serious problems of declining fiscal resources, growing populations, worsening pollution, low efficiency in service provision and growing demands from local inhabitants. Each is under pressure from local suppliers and manufacturers of vehicles and equipment. There is also the problem that each municipality has political, administrative and budgetary autonomy since there is no overall co-ordinating or governing body. What is described here are innovative schemes developed in three of these municipalities. These do not provide solutions to these problems, but illustrate alternative ways of rethinking the issue of urban maintenance in its totality rather than as a patchwork of small, poorly co-ordinated, short-sighted solutions.

Olinda – the starting point

In 1983, the municipality of Olinda selected a *favela* (low-income settlement) with 450 low-income families covering an area of 3.5 hectares – known as Triangulo de Peixinhos – for a pilot project in upgrading. The origins of the *favela* date back to 1945. In 1983, only a handful of the occupants held legal titles to the land they occupied. The settlement had no sanitation facilities and provision for drainage was inadequate or non-existent. There was no municipal garbage collection services and none of the roads were paved. Water supply was also inadequate although most dwellings were connected to the electricity network. Triangulo de Peixinhos is built in a swampy area which had previously been used as a rubbish dump. Until the project in 1983, houses were often flooded in the rainy season and the settlement's streets became mud-paths, because of no system to drain away storm and surface water. The ground water from which many inhabitants obtained their water was often contaminated with water carried by the floods from the local pit latrines and from the rubbish dump.

As part of the pilot project, 272 of the 1,350 inhabitants were tested for intestinal parasites. Results were negative in only nine of them.[11] One hundred and fifty persons had three different types of parasites while 93 had two and only 11 had one; Table 8.1 shows the prevalence of the eight parasites found in the tests. By far the most common was *Ascaris lumbricoides*, found in over four-fifths of the infected population. Since Triangulo de Peixinhos is not a unique case among Olinda's *favelas*, the inhabitants of over 50 neighbourhoods which house nearly half of Olinda's population may have comparable health problems; these too have been classified as *favelas* or irregular, low-income settlements by Olinda's municipal authorities.

Table 8.1: Prevalence of parasites among the tested population in Triangulo de Peixinhos, 1983

TYPE OF PARASITE	*INCIDENCE*	
	number of cases (per cent)	*prevalence*
Ascaris lumbricoides	212	80.6
Trichuris trichiura	90	34.2
Entamoeba histolitica	41	15.6
Giardia lamblia	17	6.5
Hookworms	5	1.9
Hymenolepis	5	1.9
Strongiloides stercolaris	3	1.1
Schistosoma	2	0.8

Source: Municipality of Olinda (1985).

Faced with such problems, the project team realized the need for an intervention which would involve the local community and at the same time provide simple but effective solutions to the lack of basic infrastructure. First, a drainage system was installed for the whole settlement and then the team decided to tackle other areas in need of urgent action such as latrines, individual house-upgrading and the paving of roads and access paths.

Before the project, only part of the household refuse was placed in a skip nearby. The rest would usually be left to rot in the streets or would be dispersed by the wind and rain close to the inhabited area. The Director of Olinda Waste Management, Engineer Rodofo Aureliano, designed a small composting and recycling plant, located in the same 25-hectare plot of land as the skip. After 18 months of hard work with the help of the inhabitants, the plant began operations. This relatively small plant offered clear advantages over a centralized system of rubbish collection for the whole city: first, a large number of unskilled labourers were given employment during construction; and secondly, running costs were comparatively low, partly because the community was involved in the everyday running of the plant.

The composting plant was the third major cleaning action in which the community took part. The first had been a general spring clean of the whole settlement. With the help of the municipality, the garbage which had accumulated in different parts of the *favela* were collected while every household got rid of discarded objects and pieces of furniture. Altogether, some 50 tons of rubbish were collected.

A second, more regular and permanent initiative followed with the daily collection of refuse using a simple hand-pushed cart, operated by one person, with a capacity to carry up to 180 litres of rubbish. This cart – a light-weight steel structure with two bicycle wheels – was designed and constructed by a local firm, with the support of the municipality of Olinda. The cart's design makes it ideal for this type of work as it combines a sturdy yet light body with a relatively large capacity and ease of maintenance. In addition, its small size allows it to reach houses only accessible through the narrowest of streets and alleys.

The composting plant was constructed with an operational capacity of one ton per day. The technology used in building the plant was an extension of the simple techniques and materials used in the upgrading of the *favela*. For instance, a soil-cement mixture was used for paving the site of the plant.

The composting plant operates in a series of steps as follows:

1. All rubbish is collected in an open 2 metres x 3 m x 0.5 m tank at ground level.
2. The re-cyclable matter (glass, paper, plastic, etc.) is removed by hand and placed in different 50-litre metal barrels, classified according to type of material, colour and texture, and finally sold.
3. The compostable waste (organic material–mainly discarded foodstuffs) is weighed on a portable scale on wheels and then piled up in heaps some 1.2 – 1.6 m high in the composting yard and covered with finished organic compost to keep off flies and other insects.
4. The water content and the temperature of the heaps is checked regularly. The piles are turned over at intervals of three to seven days and water is added as needed. The first stage in the composting process takes some 60 days. At the end of this first stage, the compost is a topsoil-like substance free from the pathogenic elements which can be harmful to humans, odourless, with a brown or ash colour.
5. The compost is then moved to a corner of the courtyard where it is left untouched for another two weeks. At the end of this period, the compost will be stable both physically and chemically.

6. The compost is then put through a sieve to take out small pieces of plastic, wood and glass, stones and other objects. The sieved matter is finally ready to be used as an organic fertilizer and soil conditioner.

According to figures gathered in the plant in 1984 – 5, between 8.9 and 14.2 metric tonnes of garbage are processed every month. Of these between 62 per cent and 73 per cent are compostable, between 3.5 per cent and 6.3 per cent are recyclable, and between 22 per cent and 34 per cent are discarded. On average, the plant received 10.5 tonnes of garbage a month between June and October 1984, and 11.6 tonnes between June and December 1985 (Table 8.2). The volume of compost produced varied greatly from one month to the next but on average the volume produced was roughly equivalent to a quarter of the garbage processed.

Table 8.2: Production of the Triangulo de Peixinhos composting plant 1984–1985 (monthly average values)

Period	*Garbage Received (kg)*	*Compostable portion %*	*Recyclable portion %*	*Discarded portion %*	*Compost produced (kg)*
June 1984– Oct. 1984	10,847	67.0	5.4	27.6	2,956[1]
June 1985– Dec. 1985	11,575	68.7	4.8	26.6	5,252

[1] Average for three months only. Compost production only started in the plant's third month of operation.

By the end of 1985, the plant was still working below capacity, as shown by the fact that the largest daily average amount of garbage handled in any given month was 595 Kilograms (Kg) (in June 1985). Perhaps not surprisingly, the *favela's* households produce less refuse (an average of 0.28 kg per inhabitant per day) than middle or high-income households in other parts of the city (between 0.5 and 1.5 kg). This is an indication of the lower levels of consumption found in the poorer area, and also of the fact that certain objects (such as tins, glass jars and bottles and newspapers) are not discarded but either kept or sold by the households themselves. The proportion of refuse that can be recycled in higher-income areas is typically of the order of eight per cent, and may go up to 15 per cent.

In the early 1980s, when the Triangulo de Peixinhos composting plant was being built, Recife's metropolitan authorities were finishing their plans for a World Bank-supported re-structuring of the solid-waste management services for the metropolitan area. These proposed an increasing centralization of the operation, involving a number of lorries of different capacities collecting and transporting refuse to a large sanitary landfill outside the built area. The metropolitan authorities were challenged by the smaller municipalities (particularly that of Olinda) where more environmentally and socially sensitive refuse-disposal projects were being put forward. Under such pressure, plans to centralize these services were soon abandoned in favour of the higher degree of local control advocated by Olinda's officials.[12]

Olinda's authorities have already produced plans for seven composting plants similar to that of Peixinhos, although in most cases much larger. By 1988, one had been built, with a capacity to process seven tonnes every day, and another was under construction and due to start operating at the end of the year, with a capacity of 60 tonnes per day. Once completed these plants will process around 40 per cent of the garbage produced every day in the municipality. The systems for rubbish collection and cleaning of streets have been designed with the areas they will serve in mind, using a combination of large compacting lorries, pushcarts and animal traction carts, the mix dictated by local conditions. In all cases, this experience has demonstrated the possibility of substituting existing complex and expensive technology with cheaper, more low-key techniques. The alternative technology has proven to be viable and closer to the needs and realities of the people it is designed to serve.

The municipality of Paulista

The problems of rubbish collection and processing in this municipality were not unlike those in Olinda. The beach area of Paulista has a resident population estimated at some 35,000 and a fluctuating tourist population, estimated at over 100,000, who come on weekends all year round to visit its 12 kilometres of beaches. Despite the importance of the tourist industry, Paulista lacks much in the way of basic infrastructure. The road system is virtually restricted to a 12 kilometre-long state highway parallel to the beach and a number of streets of which less than two per cent are paved.

A new system of rubbish collection and processing was designed and implemented by the municipality between 1984 and 1986. Sixty-five per cent of the cost was funded with a joint grant from the state government (Pernambuco), the national government and the World Bank. The municipality covered the remaining costs, which included the purchase of minor equipment and the recruitment of workers.

Faced with a large, tourist population, the local government had to determine the basis on which to calculate the resources (the number of workers and the size and type of equipment) needed to clean the beach area. The waste management service is expected to cope with the garbage generated every day by a population of 82,500 persons (the average number of people estimated to be in the beach area in any of the six days of the week when services are in operation). This, rather than the maximum number of people expected to be there in any given day was felt to be appropriate for planning purposes.

For the purposes of rubbish collection the beach area was divided into three sections. Rubbish in Section I – the area along the beach and around the highway – was initially collected by a three-person team using a 400-litre cart pulled by a bicycle. Despite its low running costs, the system did not prove very effective since the cart's bicycle wheels would get stuck in the sand and in the mud of the dirt roads. The cart was replaced by a tractor-pulled two-tonne trailer which does daily collections. Section I is served by three different teams. The beaches are cleaned twice a week by 50 workers operating in eight teams with the aid of *bangues*. These are a simple device for transporting the garbage, consisting of a box made of wire net with holes open on two sides. This box hangs from two parallel bars and can thus be carried on the shoulders of two people, one in front and one behind.

All garbage collected on the beach is gathered in eight metal skips placed along the main road which are picked up and replaced by empty ones twice a day by a lorry. Whereas running costs for the simpler collection systems described above are very low, those for the lorry (which includes a hydraulic hoist) and the skips are much higher.

Section II of the beach area which contained the highway and the dwellings and commercial premises on either side is served by a compacting lorry with a capacity of ten cubic metres (or 14 tonnes). This form of collection is carried out by a team of three workers plus the driver. Section III, which includes the remaining area (mostly residential) within the urban centre, is served by two tractor-pulled trailers and the lorry which also serves Section II. Public areas are also regularly cleaned, and overgrown vegetation on the road verges and parks trimmed by teams of municipal workers.

The composting and recycling plant designed and built under this project is located some three kilometres inland. It has a capacity of 60 tonnes per day and employs a slightly different technique to that used in Olinda. Because of the larger volumes of waste treated, the process involves more use of mechanical procedures including a conveyor belt to transport both the compostable and the recyclable matter, an electrically-powered drum and an electric hammer to mix and homogenize the compost.

The monthly running costs of this plant (not including capital costs and depreciation) amount to some US$3,500 while monthly earnings from the sale of the compost and recyclable material fluctuate between $4,000 and $4,500. Detailed costings are not yet available but provisional figures suggest that this system has already reduced rubbish transport costs by 40 per cent in relation to the old, more conventional system.

Lastly, the dramatic expansion in the coverage and volume of the waste management services between 1983 and 1988 in Paulista is illustrated by the fact that the total number of vehicles used for these services increased from 5 to 18, while the number of staff – particularly refuse collection workers – grew nearly fourfold. These are regularly given proper training, guidance and support by three engineers and four supervisors. What used to be an irregular service has become a daily feature in most parts of the municipality. The Waste Collection Department now runs its own garage for the regular maintenance of its vehicles. And more importantly, garbage is disposed of in an environmentally sound and cost-effective manner.

The municipality of Recife

The experiences of Olinda and Paulista proved important in designing a programme of rubbish collection for the much larger municipality of Recife. The scale of problems in this, the largest municipality in Greater Recife, greatly exceeds that of the two smaller municipalities. For the municipal department in charge of street cleaning and garbage collection, the problem is not simply one of collecting and disposing of the rubbish produced by a population of

1.3 million. Even though in relative terms the rich neighbourhoods (where ten per cent of the city's population live) and the downtown area are the biggest generators of solid waste[13], collection is actually more of a problem on the steep hills where many of the poor live. Within the boundaries of Recife municipality, 195 neighbourhoods were classified as *favelas*, in 1985/6. These covered an estimated 15 per cent of the city's inhabitable area and housed around half of the city's population. Some 75 per cent of the households in these settlements earned less than $150 a month.[14] Difficult terrain in many of these *favelas* makes the operation of conventional equipment particularly cumbersome. As the poor cannot afford to cover the real costs of collection, rubbish is usually left uncollected with undesirable health and environmental consequences.

Despite a considerable expansion in the number of staff and specialized equipment working in the collection and disposal of refuse since the early 1960s, an estimated 30 per cent of the total volume of rubbish is still left uncollected. Collected refuse is disposed of by means of a ten tonne per day anaerobic composting plant in operation since 1962, a 40 tonne per day composting and recycling plant similar to that of Paulista, in operation since 1986, and a large rubbish dump located 20 kilometres from the city centre.

The planning team started a pilot project in a *favela* with a population of 15,000, located in the hill known as the Morro da Conceicao, in the north of the city. As in most poorer areas in the city, rubbish had been collected in a skip located in the highest and most central point of the site. The skip was emptied once a day and people were expected to deposit their refuse there. For those living farthest from the collection point and in the lower parts of the hill it was often more convenient to throw the garbage in the open storm sewers to be drained downhill or simply to leave it any place at hand. Apart from the obvious health hazards, there was often a danger that rubbish accumulated to the point of blocking the sewers thereby producing floods in nearby areas.

A pilot scheme was devised to ensure effective collection of refuse from every house. The first stage involved developing a piece of equipment appropriate for rubbish collection in the particular conditions of the terrain. This consisted of a basket hanging from two poles held at either side by one person. The basket hinges upon the two poles in such a way that its bottom remains horizontal even if carried uphill or downhill. This was an adaption of the *bangue* used by the municipality of Paulista.

The next step was for the municipality to train and contract local workers to collect the rubbish with the help of the basket. Collection routes were defined in such a way that the two-person team would always carry the basket downhill. A plastic bag is placed inside the basket so that the rubbish thus collected can be deposited in small skips placed in strategic points around the settlement, from where it is collected by a lorry.

As this system is very labour-intensive, it is comparatively expensive. None the less, it has proven very effective for an adequate collection of refuse in the rough topographical conditions of Morro da Conceicao. There were various benefits arising from the new system. The volume of garbage collected increased from three tonnes per day with the old system to six tonnes with the new one. The higher collection rate has considerably reduced health hazards for the local inhabitants – especially children – as people have ceased disposing of their refuse in open spaces. Health and structural hazards have also been considerably reduced as rubbish is no longer left to accumulate in storm sewers or washed downhill during the rainy season.

Finally, although the new system involves higher running costs than the old one (especially to cover staff wages), it has generated employment among local residents. The settlement is now served by a staff of 18, including a lorry driver and a supervisor. There is one staff member for every 833 inhabitants which compares favourably to Recife municipality as a whole with one garbage worker to every 382 inhabitants.

With the positive results from the pilot project in Morro da Conceicao, the municipality decided to expand the collection system to cover similar poor and hilly settlements throughout the city, with a potential coverage of some 200,000 of Recife's poorest inhabitants. The collection system will be complemented with the installation of manually-operated composting units in each of these settlements. It is hoped that this expansion of the system will combine the goals of generating employment, eliminating (or at least reducing) garbage transport costs, cost recovery through the sale of recycled materials and organic compost and, in general terms, reaching a more appropriate solution from a sanitary, environmental and cultural point of view.

Conclusions

Many of Brazil's urban areas have similar problems to those evident in Recife. On the one hand, there is the large local authority where waste management is in the hands of a highly centralized and costly public institution whose range of action is often restricted to most (although rarely all) areas within the municipality's boundaries. Refuse collection and disposal is often non-existent in the poorer and most distant neighbourhoods and nearby rural areas (even if these are within the jurisdiction of the local authority).

In many cases, the largest municipalities are served by private enterprises under contract to the local authority. Although this may represent a small reduction in the cost of collecting and transporting a given volume of refuse in relation to a public enterprise, particularly as these enterprises operate on a profit basis generally with a slimmer and more efficient organization, this system may have higher operational costs than cheaper, more modest technological alternatives. Public service contracts with local authorities are undoubtedly becoming more and more profitable for the private sector. This has led many of these enterprises to form influential pressure groups with vested interests in inhibiting any change towards cheaper and less centralized technological models.

On the other hand, the smaller municipalities with fewer resources and weaker administrative structures are faced with the alternative of imitating the centralized model used by the larger municipalities or searching for new solutions to an often growing problem of refuse collection and disposal. The case of these smaller municipalities has inspired many to look for viable alternatives. There is little doubt that both alternatives have drawbacks: whether lack of resources to manage a large and centralized system or lack of appropriate technological models to implement at a smaller, more decentralized level. The experiences described here will, one hopes, prove a source of inspiration in promoting the development of smaller-scale, locally run options.

The case of Ambassatna Nadif: lessons from an experimental household waste collection project in N'Djamena

Ambassatna Nadif is a household-waste collection project jointly initiated by N'Djamena town council and Oxfam.[15] The project illustrates the difficulties in developing a grassroots initiative to address a communal problem (in this instance the collection and disposal of household wastes) which is conventionally handled by an outside agency.

Ambassatna is one of the old areas of N'Djamena, with a population of about 11,300 in 1987. Administratively, the area is subdivided into squares. Each square consists of a number of blocks, which themselves are made up of plots, locally known as concessions. In Ambassatna, there are ten squares and 797 concessions. Each concession has on average three families – 14 people – living on it.

The project involved the following steps. First, Oxfam funded the manufacture of dustbins (a third of a barrel with a lid) and the provision of tools and materials (push carts, spades, rakes, boots, etc.). Then each concession was given one or two dustbins, according to the number of families living there. A collector with a push cart goes to each concession at least twice a week to collect the garbage and take it to a designated dumping ground. The town council is then responsible for the regular collection of wastes from these dumps. The recurrent costs are met by the population, with each concession making a monthly payment of 200 CFA francs (the equivalent of around US$0.60).

To initiate this process, a waste-disposal committee was formed for each of the ten squares. The committee's role includes the organization of the refuse collection and making people aware of it. It also includes responsibility for the collection of the monthly contributions; the recruitment and payment of the collectors; and the upkeep and renewal of project materials.

The committees must also ensure that the cost of the dustbins is recovered from the local people. The dustbins are manufactured locally by a craft co-operative also funded by Oxfam. They are then resold to the population at a subsidized price. Funds obtained from the sale of dustbins in any square belongs to that square as a rolling fund put at its disposal by Oxfam. This money may be used for other projects.

The project began in September 1987, with the delivery of the first dustbins to the first square. After two years in operation, what are the lessons to be learnt from this pilot project? First, the collection of household waste still takes place in some squares, but irregularly. The collectors responsible for emptying the dustbins are still doing their job, but some are being paid each time they collect the garbage instead of a monthly salary from the committee, derived from the contributions paid by the people.

In addition, the committees have become mere figureheads and do not meet. There is little interest by the organizers to revitalize the committees. Local inhabitants are increasingly unwilling to pay the 200 CFA francs monthly contributions for only irregular collections.

So far, only a portion of the cost of the dustbins has been recovered and any rolling funds have not produced any other income-generating activities. Nevertheless, some squares have restored the public taps and repaired the streets. Crucially, the project has not been taken over by the beneficiaries. Some see Oxfam as responsible for the project, others the government. How did this situation arise?

Lessons to be learnt from the project

We are not sure we have uncovered all the causes or reasons, let alone the main problems. Yet, certain facts are significant: in particular, the origins and conception of the project, the use of urban volunteers and the heterogeneity of the social groups making up this area of N'Djamena.

In this instance, the idea of a household waste collection project did not come from the community. It was involved later on, but there was minimal participation in the conception of the project. In fact, it was following a letter from Oxfam to the Ministry of Planning and Co-operation, expressing an interest in involving itself in N'Djamena, that it was suggested that Oxfam look into this question with the town council. The town council, faced with the problems of keeping the town in a suitably healthy state, suggested waste disposal and public health as a possible area of intervention, and Ambassatna was chosen as a pilot area. This is how the Ambassatna Nadif project emerged. Surveys were then carried out, and public meetings organized to seek local support.

To set up the committees, meetings were organized with the people, square by square, to elect members to their waste disposal committee. Generally, it was the square leaders, the well-known figures and a few people influential as a result of their social position (tradesmen or politicians), who were elected. In two cases, it was members from the sub-section of the political movement (UNIR) who were elected. Young people and women were under-represented.

The fact that the committees were mainly made up of influential people did not turn out to be a sufficient asset, especially as the stakes had not been understood. These people were not used to consulting the masses; on the contrary, it was up to the people to approach them. The tasks assigned to the committees could not be undertaken by these people. Only the square leaders showed a certain commitment as their position as leaders could thus be re-inforced. For some inhabitants, however, to be part of a committee was seen as an honorary position.

The organizer of the project had to take on the work of the committees to make the project work. From being the enabling person, he became the main actor: convening the committee meetings, meeting with the inhabitants, the collectors, the crew leaders of the refuse collection teams and so on.

This raises the issue of voluntary commitments in an urban environment. In a rural environment, the problems are generally communal, for example: a lack of water or poor soil. Overall solutions can be found from which all can benefit. In an urban environment, the situation is different: problems are personal and people's survival strategies are individualistic. Promoting collective self-help is a risky and ambitious enterprise. This is even more difficult when a project requires a disinterested, voluntary commitment.

In this project, the committee members only had obligations vis-a-vis their community; their reward was to have been the satisfaction of seeing their environment improve. However, it later transpired that some committee members, especially the younger ones, had hoped for a material gain. "At the end of each month, we have to go from concession to concession to collect, with difficulty, the contributions; people don't want to pay, and we get nothing out of it".

In reality, the committees did not work because the active members with professional activities did not have enough time to devote to them. Only the unemployed did. And for those people, the main daily preoccupation is to try and find work. On the other hand, the collectors had always done their job, although maybe inadequately, because they were paid for it; they had a monthly income. Even when the committees could not pay them regularly, they continued to work, and some had even become self-employed by getting the inhabitants to pay them directly.

Should the committees' members have been paid? Who would

have provided the money: Oxfam or the community? What will become of participation? These are issues we have considered without finding a satisfactory answer.

The role of women

In Chad, as everywhere in Africa, it is the woman who is most interested in the upkeep of the house and the yard. Cleaning the yard is usually the first daily task; she sweeps, clears away and, with or without help from her children, will remove refuse from the concession.

In the Ambassatna Nadif project, the role of the women was limited to the cleaning tasks because it was their duty. They were not involved in running the project. In fact, of all ten committees, only one has a woman member. Particular efforts have been made by Oxfam to identify groups of women in the area, whether organized or not, who could support their initiatives. Similar steps were taken in collaboration with the area's social centre, who provided various organizers for the project. Unfortunately, these efforts did not produce very convincing results.

It appears that sharing a common neighbourhood is not a strong enough base around which to organize a communal activity. Women prefer to work alone, or on the basis of a personal relationship (through friendship, family, or coming from the same region). The fact that one lives in the same area does not necessarily mean that a network of interdependence or solidarity develops. Thus, only one group (embroiderers and small shopkeepers) developed, and this a year after a socio-economic survey was undertaken in a few of the squares. The survey's target was women, and the results were not very encouraging. Most of the women employed in the informal sector make local beverages, which is very profitable. In addition, neighbourhood relationships are very precarious because of the mobility of people within towns and the number of people who are tenants.

Oxfam, which forbids any involvement with alcohol, and only wishes to work with groups, found it impossible to undertake anything with these women who were fighting for their subsistence. It is interesting to note the suspicion the women showed during the survey. This stems from the fact that they likened Oxfam to the government, which had never granted small loans to poor women. One unresolved question is – should we have persisted in trying to create women's groups? Especially when dealing with money in an urban environment, it is very difficult to overcome mutual suspicion and competition, and to forge mutual objectives. This is the main reason for refusing to group together with one's neighbours.

Identifying the needs

From the beginning, everybody's needs should have been clearly identified. Oxfam's need at the outset of the project was to find a way to get in touch with the population. In 1987, the organization had only been present in the country for about a year and consequently was hardly known to the general public. In N'Djamena, as in the rest of the country, the collective self-help organizations are very young and most of them are still unfamiliar with ways of co-operating with foreign Private Voluntary organizations. They therefore had to be encouraged.

For the city authorities, the justification of the project was self-evident: waste disposal had always been a problem and any positive steps in this direction were to be encouraged. Furthermore, as the deputy mayor pointed out at a meeting in June 1987, there were other considerations :"During the civil unrest in our country, certain taxes were abandoned and we intend to reinstate them. What we are interested in at the moment is to see a project being carried out and, if it is well conducted, we will be able to see what kind of tax the population can bear".

The needs of the population, however, were never investigated or identified.

The concession: the cornerstone of the project

The fundamental element on which the project's strategy relied is the concession or, more precisely, the yard. Yet, the problem of household-waste accumulation is more acute in the street than in the concession. Generally, people are quite preoccupied with the cleanliness of their yard; on average, the women sweep it twice a day (morning and evening) and then dispose of the refuse just in front of the house (which is usually the street). This is either because the public dumping ground is too far away from the house or because it is too full. However, one of the main reasons for this behaviour lies in people's perceptions. It is not a question of wanting to live amidst refuse, just that the upkeep of the streets is perceived as the responsibility of the town council.

The population only participates in street cleaning on waste disposal days. The project would have been more efficient had the streets been taken into account. The fact that only the yards and the dumping grounds were considered meant that tangible results were not obtained. The yards are clean, as they have always been. In the same way, the streets have remained unhealthy. At first sight, there doesn't appear to be any improvement on the previous situation.

Certainly, the project has helped towards making household tasks easier and the cost of removing the refuse cheaper (200 CFA francs a month instead of 50 or 100 for each collection by private enterprises). This is much appreciated by the inhabitants who constantly express their satisfaction to any visitors: "it's a good project; it must be extended to all of the town". But the impact is limited compared to the project's objectives.

In the last six months we have withdrawn, by removing the organizer, whilst maintaining a close follow-up. The aim was to break the strong linking of the project with Oxfam but also to see if we can produce some idea in community of really taking on the project. Our dilemma is whether to go on or to stop. To continue organizing, as things now stand, would simply be to propose alternative solutions to something which might appear to be a problem in our eyes, but not in those of the community.

Chapter Nine

THE ROLE OF HOUSE DESIGN IN LIMITING VECTOR-BORNE DISEASE

C. J. Schofield, R. Briceño-Leon, N. Kolstrup, D. J. T. Webb and G. B. White

Introduction

Definitions of adequate or inadequate housing are often a source of confusion. What is adequate for one family may be inadequate in the eyes of the city architect or town planner. Here, inadequate housing implies houses that do not meet the minimum requirements of low-income families, do not satisfy building regulations and pre-dispose the house to pest infestation and the inhabitants to illness.[1]

The need to improve low-cost housing is increasingly recognized, both as a developmental goal in itself and also as an important contribution to improved health through improvements in hygiene and sanitation, reduction of domestic vectors of disease and reductions in the stress and dissatisfaction associated with overcrowding and squalid living conditions. This chapter discusses the control of disease vectors in or close to the home, with a special concentration on low-cost measures for their control.

Most common household pests are arthropods, a group which includes insects, spiders and mites. This chapter focuses on arthropods and does not discuss vertebrate pests such as birds and rats. Some arthropods can carry diseases between one person and another, or between animals and humans; these are called vectors of the diseases. The disease is not strictly caused by its vector, but by a micro-organism known as a pathogen which invades the body, usually when the infected vector bites its victim. Each pathogen can only be transmitted by certain species of vector, so the precise, Latin names for them have been used in this chapter. Some arthropods, such as lice and fleas, live on the body of their human or animal hosts, and are known as ectoparasites. Before many types of insect emerge in their final, adult form, they spend some time as *larvae* – sometimes known as grubs or maggots – and then as pupae.

Vector-control activities sometimes concentrate on the larval stage to prevent breeding of the vector; insecticides used for this purpose are known as larvicides.

Table 9.1 lists the arthropods of medical importance within the domestic environment or its immediate surrounds (known as the peri-domestic environment) and the health problems with which they are associated. The arthropods are divided into four categories: those that breed on the body; those that breed in the house; those that breed peri-domestically and/or in containers and sewerage; and those, which are termed "adventitious", who enter the house to feed.

Table 9.1: Summary of domestic and peridomestic arthropods of medical importance

A. BREEDING ON THE BODY:	CAUSE OR CARRIER OF:
Head lice[1]	
Pediculus capitis	head louse infestation
Body lice[1]:	
Pediculus humanus	typhus: *Rickettsia prowazeki* trench fever: *Rickettsia quintana* relapsing fever: *Borrelia recurrentis*
Pubic lice[1]:	
Phthirus pubis	phthiriasis
Scabies mites[2]:	
Sarcoptes scabiei	scabies
Follicle mites[2]:	
Demodex folliculorum	*Corynebacterium acnes?*
B. BREEDING IN THE HOUSE	
Fleas[1]:	
Pulex irritans	bites only: not vectors
Ctenocephalides spp.	
Xenopsylla spp.	plague: *Yersinia pestis* typhus: *Rickettsia mooseri*
Cockroaches[3]:	
Blatta orientalis	shigellosis: *Shigella dysenteriae*
Blattella germanica	salmonellosis: *Salmonella* spp.
Leucophaea maderae	and other enteric infections;
Periplaneta spp.	viruses: hepatitis A, poliomyelitis, etc.
Supella spp. etc.	Legionnaire's disease: *Legionella* etc.
Bedbugs[1]:	
Cimex hemipterus	viral hepatitis B?
C. lectularis	

Table 9.1: (continued)

Triatomine bugs[1]:	
Panstrongylus megistus	
Rhodnius prolixus	Chagas Disease, *Trypanosoma cruzi*
Triatoma infestans	
Soft ticks[1]:	
Ornithodoros spp.	relapsing fever, *Borrelia duttoni*
Argas spp.	bites only: not a vector of human disease
Dust mites[2]:	
Dermatophagoides spp.	house dust allergy
C. BREEDING PERI-DOMESTICALLY and/or IN CONTAINERS AND SEWERAGE:	
Jiggers[1]:	
Tunga penetrans	jiggers
Midges:	
Culicoides furens	
C. phlebotomus etc.	*Mansonella ozzardi, M. perstans*
C. austeni	
C. grahami	*M. perstans, M. streptocerca*
Mosquitoes[1]:	
Aedes aegypti	
Ae. albopictus	dengue, chikungunya
Ae. aegypti	
Haemagogus equinus	yellow fever
Ae. scutellaris group	subperiodic Bancroftian filariasis
Culex pipiens group	urban periodic Bancroftian filariasis
Cx. tritaeniorhynchus	
Cx. gelidus etc.	arboviruses, e.g. CHIK, JE, WN
Anopheles stephensi	malaria: *Plasmodium* spp.
Armigeres subalbatus	bites only: not a vector of human disease
Sandflies [1]:	
Lutzomyia spp.	sandfly fever
Phlebotomus spp.	visceral leishmaniasis: *Leishmania donovani* complex cutaneous/mucocutaneous leishmaniasis: *L. braziliensis, L. tropica*
Mothflies[3]:	
Psychoda spp.	allergy to moth
Telmatoscopus spp. etc.	flies
Blowflies[3]:	
Calliphora	intestinal myiasis, dysentery:
Lucilia	*Clostridium, Salmonella, Shigella* etc.
Chrysomya	
Houseflies[3]:	
Musca domestica	dysentery: *Clostridium, Entamoeba, Salmonella* etc. viruses: hepatitis A, poliomyelitis etc.

Table 9.1: (continued)

Latrine flies[3]:	
Fannia spp.	dysentery?
Face flies[3]:	
Musca sorbens	yaws: *Treponema pertenue* trachoma: *Chlamydia trachomitis* septicemia: *Clostridium, Staphylococcus, Streptococcus* etc. infective dermatitis: *Candida, Staphylococcus* etc.
Stable flies[1]:	
Stomoxys spp.	bites only: not a vector of human disease
Poisonous spiders[3]:	
Atrax, Latrodectus, Loxosceles, Lycosa etc.	spider bites
D. ADVENTITIOUS – ENTERING THE HOUSE TO FEED	
Mosquitoes[1]:	
Aedes spp.	arbovirus, e.g. CE, JE, RVF, VEE subperiodic Bancroftian filariasis
Anopheles spp.	arboviruses, e.g. JE, ONN, malaria: *Plasmodium* spp. periodic Brugian filariasis rural periodic Bancroftian filariasis
Coquillettidia spp.	arboviruses, e.g. BSQ, COT, CVO, MAY, MUR, TEN, WN
Culex spp.	arboviruses, e.g. CHIK, CE, EEE, GMA, JE, RVF, SIN, WN
Mansonia spp.	arboviruses, e.g. ILE, RVF, VEE sub periodic Brugian filariasis
Sandflies[1]:	
Phlebotomus spp.	cutaneous leishmaniasis: *L. aethiopica, L. major, L. tropica* visceral leishmaniasis (kala azar): *L. donovani, L. infantum* sandfly fever
Scorpions[3]:	
Androctonus, Buthus, Centruroides etc.	scorpion stings

[1]blood sucking [2]dermatophagous (eating skin) [3]scavenging

Source: Adapted from C.J. Schofield and G.B. White, "House design and domestic vectors of disease", Transcript of the Royal Society for Tropical Medicine and Hygiene Vol. 78, 285, 1984.

House Design

To satisfy the requirements of low cost, ease of construction, permanence, comfort and acceptability to the householders concerned, housing materials and design should make use of non-imported materials coupled with techniques and designs that are already familiar in the area. Rather than capital-intensive programs – for example using prefabricated units which impose unacceptable design constraints – construction techniques should emphasize labour-intensive systems making best use of the local labour force and locally-available materials. [2] In Third World nations where the marginal cost of imported capital and materials may be particularly high, emphasis on labour-intensive systems can be a key factor in minimizing costs as well as increasing the local acceptability of the techniques. The use of imported materials must be minimized in order to keep costs low (in many nations, cement, steel and glass are imported), and energy-expensive materials such as fired-clay bricks and concrete should also be discouraged since they can add considerably to material production and distribution costs.

Frequently, the constraints of cost, materials and technique, design and cultural acceptability, lead to an optimum solution in the form of existing traditional styles of housing.[3] Generally, traditional styles of housing use locally-available materials, constructed with proven local techniques, and follow a style already compatible with the cultural aspirations and social requirements of the householders (even though they may not follow legally-defined building regulations). This is often true of traditional rural housing, but less apparent for more recent urban illegal or informal settlements where shelters may be prepared using the most precarious of materials – packing cases, cardboard boxes, old planking, corrugated iron and so on. In most cases however, given land tenure and adequate services such as drainage, water, vehicular access and, if possible, electricity, the poorer urban settlements can be upgraded using techniques developed for rural areas.

In addition to their technical, material and cultural aspects, traditional styles of housing usually offer other advantages that may be difficult to replicate using other designs.[4] The most important of these are their suitability for the local climate and its fluctuations. The elegant studies of Kroeger on rural housing in Ecuador[5] demonstrated the advantages of traditional earth-walled, thatch-roofed houses in maintaining a cooler daytime climate within the house.

Similarly, traditional houses in Africa and the Middle East are designed to provide daytime shade and, in drier areas, to preserve atmospheric humidity,[6] while raised houses of slatted bamboo in humid coastal regions of Ecuador and South East Asia allow welcome cooling ventilation, as do the pole-walled houses of the Mayans in Central America. In any attempt to improve traditional styles of housing it is therefore important to identify and preserve these useful characteristics.

In both tropical and temperate areas however, traditional and modern housing can offer a range of habitats that may be exploited by arthropod pests and vectors of disease (Figure 9.1). Of the vast range of vector-borne pathogens, there are relatively few for which the household environment does not offer an important site for transmission to humans.[7] Indeed, for many vectors, it is their close association with the human domestic environment that has altered them from agents transmitting disease among animals to vectors of significant medical importance.

Good house design, and use of appropriate materials, can minimize the risk of pest infestation. In most cases however, designers and builders, both of traditional and contemporary houses, either ignore the possibility of pest infestation, or concentrate only on those pests that threaten the structural integrity and function of buildings and their services. The risk of direct structural damage due to rodents, ants and termites, or indirect damage due to birds – for example by their droppings or by blockage of drains and gutters by their nests – is fairly well recognized.[8] However, even in Europe and North America, the risk to human health by pest-contamination of catering facilities, foodstores, and hospitals is generally ignored at the design and construction stage – while even subsequent remedial action may be lacking or grossly inadequate.[9] In temperate and tropical countries alike, appropriate house design to minimize pest problems is generally given even less priority.[10]

The domestic vector problem

The environment in and around human dwellings offers an important habitat for a wide range of arthropods. Obviously, our homes are widely distributed throughout temperate and tropical areas. They offer shelter from extremes of climate, often allowing inhabitants to survive in regions that would otherwise be inhospitable. For

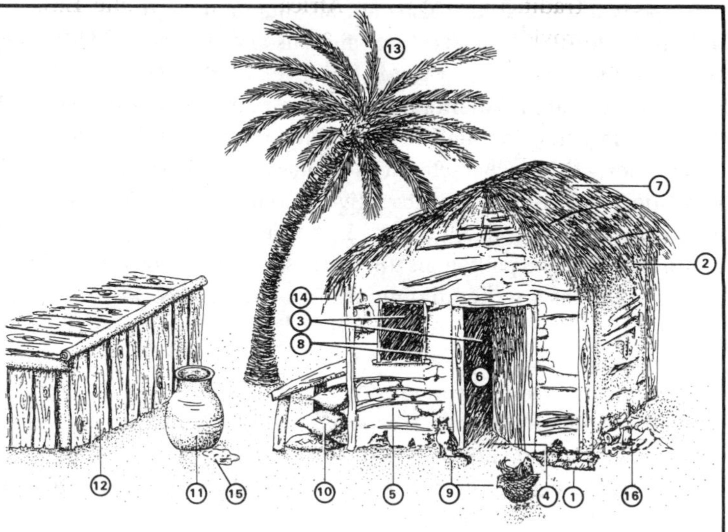

Figure 9.1: Factors which predispose the domestic and peri-domestic environment to colonization by arthropods of medical importance

Figure 9.1: numerical key

1)-inadequate foundations, and inadequate protection of the base of the wall against water erosion, causing damage to footings of wall, allowing entry of crawling pests. 2)-open, unscreened eaves, with no internal ceiling, allowing entry of flying insects into living space. 3)-open, unscreened window and door allowing entry of flying insects. 4)-cracked uneven floor providing refuge for ticks, flea larvae and other insects. 5)-unrendered, cracked walls providing refuge for cockroaches, bedbugs, triatomine bugs etc. 6)-dark, poorly ventilated interior favouring arthropods that rest during the day. 7)-roof of thatch allowing resting places for insects. 8)-shrinkage cracks at junction between wooden frames and walls of other material. 9)-domestic animals offering food source for blood-sucking arthropods, and may also act as reservoirs for parasites and pathogens. 10)-stored products in or near the house attracting rodents and other pests. 11)-unscreened water storage vessels providing breeding sites for mosquito larvae. 12)-animal enclosures near house providing additional refuge and food source for insect pests. 13)-shade tree maintaining roof fabric cool and more suitable for insects, and also offering refuge for some peridomestic insects. 14)-inadequate roof overhang does not protect wall from rain, causing erosion and cracking. 15)-water seepage providing moist breeding grounds for mothflies and other species. 16)-organic refuse providing breeding grounds for houseflies etc.

arthropods, these habitats also offer an abundant source of potential food in the form of humans, their animals and products. Moreover, the domestic environment tends to be relatively stable over time. Even the temporary shelters of nomadic peoples offer a degree of stability compared to much of the outside environment.

Together, these characteristics make the domestic and peri-domestic environment an attractive habitat for a wide range of arthropods – many of which are important as carriers or vectors of human disease pathogens (See Table 9.1). Amongst the best known examples are the ubiquitous houseflies and cockroaches, the triatomine bugs of Latin America that live in cracks and crevices of poor-quality rural houses and whose painful bites can transmit Chagas' disease, and the domestic *Ornithodoros* ticks, vectors of a range of rickettsial fevers especially in parts of Africa. Other domestic arthropods are better known for their direct effects, such as the widespread bedbugs implicated in chronic iron-deficiency anaemia and possibly hepatitis-B transmission, or the housedust mites (*Dermatophagoides spp.*) which are important causes of asthma and other allergies. In some areas, venomous spiders such as *Atrax robustus* (Australian funnel-web spider), *Latrodectus mactans* (the "black widow") and *Loxosceles reclusa* (the "brown recluse spider") are important domestic pests.

Some domestic arthropods go further, colonizing humans or their domestic animals. Well-known examples include head and body lice, scabies and follicle mites, and various species of flea whose larvae live in the accumulated debris around the house while adults spend much of their time on the surface of their chosen hosts. Other medically important insects – particularly mosquitoes and certain species of sandfly – enter the domestic environment to feed but use breeding sites that may be close to or distant from the house.

With the exception of houseflies and some of the *Aedes* mosquitoes, most domestic arthropods are active at night when their vertebrate hosts and potential predators are resting. During the day these arthropods rest, seeking dark undisturbed crevices that offer protection from predators and climatic extremes. In the case of *Triatoma infestans* for example, studies of their daytime vertical distribution in the cracked walls of houses in central Brazil show that they tend to congregate in crevices at the upper levels, which is interpreted to represent avoidance of the predatory behaviour of domestic chickens.[11] Moreover, since these bugs depend exclusively on a diet of vertebrate blood, and their population size is regulated by access to that blood, their nocturnal feeding behaviour is interpreted to be an important adaptation to minimize disturbance while feeding off their resting hosts. By contrast, some other species of triatomine bugs that might feed on nocturnal animals, tend to be more active during the day.[12] Similar adaptations are shown by other blood-sucking insects, representing a balance between minimizing their risk of predation, avoiding climatic extremes, and acquiring adequate blood meals.[13]

In terms of vector-borne diseases, the greatest problems are apparent in tropical areas, where higher temperatures unrelieved by extreme winters allow vectors to reproduce more quickly and often permit disease transmission throughout the year. Some problems are particularly associated with cities, where blocked drains and inadequate sewage disposal can provide breeding sites for mosquitoes such as the vectors of filariasis, while accumulated refuse promotes housefly breeding and an abundance of water containers can encourage the breeding of nuisance and vector mosquitoes such as *Aedes aegypti*, *Ae. albopictus* and *Armigeres subalbatus*. Such problems can best be dealt with by improved urban services aided by appropriate legislation – as for example in Bombay,[14] Singapore[15] and urban areas of Malaysia and Cuba where fines can be imposed on householders who allow mosquito breeding sites on their property. Local authorities that refrain from such legislation, or from its effective enforcement, do a disservice to the community. For example in the USA lax legislation concerning the control of *Ae. aegypti* infestations has led to recent outbreaks of dengue in Texas.[16] In addition, many features of the design, construction, situation and maintenance of individual houses – both in urban and rural areas – can also help to minimize these problems as well as inhibit vectors that actually breed in the domestic and peridomestic environments.

Four aspects of household pest and vector control

There are four key features of the domestic environment that promote access or multiplication by arthropod pests and vectors of disease. The first relates to the position of the house within areas where a given pest species is known to occur. Siting a house close to known or potential breeding-sites of mosquitoes or other vectors will clearly increase the risk of house invasion by these species, and will therefore require more careful measures to avoid them. Similarly, siting a house distant from any potential source of vectors implies that less rigorous measures may be adequate. The second feature is the likely mode of entry of the vectors. Entry can be by crawling or flying, which may be inhibited by physical barriers such as window screens, or it may involve being carried passively into the house on humans or animals, or on materials brought into the house such as food and furniture. The third and fourth features relate to the restriction of vector access to potential food-sources and to the physical elimination of potential resting and breeding sites within the domestic and peri-domestic environment. Effective pest or vector control may require action on any or all of these features.

Location of the house

The risk of vectors and vector-borne disease rarely influences the decision on where to site a house, although settlement plans have been disrupted by vector-borne diseases in some areas – for example some new settlements in the Amazon region have been discouraged by the high malaria risk,[17] and some parts of West Africa have, in the past, become depopulated due to the high risk of river blindness (onchocerciasis).[18] Clearly however, the risk of invasion will influence the stringency of measures that should be applied to avoid vector invasion or colonization of houses.

Because water is needed for drinking and washing, houses must either be provided with a piped supply, a well or rain-water collection system, or else dwellings must be sited near a suitable source such as a communal stand-pipe, well, pond, stream, lake or river. Where these sites are also favoured by human-biting mosquitoes, biting midges (*Culicoides*, *Leptoconops*) or even blackflies (*Simulium*), it is unwise to locate houses within the flight range of these insects, unless the houses are adequately screened against mosquitoes or the breeding sites are controlled by insecticides or environmental methods.[19] Exposed water of any type is likely to serve as a breeding site for a range of insects and some, even though not blood-suckers, may become an abundant nuisance, especially moth-flies and midges whose cast pupal skins may provoke allergies. [20]

Different mosquito species tend to be associated with particular types of water. Some are efficient colonizers of even the most temporary rainwater pools, completing their development from egg to adult in as few as seven days. Others prefer more permanent waters such as the margins of larger ponds and lakes. Generally, during the development of human settlements, the nature of exposed water bodies changes, often promoting a succession of mosquito species of different habits and different capacities to transmit disease. In the Amazon region for example, new settlements have arisen at points where inadequate drainage of transverse streams and borrow pits along the highway have resulted in extensive shallow pools. Such pools have become good breeding sites for *Anopheles darlingi*, with a consequent rise in malaria transmission.[21] However, around older settlements, where exposed waters have become successively more polluted through human activities, fewer *An. darlingi* are now found by comparison with other mosquito species.

Despite the tendency of females of most malaria vectors to enter houses at night in search of a blood meal, and often to rest indoors during the day, nearly all these mosquito species breed in pools and swamps some distance from houses. Thus it is usually people living in rural areas or on the outskirts of urban centres who are most vulnerable to the nightly immigration of these mosquitoes. An exception is *An. stephensi* in urban areas in the Middle East and India, which has adapted to breeding in wells and water-storage tanks both indoors and outdoors, giving rise to an increase in malaria incidence in cities such as Bombay and Karachi. Strict surveillance supported by legislation has proved effective in compelling householders in affected areas to cover water tanks and to treat wells with larvicides to eliminate mosquito breeding-sites.[22] The larvicides should of course be non-toxic if the wells are still in use. The versatile malaria vector *An. arabiensis* may also be adapting to urban conditions in some West African cities,[23] a process which could be retarded by appropriate house design.

Restricting access of vectors

Table 9.2 summarizes some of the factors affecting mosquitoes biting or resting indoors.[24] The tendency of most flying insects, especially mosquitoes, to fly upwards on encountering an obstruction such as a house wall, means that the eaves under a roof – as well as holes in the wall, open windows and doors – are important points of entry into a house. These can be screened to prevent entry of flying insects, but efficient screens can severely restrict ventilation and, for this reason, are not generally used except in houses with alternative means of air-conditioning (as in parts of the southern USA) or in areas with constant year-round problems of mosquitoes and high incidence of mosquito-borne disease. For efficient screens, mesh apertures must be less than 1.2 millimetres (mm) to keep out mosquitoes, but the smaller biting midges and some sandflies can penetrate much finer screens down to 0.2 mm aperture. Cotton netting, which is most efficient but prone to damage, can restrict airflow by up to 70 per cent. Metal screens are less restrictive of airflow, but in humid areas they can corrode rapidly (except for stainless steel mesh, which is prohibitively expensive). Plastic mesh is better for window screens, but still reduces airflow by up to 35 per cent.[25]

Table 9.2: Factors increasing (+) or decreasing (–) the likelihood of mosquitoes biting and resting inside houses

	Anophelines	*Culicines*
Elevation	+	–
Isolation of house	+	–
Water containers indoors	–[1]	+
Proximity to streams/lakes	+	+
Windows open/unscreened	+	+
Eaves open/unscreened	+	+
Walls open/damaged	+	+
Ceiling present	–	–
Bednets in use	–	–
Woodsmoke indoors	–	–
Pyrethrum burning	–	–
Use of other insecticides	–	–

[1]+ for urban *Anopheles stephensi* in Middle East, India, Pakistan

Source: Based on G.B. White, "Factors influencing densities of mosquitoes resting indoors", Annual Report of the East African Institute of Malaria and Vector-borne Diseases, 1969, p. 37.

Where the eaves of a house cannot be blocked or screened because of the need to ventilate the roof space, an alternative is to fit some form of ceiling. Even where the house structure or personal preferences of the householder would not permit construction of a solid ceiling of wood, or of sticks and clay, an effective alternative is to fit a lightweight ceiling of hessian-type cloth or woven matting. This can bar mosquitoes from access to people sleeping in the room below – acting, in a sense, as a permanent communal bednet.[26] In houses with corrugated metal roofs, ceilings have the added advantage of reducing the heat radiated inside from the roof. In contrast, a ceiling can make a thatched house less comfortable by reducing ventilation. In a survey of 475 villagers in Tanzania, several other advantages and disadvantages of ceilings were given, with 86 per cent of those who had fitted some form of ceiling citing exclusion of mosquitoes as one of the reasons for constructing it.[27]

However, if the ceiling is of fairly solid construction – such as plywood or board, or sticks sealed with rendered clay – this can transform the roof space into a habitat for birds and small mammals such as rats, mice, opossums, bush-babies and bats. These are inconvenient and can cause structural damage to the house, as well as acting as reservoirs of disease and as additional food sources for blood-sucking insects. In Latin America, unfortunately, the roof space above a ceiling can also provide an excellent habitat for triatomine bugs.

Many domestic arthropods can also be carried into the house on other animals, with baggage, or with items of food or furniture. Ectoparasites such as fleas, lice and follicle mites (*Demodex*) gain access by their close association with domestic animals. In Latin America, triatomine bugs can gain access to houses by active flight,[28] by passive carriage as small nymphs and eggs amongst the feathers of birds such as house sparrows,[29] and by being carried in the luggage and clothing of people visiting from other areas.[30] Bedbugs can also be transported in the sleeping mats of visitors, and – even in temperate climates – can be passed from house to house in cracks in second-hand furniture. Bedbugs (Cimicids) and Triatomine bugs can both survive for several months without feeding. As a result, they can disperse through the sale of second-hand furniture from infested premises, and may even spread in furniture stores amongst different items offered for sale.[31]

Restriction of food sources

Those insects and mites that live in permanent contact with their vertebrate hosts, such as mites and lice, are best treated as medical conditions. Prevention of further infections however, will be assisted by provision within the house of suitable washing facilities, and by provision of adequate sleeping quarters such that, for example, children are not required to share the same bed or sleeping mat. Overcrowding, leading to close physical contact while ectoparasites are at their most active, can facilitate the transmission of arthropod ectoparasites between family members. However, most ectoparasites are not actually transmitted on clothing or bed linen, because they survive for only a very short time away from their hosts.[32]

For other domestic and peri-domestic arthropods, restricted access to food sources is an important way of minimizing their numbers. For scavenging insects, it is particularly important to disallow access to stored foodstuffs and to provide adequate disposal for organic wastes, because scavenging insects – especially houseflies and cockroaches – can readily transmit disease pathogens from one to the other. Pathogens from faeces carried by houseflies and cockroaches probably contribute significantly to health problems such as childhood diarrhoea, a major cause of child mortality in many countries. In more affluent communities these hygienic measures can be achieved by the use of refrigerators and screened foodstores with insecticidal fumigation where appropriate, and the provision of closed refuse containers (protected from physical damage by rats, mice and other animals) and well-maintained toilets.[33] Such measures, combined with vigorous public health advertising, contributed to the decline in housefly populations in Europe during the 1950s. Elsewhere, traditional styles of housing and lower family income levels may limit the possibilities for pest control by these methods, but community health programmes should inform and encourage householders to minimize insect pests by preventing access to both food and waste.

In agricultural communities, protection of stored products is primarily to prevent climatic damage and losses due to birds, rodents and other small mammals. These small animals often act as reservoirs of disease, and are often associated with insects which can bring these diseases into the domestic environment. Important examples include bubonic plague transmitted by rat fleas, and some forms of Chagas' disease transmitted by triatomine bugs in Latin America. It is clearly desirable that stored products be adequately protected, and should preferably be sited in outhouses away from living quarters.

Domestic animals should also be housed away from the house itself, thus removing one source of litter and waste from the house and also reducing the number of blood sources in a house available for blood-sucking insects. Care must be taken that the outhouses and animal enclosures do not also become resting and breeding sites for pest insects. For goat corrals in the Argentine *chaco* for example, wire-fencing should be preferred to traditional brushwood because the latter can provide a good habitat for blood-sucking triatomine bugs.[34] In Latin America, domestic populations of triatomine bugs are primarily regulated by the size and numbers of available hosts, and removal of each domestic animal is likely to cause a corresponding reduction in bug population size.[35] Domestic cats and dogs also serve as reservoir hosts for the pathogen which causes Chagas' disease. Provision for these animals to sleep outside the house is therefore likely to reduce both the size of the bug population and the proportion infected with the disease.

The regulation of mosquito populations is less clearly understood, and it may be that most species are regulated primarily by access to bodies of water in which they can breed rather than to sources of blood. Moreover, it is not clear if reduction in the number of hosts within a house would reduce the number of mosquitoes attracted to feed in that house. However, it is sometimes possible to exploit the host preferences of some mosquito species for cattle and other livestock, and thus reduce the frequency with which they bite people. This tactic, known as "zooprophylaxis" is insufficient to interrupt transmission entirely, but can lead to reduced transmission of some mosquito-borne diseases. For example, many vectors of malaria are strongly attracted to cattle (e.g. *An. arabiensis* in Africa; *An. annulatus*, *An. culicifacies* and *An. maculatus* in South Asia), so rates of transmission fall significantly when more livestock are present as alternative hosts to humans. Some sandfly vectors of leishmaniasis are also less likely to enter the house to bite people if their preferred animal hosts are kept outside the house. Examples include the Indian species, *Phlebotomus argentipes*, which is attracted to cattle, as well as *Phlebotomus papatasi* and the South American *Lutzomyia longipalpis*, which are attracted to chickens and may breed in chicken houses.[36]

Screens, and mosquito nets over beds at night, can also be effective in preventing host access by nocturnal flying insects such as mosquitoes. Their effectiveness can be improved by impregnating the nets with insecticides such as permethrin. However, screens and nets are generally ineffective against insects that inhabit the bed or that gain access by crawling (such as argasid ticks or triatomine bugs). Such pests can be inhibited by hanging sleeping mats and bedclothes outside in the sunlight during the day, since many are unable to tolerate direct insolation.

Restriction of hiding places

All domestic arthtopods require a shaded undisturbed resting site within the house for part of their lives. Even for mosquitoes which normally bite outside the house, such as *An. darlingi*, at least a few minutes are spent resting on an interior surface before and after feeding.[37] Other domestic insects and ticks rest during their inactive phases in dark crevices in the floor, walls, roof, or under debris or in a similar type of habitat. In all cases, control campaigns may include fumigation or spraying the internal surfaces with residual insecticides, an approach which can be helped by the use of housing materials that offer a good non-absorbent surface for the action of such insecticides. Walls of unrendered earth, for example, tend to absorb the active ingredient very quickly, causing a rapid loss of insecticidal activity at the surface where the insect rests.[38] Similarly, thick roofs of thatch or brushwood can provide an open structure within which insects can rest but where insecticide sprays cannot reach. Some types of earth used in house walls, due to their extreme acidity or alkalinity, have the additional disadvantage of provoking chemical breakdown of some sprayed insecticides.

In areas of high risk for vector-borne diseases, where insecticide spraying campaigns may be required, housing materials and construction methods should be chosen to provide non-absorbent surfaces suitable for the insecticide, and to minimize areas where insecticide sprays would be unable to penetrate. The presence of domestic arthropods can also be discouraged directly by the use of materials that do not crack to provide resting sites, ensuring close fitting junctions between dissimilar materials, and allowing easy maintenance such as plastering over any cracks or holes that subsequently appear. Moreover, since most domestic arthropods are nocturnal and so require dark crevices in which to hide during the day, houses that are well ventilated and well lit – for example by adequate window openings – will discourage indoor resting insects. These design considerations apply equally to all parts of the house.

Low-cost design and construction

Attention to the design and construction of house foundations and floors, walls and the roof can help address problems with disease vectors.

A primary defect in many traditional houses is the absence of secure foundations. This imposes limits to the height and weight of wall and roof that can be supported, resulting in low houses with inadequate ventilation and dark interiors favouring domestic pests. Overweight walls and roofs may shift, causing damage or partial collapse – although paradoxically this can sometimes discourage domestic insects because of the resulting increase in ventilation and illumination. However, rainfall damage concentrated at the base of a wall can open up crevices, through which rodents and other pests may enter, and may undermine the walls suffiently to cause total collapse.

Foundations serve two main functions. They transfer load from the walls and roof uniformly to firm ground, and they serve as a shield preventing water damage to the base of the wall and the floor. To some extent, they may also inhibit termites. Wall foundations would probably be the single most important improvement to traditional houses, making the buildings more permanent, structurally safer, and so encouraging householders to make other improvements. Foundation footings should be embedded deep enough to reach root-free soil which will not be washed away by water. Usually, 30-40 centimetre depth will suffice for a single storey building, but in areas prone to water erosion and soil swelling a depth up to 1 metre or more may be required. Materials for footings can be compacted stones, soil-cement mortar, anthill or termite mound mortar, fired-clay bricks or compressed earth blocks (see below).

Good foundations will also allow a firm and level floor. In many styles of traditional house the floor is of beaten earth. This is cheap, easy to construct, and has some functional advantages such as absorption of spilt liquids. Cracked and uneven earth floors can provide refuges for house dust mites and flea larvae amongst the debris that accumulates in the cracks, and for argasid ticks (especially under sleeping mats). In Central America, *Triatoma dimidiata* – an important vector of *Chagas' disease* – also occurs commonly in cracks in the floor, and replacement of mud floors with smooth cement can significantly reduce house infestation with this vector.[39] In areas where wood is readily available, floors may be made of wooden planks – often raised on stilts to avoid flooding as in coastal parts of South-East Asia. The space under the floor, which is often used for storage, can provide refuge for small mammals, snakes, scorpions, spiders, cockroaches and other pests. In these cases, the underfloor space should be kept clear of stored products and debris, while the floor itself should be made of very close-fitting slats, or slats with ventilated spaces more than one centimetre wide which are unsuitable for resting insects.

Materials for house walls depend on the lifestle of the householders, their income levels, and on availability of local materials. Temporary shelters of nomads – such as the grass tents of some Amerindians or the leafy huts of West African Fulani – are rarely colonized by arthropods because of their temporary nature, but they provide little protection against insects such as houseflies and mosquitoes. Dwellings of a more substantial and permanent nature often provide a range of habitats for residential arthropods. In the high Andes of Chile and Bolivia, stones and earth are commonly used for the walls since timber is not readily available; the spaces between the stones are often occupied by cockroaches, spiders and triatomine bugs. Similarly, houses of split palm logs in the humid *chaco* of Paraguay offer excellent habitats for triatomine bugs within the fibrous inside of the logs. In Ecuador, houses of split bamboo suffer the same problem, as do houses in parts of South-East Asia which are sometimes colonized by *Triatoma rubrofasciata* (although Chagas' disease is not transmitted outside the New World).[40] In contrast, houses with walls formed entirely from wooden poles – as with those of Mayans in Central America – are rarely colonized by arthropods. This is probably because the poles are too widely spaced to offer suitably dark crevices for bugs and cockroaches, and also allow very good ventilation and good daytime illumination to the inside of the house. Darker houses of hewn planks or overlapping boards do provide good refuges for arthropods.

But the most widely used material for the walls of traditional–style houses is earth, either as mud pressed onto a framework of sticks and poles, or as adobe mud blocks held in place by a mud-based mortar. Such houses, common throughout savanna areas of Africa and Latin America, are very prone to cracking as the earth dries and shrinks, pulling away from wooden supports and the frames of doors and windows. This provides a multitude of dark, undisturbed cracks and crevices where insect pests and vectors thrive. Where the wall is otherwise sound, cracks can be filled and the wall rendered smooth with cement or lime-based plaster – often mixed with cow dung, sisal, straw, cotton waste or other fibre to give added resistance to cracking and powdering-off. Use of fresh cow dung in the mixture is traditional in the Indian subcontinent, and minimizes the requirement for water in the mix, but in experiments in Brazil it was found that this could give problems during certain seasons as dung beetles later emerged from the plaster leaving substantial holes.[41] Also, in experiments in Argentina, goat dung was found to be inferior to cow dung as an additive to low-cement plaster.[42] In addition to eliminating cracks in walls, plaster or other rendering can improve the aesthetic appearance of a house; light-coloured plaster will both reduce the rate of heat absorption on exterior surfaces as well as improving reflected illumination inside the house. Plaster also protects the wall surface from rain and wind, but for this reason is generally made of stronger material than the wall itself (e.g. with higher cement content). This means that the plaster and the wall will have different rates of movement in response to changing humidity, tending to cause the plaster to crack and flake off. Plaster rendering should therefore use material of a similar strength to the wall material, applied in two coats (with the first allowed to dry before applying the second). External plastering should also be protected from rain by an overhanging roof – as a rough guide, the roof overhang will protect down to three times its total width.

Where walls are unsound they should be replaced. Fired bricks and cement mortar can be used where available, and when income levels permit their purchase, but such materials are energy-expensive both in terms of fuel for the firing, and in terms of distribution cost. There are several alternatives, such as using lightweight sticks and mud rendered with heavy duty plaster – as in the improved *bahareque* in low-cost Venezuelan houses – or using stabilized earth methods.[43]

Earth used in construction must contain clay for cohesion, sand as a filler, and silt to provide fine particles. However, the clay portion of a soil will swell when taking in moisture and shrink when drying out, causing cracks to occur. For house construction, the earth can be stabilized against erosion, cracking and shrinkage by the addition of bitumen (to make asfadobe), cement (to make soil-cement), or lime. Stabilized earth can be further improved by compaction, either *in situ*, or to form blocks using a mechanical press.[44] *In situ* compaction is achieved by ramming successive layers of earth with wooden mallets between wooden formers, as in the French *pisé de terre* – widely used in parts of France, Spain and North Africa. A similar technique, known as *pisa tapial* or *taipa pilão* is also used in parts of Latin America – often with milk or animal blood added to increase cohesion of the rammed earth. In parts of France, especially around Grenoble, houses of two or three stories dating back a century or more testify to the usefulness of this technique – even in regions of high rainfall and winter frosts.

Block-making presses also produce building materials of a very high quality. All block-making presses follow a similar principle: sieved earth with up to 25 per cent clay content stabilized with a small proportion of lime or cement is loaded into a steel mould and compressed by the action of a hand-operated lever. Some versions allow power-operated levers. One of the earliest and best known hand-operated block-making press is the CINVA ram, developed in Colombia, which produces blocks of a standard size (290 x 140 x 100 mm) that can be used in construction in the same way as adobe blocks. More recently, the UK Building Research Establishment has developed an improved press, known as the BREPAK, in which compression exerted by the hand-operated lever is hydraulically assisted to produce a higher compaction pressure. The resulting blocks, of the same size as adobe blocks but considerably heavier, actually exceed minimum British Standard Specifications for fired clay bricks, in terms of load-bearing strength when wet.[45]

The superior performance of compressed soil blocks, and their ease of manufacture in local communities, could bring about considerable improvements in the quality of rural and urban housing throughout the world – both in arid and humid climates – and extensive field trials are now being conducted in several countries. Moreover experimental work suggests that by changing the type of mould in the press, blocks could be made of a size, shape and hardness suitable for floor and roof tiles, and for the liners of pit latrines and irrigation canals.[46] Used in wall construction, the blocks do not crack, and they bind well to soil-cement mortars to produce a structure without crevices where domestic pests can hide. Even where insecticides must be used against mosquitoes and other insects flying into a house to feed, the non-porous nature of the compressed soil blocks appears to offer a greatly improved surface for the action of residual insecticides, compared to adobe blocks made from the same material.[47] Inexpensive presses such as the CINVA ram and BREPAK are ideally suited to small-scale business enterprises or community co-operatives, where they can be moved from site to site to produce the blocks required for each building.[48] This is both simpler and cheaper in transport than distributing bulky construction materials from a central production site.

In regard to the roof, traditional styles of housing with an earth roof are still favoured by some communities, especially in the arid Sudan savanna and Sahelian belts of Africa. Like the earth walls, such roofs are prone to cracking, providing dark crevices that can be occupied by insect pests. More usually however, a timber framework supports a roof of thatch, tiles, or corrugated metal or fibrocement sheets. Thin unshaded roofs, exposed to direct sunlight, can heat up considerably during the day. This discourages insects although it can also make the house intolerably hot for the householders.

Thicker roofs of thatch offer better insulating properties but also provide good resting places for insects. A favoured hiding place for many house-resting and human-biting mosquitoes is within the exposed strands of thatch under an unlined roof. These hiding places closely resemble those amongst straw and leaves outside the house, but offer greater climatic protection and proximity to blood sources. Omer and Cloudsley-Thompson reported that in Sudan, females of *An. arabiensis* could survive for up to nine months during the extended dry season, sheltering in the roofing thatch during the day when outdoor temperatures were too high for them to survive.[49] In more northerly latitudes, some malaria vectors could winter indoors by resting on rafters, walls or under thatch, with intermittent blood-feeding that gave rise to the phenomenon of winter malaria in Europe before improved housing eliminated such problems.

In Venezuela, traditional roofs made of palm thatch pose a particular problem since the eggs of the Chagas' disease vector *Rhodnius prolixus* are often stuck to the palm fronds used in thatching. This can be an important source of domestic infestation and replacement of palm thatch with corrugated metal roofs has been an important factor in Chagas vector control in Venezuela.[50] In the Argentine *chaco* and parts of Bolivia, where nighttime temperatures can drop below 5°C, the traditional flat roofs are made from poles piled with brushwood and packed with earth. The resulting thick porous structure provides an ideal habitat for *Triatoma infestans*, into which insecticides cannot be sprayed even using motorized mist-blowers. Corrugated metal sheets are not favoured because in addition to heating up intolerably during the day, they provide no protection from the cold at night. Insulating layers of earth over the metal offer no solution because rapid corrosion results. A possible compromise would be the use of locally-made ceramic tiles of the type favoured in Brazil and lowland parts of Bolivia and Peru. The increasing use of such roofing tiles was an important part of the progressive improvement of housing which contributed to the decline of malaria transmission in Europe.[51]

Constraints to improved low-cost housing

As noted earlier, the necessity to improve low-cost housing is increasingly recognized, both as a developmental goal in itself, and also as an important contribution to improved health. In parallel, there have been welcome technical advances such as the use of compressed, stabilized earth-blocks for walls and floors, and fibre-reinforced sheets for roofing. A few selected examples have been given, but these factors do not complete the full spectrum of constraints to large-scale improvements to housing. Cost is a major factor, and with this is the question of who will pay. Here, key questions concern the perceptions and priorities of individual householders, and their relationship with state organizations which must motivate and assist in anv large-scale housing programme.

Human perceptions rarely differ in the generalities of what constitutes an ideal house, but often, low-income householders may feel that such standards are inappropriate or unobtainable for them. With this concept, they may accept their current living standards as appropriate to their particular class, and so lack motivation for their own role in improving living standards for themselves and their families. This is often reflected in perceptions of disease, where, for example, disease agents may be recognized but accepted within the natural order as inevitable, or not worth the investment or change in lifestyles required to avoid them.[52]

Studies in Venezuela on the role of house improvement as a means to limit domestic infestation by triatomine bugs show that the most important factor is to generate the belief in affected communities that they themselves can contribute to the improvement – that this is not merely a state intervention as represented by large-scale prefabricated constructions, or by periodic visits by sprayers to apply insecticides to control the bugs. The first task is to establish what are the main perceived requirements of the local communities – which might not include vector control or improved housing as key factors – and then to design participative programmes which satisfy perceived needs while incorporating those activities useful for health improvement. During the course of such programmes, health education can be carried out, leading to changes in perceived needs and greater emphasis on the health requirements. At the same time, those responsible for such programmes will then be satisfying the beneficiaries, rather than imposing a preconceived model of what ought to be done.

The role of the state in large-scale house improvement programmes for low-income communities is threefold: to establish secure tenure of land on which such programmes can be based, to mobilize teachers and community workers trained to respond appropriately to this level of development, and to open accessible lines of credit to those involved. One of the greatest barriers to progress at this level however, is the established approach of many bureaucracies which fail to accept this type of community programme. Often, the concept of large-scale authoritarian state intervention is preferred, with emphasis on the most "modern" of styles and materials. Such emphasis is often re-inforced by the interests of industrial cartels because profits are made from the manufacture or import of inappropriate materials such as steel and concrete. The result in many regions is that traditional skills of house design and construction may be lost, while innovative techniques using such materials are discouraged.[53] For similar reasons, the potential of low-cost house improvement for limiting vector-borne diseases and other health risks may also be dismissed by many poorly informed bureaucrats.

Some of the difficulties in sustaining effective vector control by insecticide spraying alone reflect the fact that no lasting change has been made to the environment exploited by the target insects. The finding of insects or other arthropods in a domestic or peri-domestic environment indicates clearly that the environment is appropriate for them. A transient change, such as making the environment toxic with insecticides, may inhibit the insect populations, but if that change cannot be sustained, then those insects will have the opportunity to return.

For vector-borne diseases such as Chagas' disease, where transmission is absolutely linked to the domestic environment, the potential of house improvement for vector control has long been recognized. Carlos Chagas himself raised the importance of this approach 80 years ago, soon after he first described the disease and its vectors. Similarly, house screening and personal protection with nets has long been recognized as a primary defense against mosquitoes[54] and against malaria,[55] while the idea of "building out malaria" was strongly advocated by Wilson in 1957 for malaria control in tropical Africa.[56] Techniques are now available to improve, at very low cost, the quality of urban and rural houses. The impact of such improvements on vector-borne diseases and other health indices has been demonstrated in numerous studies, and sociologists are now tackling the political and social constraints to large scale implementation of such developments. The emphasis must be on technical, state, and community participation – a process that is already exemplified by collaboration between vector-control specialists, sociologists, economists, epidemiologists and engineers. House improvement, at least on a large scale, is difficult to justify on the basis of disease control alone, but there can be no doubt that house improvements can contribute substantially to the control of a very wide range of diseases.

Chapter Ten

LIFE SAVING SERVICES

Greg Goldstein

Introduction

Only a small proportion of the Third World's urban population can obtain an ambulance in an emergency. Most cannot obtain rapid treatment from trained health personnel if they have some accident such as a burn, cut or scald, although the right kind of prompt treatment often saves lives and almost always greatly diminishes the extent of the injury or ill-health. In the event of a fire, a rapid public response with fire-fighting specialists and fire engines is rarely forthcoming, especially in illegal settlements. Meanwhile, most low-income people live in houses and settlements where serious accidents and emergencies are much more common because of the lack of infrastructure and services, the poor quality and overcrowded housing, and poor quality sites. Low-income people generally face the dual burden of housing and living environments which make them far more vulnerable to accidents and injuries, combined with little or no provision for emergency services in response to accidents.

As described in earlier chapters, high mortality and disability affects all ages from infancy to the elderly in low-income settlements. A major part of the high mortality and disability is related to accidents and injuries. Typical accidents and emergencies for any urban authority are fire, building collapse, violence, floods, motor vehicle crashes, and land or waste-slides. There are many instances where emergency interventions – medical personnel, rescue teams, fire-fighting or civil defence – could intervene to reduce the mortality and ill-health.

It can be argued that the emphasis in poor communities should be on preventing accidents rather than emergency services to deal with them when they do happen. The emphasis here on the importance of emergency services should not be construed as a bias against preventive measures, since both are needed. The high cost of emergency services to cope adequately with increasingly frequent small-scale accidents (collapse of dwellings, waste slides, traffic accidents, urban violence) has to be balanced by attention to improving social, economic and physical conditions to reduce people's vulnerability to accidents. Earlier chapters have stressed the improvements needed in physical conditions – major improvements in water, sanitation, drainage, garbage collection and control of disease vectors. But the very nature of most low income settlements means that there will always be a high risk of various accidents and emergencies, even if preventive measures are successfully implemented. Unexpected and sudden deaths have a demoralizing effect on a community that can undermine development efforts. Feelings of insecurity and anxiety are created by a lack of access to instant help when and where it is needed.

The high vulnerability of low-income groups

High vulnerability is a term for a high risk of death or disability.[1] It is associated with three factors: the site of the settlement; the physical environment; and the social environment. These are inter-related, and their importance varies from settlement to settlement. We shall see that the degree of access to emergency and medical services is related to all three factors, and to vulnerability. Box 10.1 lists various hazards ranging from earthquakes and landslides

Box 10.1: Local diagnosis of hazards and vulnerability

HAZARDS	FACTORS INFLUENCING VULNERABILITY
Earthquake	*Local conditions*:
	Location
	Topography/declivity
Landslide	Hydrography: water courses: tides, rates of flow
	Climate: rain and wind
	Ground: composition/stability
Storm	Ground cover (including forestation/vegetation)
	Built environment: landfill, industrial waste; fire ducts; water mains; culverts; pipelines (gas); electricity cables
Cyclone	

Box 10.1: (continued)

Disease Epidemic Sudden or severe illness Childbirth Falls Cuts Bites and stings Fights Terrorism Mugging Knife wounds Gunshot wounds	*Construction quality:* Slope management Building location Building: foundation and site structure; materials used; age and condition; maintenance Density of occupation (persons per room) Rooms per dwelling Facilities for cooking and storage *Infrastructure and Service Provision:* Electricity Cooking fuel Water supply Stormwater drainage Sewage disposal Garbage collection Emergency services (doctor, ambulance, fire) Access ways (both pedestrian and motor vehicle) Midwifery and community health Communications (e.g. telephones) Education and training *Social and economic factors:* Age Gender Income/employment Organization: groups and associations (including cultural groupings) Dangerous occupations or work areas (and protection practices in these) Familiarity with surroundings

to disease epidemics to falls and cuts and the factors that influence the population's vulnerability.

In rapidly growing urban areas, the availability of land is severely limited, especially for housing affordable by low-income groups. Many settlements develop on dangerous land-sites because such land is unsuitable for commercial or industrial developments and undesirable for wealthier social groups. This explains the large number of settlements which develop on land prone to flooding or tidal inundation (for instance Bombay, Delhi, Port Moresby, Bangkok, Guayaquil, Recife, Monrovia and Lagos), on hillsides prone to landslides and rock falls (Rio de Janeiro, Guatemala City, La Paz, Hong Kong, Medellin, Caracas), and on sandy deserts (Lima, Khartoum).

Box 10.2: Fire

Causes of fire include upset cooking-stoves, spilt gasoline or kerosene (used for cooking, heating or lighting) or leaking gas cylinders, and the tipping over of candles used for lighting or religious practices. Vulnerability to fire is extremely high in dwellings constructed of flammable material (wood, cardboard, plastic, canvas, straw), where uncollected waste material may be piled in open areas and burnt for clearance, and where dwellings are constructed very close together.

Chapter 1 outlined how a high proportion of low-income urban inhabitants live in settlements which developed illegally. In these (and in some legal housing developments) the buildings may be constructed with no consideration of the overall capacity and layout of the site. The result is often a very dense settlement, with the houses crammed together, a lack of recreational space, narrow paths or streets as the only means of access, inadequate provision of drainage and water supply, and inadequate street lighting. Pedestrian access may be limited to narrow spaces between buildings; vehicular access may be severely restricted or impossible. The only public utilities available may be those arising from illegal connections – for instance to overhead electricity cables or to water mains. These conditions increase the risks of falls, burns, cuts, bites and accidental poisoning.

The risks are further increased by poor construction quality, inadequate slope management in hillside settlements, inappropriate building materials and methods of construction, and reliance on open fires or unguarded stoves for lighting and cooking. Many low-income settlements have no service to remove garbage and this often means an accumulation of waste heaps which can lead to waste-slides and increased problems of flooding as the wastes block drainage ditches.

Box 10.3: Building collapse

In Rio de Janeiro, 40 per cent of accidents attended in the *favelas* (illegal settlements) are caused by building collapse and another 30 per cent by landslides. Many of Rio's *favelas* developed on the steep slopes of rocky outcrops which are common within the city. Building collapse is endemic in low-income areas. Dwellers who have migrated from rural areas where they built on flat sites are ill-informed about building techniques needed for urban sites on steep slopes. A dwelling owner in Rio may sell the roof slab of his house for the construction of another dwelling, and this owner in turn will sell his roof for another, and so on. There has been one case of nine dwellings built against a steep hillside in this way. Dwellers lack the knowledge to deal with problems such as surface water drainage, pedestrian access, and danger of collapse in construction of dwellings built on the roofs of other dwellings.

Recently, attention has been drawn to a third aspect of the vulnerability of urban low-income communities, namely social deviance, criminal behaviour and mental illness, which are manifestly more common than in wealthier areas of the city. The cause of these problems is complex; they cannot be attributed only to poor housing or environmental conditions, although these certainly contribute to these problems. Alleviation of poverty and an improvement in the urban environment would not solve these problems, but could be expected to reduce them. Street violence is a major health issue in many settlements and accounts for a substantial proportion of injuries and medical emergencies. While all injuries require

Box 10.4: Landslides

Landslides may themselves be induced by inappropriate construction and land formation techniques. Low-income households' anxiety to find sites for dwelling construction often lead to house construction on steep slopes. But this is often done with inadequate site preparation and with site excavation and filling which breaks

Box 10.4: (continued)

the natural balance of slopes and which causes instability, and eventually landslides. Such landslides often involve several dwellings at a time. This process is made worse over time by the action of surface water. Another form of landslide is that caused by unstable waste accumulation which may accrue over many years in the absence of a removal service. Eventually the waste heap slides down the slope, causing property damage, injury and death.

treatment without excessive delay, rapid treatment for penetrating knife or bullet wounds is particularly vital, and the time between injury and treatment is often literally a matter of life or death.

Access to services

Compounding all the above problems are inadequacies in first aid and in emergency and medical services. Often the main cause of death is the delay in moving the injured to hospital. All too often, inhabitants of low-income urban areas find that access to life-saving services is difficult or restricted, for a range of physical, logistic, financial, legislative, social or cultural reasons. Compared to a promptly treated injury, any injury that does not receive prompt attention, whether it is a minor burn, cut or sting, or major road trauma, gunshot, knife wounds, or electrocution, is of greater significance and threat. It results in greater mortality, slower recovery, and greater chance of long term disability. In this way the neglected

Box 10.5: Floods

Floods in urban areas can be caused both by abnormally high rainfall in areas with properly constructed drainage systems, and by less abnormal rainfall in areas without such systems. Tidal flooding, storms or high tides, and river flooding, extend the range of areas subject to flooding. The increased vulnerability to flooding for many low-income groups is a result of their settlements developing in areas prone to flooding, which would be better left unoccupied. The fact that so many low-income groups are priced out of the

Box 10.5: (continued)

legal real estate market leads to illegal housing developments on sites prone to flooding. This in turn can lead to the construction of river banks to protect these which can then cause overflow in other areas, with consequent backing up of sewage outfall, drains and culverts. Maintenance of the river and river banks may be impeded by riverside settlement construction. The disposal of solid wastes into rivers may cause obstruction of flow. Lack of adequate solid-waste collection and disposal is a major factor in local flooding in many cities because a substantial amount of the uncollected waste enters and clogs the drains. Floods not only cause drownings and property damage, but also bacterial contamination of clean water supplies and food, and are commonly associated with outbreaks of infectious diseases.

injury is of greater threat to family livelihood and food security.

It is often difficult or impossible for medical, ambulance or rescue crews to reach the site of an accident. Houses are often built in such close proximity to each other that only pedestrians can pass between them. Road vehicles may not be able to reach settlements built on steep slopes or in areas prone to flooding which have no internal all-weather roads and often no all weather roads connecting them to the city. Ambulances cannot attend a critically ill person, fire services cannot get close to fires and police vehicles are impeded. Sometimes access is restricted because of social barriers – for example different social or ethnic groups may be excluded from a particular service. In illegal settlements, the responsible government authority may not wish to supply services of any kind because to do so would imply official acceptance or recognition of the settlements. Or services may only be available at a price which is beyond the means of the patient or his or her immediate family.

Box 10.6: Industrial disasters

Industrial development may bring many bonuses, but it also opens up new possibilities of accidents involving transport accidents,

Box 10.6: (continued)

chemical spills, fires and explosions, toxic wastes (including gases), and mass poisonings. A few dramatic events of recent years, including the accidental release of chemicals at Bhopal (1984) and Seveso (1976), the gas explosions in Mexico City (1984) and the explosion of the nuclear power station at Chernobyl (1986), as well as many other close calls, have served to draw public, governmental and expert attention to the growing problem. In all countries, industry is using larger quantities of dangerous raw materials in more advanced and complex production systems. Increasing quantities of explosive, toxic and radioactive materials, whether manufactured locally or imported, are stored, transported, used in industrial processes and then disposed of. The use of these materials is important for economic growth and development, but poses serious additional risks to the health and safety of nearby populations, as well as to the natural and human environment. These risks are in addition to the danger of extreme natural events (floods, earthquakes and the like) with which they may act synergistically. It is in the Third World regions with rapid urban population-growth that urban planners face the greatest problems in managing urban expansion and in so doing, limiting the risks arising from the close proximity of people, industrial production and pollution, risks accentuated by poverty.

Reduction in vulnerability

A reduction in vulnerability requires both environmental improvements and the improved availability of emergency life-saving services. A key requirement in both cases is a programme of what may be termed urban regularization involving (a) improvement in the security of tenure for the inhabitants of low-income settlements, with more recognition by local authorities of the rights of the inhabitants to basic housing; and (b) the provision of basic infrastructure and services. As other chapters have outlined, there are many cost-effective ways to improve this provision through community organizations and local governments working together.

The legal provision of electricity to low-income settlements by the electricity authorities, rather than inhabitants illegally tapping overhead cables may bring a reduction in the number of fires. Garbage collection may reduce the number of outbreaks of disease, as well as the scale and number of waste heaps and the frequency of waste slides. Sewers and storm-water drainage, essential for slope stabilization and flood control, can be constructed jointly by the community and the authorities if the inhabitants acquire secure tenure, and thus feel that it is worth their time and effort to improve the site.

Community provision of emergency services

Residents in crowded urban settlements often organize themselves to take immediate action against fires. Such effective self-help may be extended to the provision of other services. In Cebu City, the Philippines, a volunteer group serves as an emergency bucket brigade to control fires, and also provides first aid for accidents such as cuts and falls, and to victims of electrocution. In the control of fires, the first three minutes is the most critical period, for fires can usually be controlled at this stage by two or three persons. After 15 minutes the group reports that a fire may involve entire houses and require a whole community to control it, using a bucket relay. An early fire-alarm system and the prompt use of a bucket brigade can be more effective than a delayed response with fire trucks and heavy pumps.

But regularization and community participation alone may not be sufficient to reduce vulnerability. What is needed is the establishment and continued operation of an institution dedicated to the provision of access to life-saving services.

Box 10.7: Types of emergency by initiating event and the role of paramedics

Initiating event	Health consequences	Importance of paramedic role[1] (+=low; 3+=high)
A. Individual emergencies		
Falls	Head injury	+
Road accidents	Spine injury	2+

Box 10.7: (continued)

Knife wounds Gun shot wounds	Abdomen injury	+
	Chest injury	2+
	Fractured limbs	2+
	Laceration and haemorrhage	2+
Fire, heat and smoke exposure	Scalds	2+
	Burns (graded by percentage of body affected)	2+
Diseases	Coma, metabolic and severe infections	+
	Respiratory failure	+
	Circulatory failure	+
Childbirth	Obstetric emergencies	2+
Poisoning	Coma, fits, etc.	3+
Drowning	Cardiac, respiratory arrest	3+
Electrocution	Cardiac disturbance	3+
Bites (dogs, wild animals, snakes)	Laceration, envenomation, infection	2+
B. Mass emergencies		
Epidemics		
Natural hazards (floods, earthquakes, landslides		
Industrial and transport accidents		
Riots and social disorders		

[1]In all instances of serious injury, the paramedic has the very important role of advising whether the patient must attend hospital for emergency treatment. The rating + means it is probable that there is little, apart from referral to hospital, that the paramedic can do, while 3+ means there are key paramedic procedures available that affect the survival rate.

The organization of an urban emergency service

The following description is based upon Rio de Janeiro's experience, but it serves as a useful model that could be adapted for other cities with low income and illegal settlements, to take account of other social and cultural contexts. One of the most important characteristics of an effective emergency service is the appropriate involvement of numerous sectors and organizations, particularly in regard to the activities set out under preventive measures and rehabilitation.

In Rio de Janeiro, the emergency organization consists of three main components:

i) A co-ordination system formed by a small number of persons with some background in emergency assistance. The system operates 24-hours per day in a telecommunications office, receiving calls for assistance and relaying them to an Emergency Co-ordinator. The office serves as a central point where the community can request help for any emergency, and it activates the agencies responsible for emergency assistance.

ii) A board of representatives of all appropriate government agencies, including the municipal secretariat and executive sectors, and relevant commercial, academic and public organizations. The board activates community assistance agencies and reviews emergency plans. It is responsible for ensuring that there are satisfactory arrangements to cope with both small-scale and large-scale emergencies. For instance, if it is found that patients from a particular community requiring emergency medical treatment are being denied access to services at a local hospital, it will discuss the matter with the hospital board and/or secure alternative arrangements for the emergency cases.

iii) A Council of non-government organizations, often chaired by a representative of the local Red Cross or Red Crescent organization, which serves as a link between the government and non-government services in emergency and disaster prevention and relief activities.

An effective emergency service has four components: prevention, relief, support and rehabilitation. The scope of each component is outlined in Box 10.8. There is considerable overlap in each of these components and the actions undertaken in each re-inforce the effectiveness of the others. For example the availability of an effective emergency service provides a nucleus of people which can advise low-income households and their community organizations on preventive measures against accidents and disasters.

Successfully implementing these four components will require community participation in diagnosis, planning, implementation and evaluation. The emergency service should take a supporting role in regard to existing community efforts at prevention and not try to bypass these and start anew. Implementation of preventive measures through environmental improvement is best achieved through hiring people from within the community, who act as organizers, advisors and motivators. The benefits of large post-disaster investments are much less, per unit investment, than the benefits of long-term programmes for urban improvements in which the dweller is able to take part.

Box 10.8: The four components of an effective emergency service

1. Preventive measures for communities and for local governments

Housing and community level activities	*Local authority measures*
Raising awareness of the community and local government	Analyze, evaluate and plan: – inspection of critical areas
Public orientation campaigns	– preventive works
Distribution of books, manuals and leaflets	– removal and eradication of critical dangers
Programmes for schools and community associations to disseminate self-protection procedures and techniques	– inventory of resources – selection of shelter areas
Support for the organization of urban primary health care and similar community initiatives	– access way improvements – communications provision and maintenance (e.g. public telephones)
Maintenance, clearance and removal of obstacles in access ways.	

2. Relief and support measures for local government with community participation in the event of an emergency

Relief action	*Support action*
Rescuing affected people	Shelter for affected, evacuated and endangered people
Evacuation of endangered people	First evaluation of damage and ensuing risks

Box 10.8: (continued)

Emergency medical assistance	Clearance of access ways
Vaccination of people threatened by contamination	Support to assistance agencies
	Dissemination of information for public guidance
	Support for community participation

3. Support measures after the emergency

Community measures	*Local authority Measures*
Screening and recording	Re-establishment of essential public services
Finding of missing persons	Clearing and removal of rubble
Identification of dead and injured	Evaluation of damage
Collection and protection of goods and possessions	
Public information stations	
Medical care at hospital units	
Improvement of shelter and food provision	
Management of donations	

4. Rehabilitation measures for restoration and prevention

Restoration measures	*Preventive measures*
Restoration of public and private services	Identification and implementation of preventive measures, according to damage sustained such as:
Re-establishment of social morale	slope retention, dredging of rivers and channels, improved building construction
Re-establishment of the economy	
Housing repair and construction	Provision of public and private services
Help with legal problems (e.g. landlords, insurance companies)	Evaluation of all measures undertaken in order to improve civil defence planning for prevention and relief assistance

The interests of victims and the community must be protected both in emergencies and in preventive action. Immediately after an accident, different internal and external groups clash in seeking to profit from the situation: potential community leaders attempt to assert their authority; former landlords try to repossess property; developers seek land for the real-estate market; politicians try to gain favour with their constituents; religious leaders offer spiritual assistance; and experts demonstrate their technology and attempt to test and introduce innovations. Not surprisingly, victims' rights are often overwhelmed by these intrigues.

The credibility of emergency-service workers will be improved by their provision of protection for dwellers' belongings when accidents occur. Victims may endanger themselves through reluctance to leave the site of a flood or fire, because they fear their possessions will be stolen. There must be organized prevention of looting, with storage and protection of household belongings and identification of the owners. It is important for the emergency service to establish trust and a clear identity for any proposed assistance. Low-income settlement dwellers will primarily relate to an outsider by asking "What do these people want to take?" or "What do they have to offer?". Militarized civil defence or emergency services may be confused with the police, and create suspicion. Where services have previously acted with police support on activities such as resettlement with removal of dwellings, there may be an insurmountable loss of trust.

An emergency medical service

An emergency medical service may develop as a component of an urban community primary health care or neighbourhood health programme. There is no established blueprint for neighbourhood health programmes; different models exist in different cities and to be effective, they must adapt to local conditions. The World Health Organization has recently published a book on urban primary health care that explains some of the key characteristics of successful urban primary health care.[2] Urban primary health-care encompasses not only health services, but also organized community efforts at environmental improvements such as a secure, safe water-supply, and prevention strategies such as immunization and improved nutrition. Neither the exclusively community-managed self-help health programme, nor the paternalistic government-sponsored and imposed programme are ideal. Success is more likely with a health care system set up and run in partnership between community and government. This implies a willingness on the part of government authorities to co-operate with popular action.

Governments will usually face more problems in developing such partnerships in settlements which lack community organizations and which have a transient population. Primary health-care programmes are very difficult to organize among constantly changing urban populations for without strong links between community members, the struggle for individual survival may take precedence over collective activities for the common good of the community. Special difficulties will be encountered in areas which have a high proportion of cheap rental accommodation (for instance inner-city tenements, areas with cheap boarding houses and illegal settlements which have a high proportion of tenants). Many urban primary health-care projects have developed as an offshoot of another community enterprise: an income-generating scheme (such as small-scale stores or food sellers), water-supply schemes, a transport or food co-operative, a crêche or a health card (insurance) system for health care. Social development initiatives must identify such projects and give their implementers the skills to run them by themselves, leading to the experience of success and recognition. Primary health-care projects by themselves may dry up sooner or later unless they address issues which may have a higher priority for the community than health status.

The key to an effective emergency medical service is a health-worker, capable of giving emergency treatment of wounds, burns, and poisoning and resuscitation, and able to determine when hospital treatment is needed. Such a person should co-ordinate a stretcher service provided by the community itself, which is set up to transport an injured or unconscious patient to the nearest pickup point for an ambulance, or to a local hospital if there is one nearby. The well-known WHO publication, "The Community Health Worker", is a practical guide for the training of community workers in these techniques.[3] Liaison with a hospital is an essential component of an emergency service, and ideally the hospital emergency service should offer training in emergency first-aid to health workers and other community leaders who might organize an emergency service.

Chapter Eleven

THE FUTURE CITY

Jorge E. Hardoy and David Satterthwaite

Conditions in Third World cities are much better documented today than they were only 20 or 30 years ago. Despite great diversity between nations and cities in the scale and nature of urban change, certain problems have been shown to be common to most Third World cities: a high proportion of people with incomes too low to allow them to meet their basic needs and living in very poor quality housing with little or no provision for infrastructure and services essential for health; little or no protection for workers from unsafe workplaces and over-long working hours; high levels of air and water pollution and inadequate controls over industrial wastes, including the monitoring, collection and disposal of toxic and hazardous wastes; and a haphazard, unplanned pattern of urban expansion. Most such problems are linked to the failure of government to provide an effective regulatory and planning framework which addresses the problems of poorer citizens and protects the urban environment (and the environment in the region around the city) from contamination with pathogens and pollutants. One of the root causes is the lack of power and resources allowed to city and municipal authorities by higher levels of government, despite the fact that they have been allocated most of the responsibilities for housing, infrastructure, services and the control of pollution.

The purpose of this chapter is to consider the future city in the Third World. The broad context within which it will be constructed and the main actors in its construction are known with some certainty. Based on this, it is possible to consider the differences between an urban future with no changes in government attitudes and policies and an urban future which could result from new attitudes and approaches.

The context for the future city

Chapter 1 described current conditions and trends in urban areas of the Third World. In most nations, rapid urban growth will continue – at least in the next 10–20 years. The scale of future urban growth may have been exaggerated, as has the demographic importance of the so called mega-cities within the total urban population; analyses of recent census data suggest that most of the Third World will be less urbanized and far less dominated by "mega-cities" than that predicted by most of the general literature on urban development.[1] The growth rates for urban populations in many nations have slowed considerably in the last inter-census period compared to previous decades; the economic climate apparent in most Third World nations during the 1980s suggests their urban populations will have grown more slowly than anticipated by most governments and international agencies, when results from censuses taken in the years 1988–91 become available. Population growth rates in many of the Third World's largest cities or metropolitan areas have also slowed in recent years and new, more decentralized patterns of urban development have become evident within the core economic regions of some of Third World's more urbanized nations.[2] This implies that only a small proportion of the Third World's population is likely to live in very large cities, even looking ahead 30 years or more.

However, most Third World societies are likely to continue urbanizing; the economic, social and political factors driving the move to a more urban society are too strong to stop, even if their power may diminish. A few of the more urbanized Third World nations may stop becoming increasingly urban but this will probably be more a reflection of new urban patterns than de-urbanization.[3]

The population growth confronting many municipal, city and metropolitan authorities will also be of a scale for which there are very few precedents. Dozens of city or metropolitan administrations will be faced with populations growing by more than 100,000 inhabitants a year; only in very few instances have urban authorities in Western nations ever had to face such a scale of urban growth in one location. When such rapid growth took place in the West it was usually in national or provincial capital cities with buoyant economies and well-developed local government structures.

Hundreds of weak and ineffective city and local governments in the Third World will be faced with populations within their jurisdictions growing at between 20,000 and 100,000 inhabitants a year. Very few cities in Europe and North America face this scale of growth and again, virtually all those that do are rich and successful cities with well-resourced city governments. There are hundreds of urban centres in the Third World which have grown from a few thousand inhabitants 30–40 years ago to between 100,000 and 250,000 inhabitants today, but with local governments whose form, mode of operation and resource base has changed little to reflect the fundamental change in the scale and nature of the entity they are meant to plan and manage. In the Third World, most of the nations urbanizing more slowly (usually poorer nations suffering prolonged economic stagnation or those already predominantly urban) still have steadily-growing urban populations arising from natural increase.

A second characteristic common to most Third World nations will be a minor role for government and the conventional (or legal) private sector in the construction of new housing. It is common for between 30 and 60 per cent of the population of cities to live in houses and neighbourhoods which have been developed illegally, and in most cities between 70 and 95 per cent of all new housing is built illegally. Neither government nor the conventional private sector has contributed much to the construction of housing, to the installation of basic residential infrastructure (roads, water supply, sewers, drains, pathways) or to the provision of basic services like health care, garbage collection and street cleaning.

A minor current and future role for conventional private-sector enterprises is easily understood. Most of the population cannot afford to buy or rent even the cheapest legal house or apartment. In most cities, there is a large and varied illegal (or informal) private sector selling or renting land for housing (or housing itself) and renting rooms. In many cities, the scale of these operations, both in terms of the number of enterprises and the money involved makes them more important than legal operations. The fact that they are illegal (or extra-legal) means serious problems for those who buy or rent housing or land since their rights are not protected by law. In addition, illegal housing and land developments do not conform to building and planning codes and the quality of the houses or rooms rented or sold is usually very poor (with great inadequacies in the provision of infrastructure and services). Informal or illegal private sector enterprises often sell water, health services and garbage collection but here too, standards are often poor and unit costs high.

The minor role for government is usually the result of national governments' refusal to allow local governments the powers, resources and representative nature they need to be effective. Innovative projects have demonstrated that low-income people can be reached with piped water, improved sanitation and drainage, health services and other improvements at low per capita costs and with good cost recovery. They have also shown how poor households can afford to repay small, flexible loans for the purchase of land and the construction or improvement of housing, and how loan schemes which meet their needs can obtain good levels of cost recovery and very low levels of loan default.[4] Such innovative projects reach only a tiny proportion of those in need. Most have been carried out by community organizations or non-governmental organizations, not governments. Innovative primary health programmes in urban areas are also mostly undertaken by NGOs or international agencies.[5]

In most Third World nations, economic circumstances are unlikely to change for the better in terms of increasing the poor's capacity to pay for housing and health services. It is unrealistic to expect that most governments will increase the scale of funding for housing, basic infrastructure and services to a point where it begins to match the scale of need. Even under the most optimistic scenarios for economic recovery, most governments will continue to lack the economic and institutional capacity to provide the majority of urban dwellers with water piped to their homes, sewers, drains, paved roads and pathways, health care and emergency services. For most nations, only decades of sustained rapid economic growth could provide the potential to afford this. Building local government's institutional capacity is also a long process even with economic prosperity and the political commitment to strong representative local government.There are also special problems on the periphery of existing cities, where most urban growth takes place. These are often within the jurisdiction of suburban municipal governments who are far weaker economically, politically and technically than more central and better- established municipalities.

For the few nations whose economic performance creates the possibility of larger public investments in urban infrastructure and services, it remains uncertain whether national governments will allocate sufficient resources either to improve housing conditions or to set up the local government structure to allow its implementation. It is notable that in Seoul in South Korea, during a period when the economy underwent one of the most rapid and sustained expansions achieved anywhere in the world, housing conditions for the poorer groups deteriorated.[6]

A third characteristic of past and current urban development in the Third World, evident for more than 30 years, is a minor role for international agencies in providing the funding for urban development. The current level of funding from aid and development-assistance agencies is so small in relation to need that even if current levels were multiplied severalfold (which is very unlikely), it would still make little impact. At present, most multilateral and bilateral development-assistance agencies allocate less than six per cent of their funds to primary health-care (including improved water supply and sanitation, immunization, health education and community-level health services) and less than two per cent to other kinds of project aimed at improving housing and living conditions and basic service provision.[7] Despite the inadequate levels of government investment in urban housing and infrastructure in the Third World, this still represents around 30 times that provided by international agencies.[8]

A fourth characteristic which will continue to shape most Third World cities is legal barriers to providing poorer groups with infrastructure and services. The fact that most new housing and neighbourhoods in major cities have been built illegally on illegally-occupied or sub-divided land introduces a complication into the provision of infrastructure and services. The provision of public services would imply some legal recognition of the inhabitants' right to be there.

The main actors in building and financing the future city

To a large extent, the future city will be financed, built and shaped by people with low incomes – garbage collectors or scavengers, shoemakers, peddlers, those making clothes, foods and crafts in their homes, maids, low-paid government clerks, office messengers and drivers, low paid factory-workers, shoe-shiners, market sellers and others. These people provide the cheap labour and cheap goods and services on which much of the city's economy depends. But they are excluded from legal land and housing markets, legal health services and very often legal markets for water and transportation.

These are also the people who will manage most new city developments. The city's expansion will be much influenced by where such people can obtain land on which to organize the construction of their houses – usually through negotiation with landowners, developers or those who traditionally allocate rights to occupy land. In some instances, collective action may allow them to obtain land without negotiation – for instance, in the case of land invasions – but the political circumstances which allow these to succeed are unusual.

Much of this future city will be financed by informal loans and by the residents' own self-help efforts in building, maintaining or expanding their dwellings. Employment patterns, houses and settlements will reveal the inventiveness, resilience and ingenuity of the millions of poor people whose main skills are their capacity to survive under very difficult circumstances.

The Third World city of the 1990s will be a city of young people. In most cities, children and adolescents will make up most of the population. Many will go to work well before the minimum age established by national legislation because the incomes they earn are crucial parts of family survival. Most will not have completed primary school. The contribution that even small children working for very low returns (and often under highly exploitative conditions) can make to household income is usually of great importance for survival; Western commentators sometimes forget that this was also common practice in the richest nations little more than a century ago.[9]

Women from all social groups will come to have greater political and professional roles – and their economic roles will become more explicit. This trend has been evident for some time, although taking very different forms in different nations and cultures.

The future city will grow horizontally, not vertically. Homes and neighbourhoods built informally or illegally by an incremental building process with ambiguous tenure and limited capital do not provide the basis for multi-storey buildings.

Cities of the future will also be as diverse as the nations, cultures, societies and economies within which they develop. Research is increasingly showing the very different forms that urban change is taking within different economic, social, political and cultural contexts.

The future city without changed policies

It is possible to predict some characteristics of the future city if there are no changes in the attitudes and policies of governments, by extrapolating some current trends into the future.

There will be hundreds of millions more people living in squatter settlements or illegal sub-divisions. For a high proportion, eviction will be a constant threat. Inadequacies in the provision of infrastructure and services in their homes and settlements will be no less than that described in earlier chapters and may indeed be worse.

Cities will increasingly be made up of settlements built on dangerous sites, continuing the long-established trends whereby poorer groups illegally occupy or purchase land and develop housing on steep hillsides, flood-plains or polluted land-sites (for example, around solid waste dumps, beside open drains or in industrial areas subject to high levels of pollution). They will settle here (and try to avoid eviction) because these are the cheapest options open to them – or the options which give the best chance of avoiding eviction, because the dangers lessen their commercial value.

There will also be an increase in the number of people suffering from diseases relating to poor, over-crowded and contaminated living environments. The increase will largely be the result of the growing number of people living in settlements without adequate water supply, sanitation, drainage, health care and emergency life-saving services. In many cities, it will be exacerbated by a growth in over-crowded tenements or boarding houses as a result of increased competition among poorer groups for cheap rental accommodation within easy reach of jobs or income sources.

People's health will suffer not only from inadequate water and provision for sanitation but from high levels of air and water pollution and from exposure in work-places to toxic chemicals and other health hazards. A review of environmental problems in Third World cities suggests that the next 20–30 years will show that the health impact of pollutants in the human environment – in the air and water and through exposure in the home and work-place – has been greatly under-estimated.[10] Few urban governments in the Third World have provision to control the dumping of toxic or hazardous wastes. An increasing number of incidents are being reported of severe injury, disablement or death as a result of very high concentrations of toxic chemicals in water supplies, in work environments or in the air of certain districts (almost always predominantly poor districts).[11] There is little evidence of any government action to address such problems or, in most nations, of the capacity of existing agencies to do so.[12]

Tens of millions more children and adolescents will have to begin work at a young age. Most are likely to be exploited at work.

Many will abandon their homes and live on their own in the city streets, threatened by many forms of violence, exploitation and dehumanization.

Cities will become increasingly segregated: the poor in the worst quality, worst served and often worst-located sites with richer groups in the best located, best quality, best-serviced locations. Cities' physical growth will be defined by where poorer groups can invade or illegally negotiate for land. This will produce a pattern of urban development which makes the provision of basic services increasingly costly. One of the great advantages of a planned urban expansion is the large cost savings in the provision of infrastructure and services. New housing developments or commercial sites located to take advantage of existing roads, drains, water mains and sewers result in major cost savings in the provision of these services. Well-designed site plans also reduce the amount of road, water and sewer pipe and pavement per house site, without reducing quality. The uncontrolled process of urban expansion creates the opposite of this: large areas of land left undeveloped because the owners benefit from rising values (partly created by public investments) and a patchwork of illegal settlements wherever poorer groups found it possible to settle, scattered around the city region – many of them on swampy land or hillsides to which infrastructure and service provision are very expensive.

Without changes in the attitudes and policies of governments, the urban future for tens of millions of people will be one of constant insecurity. This problem will be most evident in cities with rapidly expanding economies with non-democratic governments. Seoul provides an example; millions of people have been forcibly evicted from their homes in the last 30 years – including many legal home owners. With growing demand from commercial and industrial concerns for well located land sites, there is increasing pressure to redevelop the better located residential areas. Such pressures often lead to mass evictions for poorer groups from inner city tenement districts or from some of the older, more centrally located illegal or informal settlements. There are fears that mass evictions will resume in Bangkok, as an economic boom increases land prices – despite the more realistic government policies in housing in recent years and the innovative land-sharing compromises negotiated between landowners and squatters.[13]

The urban future is also likely to bring a decline in the amount of public open space per capita. The deficiencies will be most evident in poorer districts. This means a major shortage in the amount of open space for play, recreation and culture. A failure today to ensure that each neighbourhood has open space for recreation and leisure and safe places for children to play, away from dangerous streets, ensures that future inhabitants of these neighbourhoods also suffer such deficiencies. Once an area is built up, it is very difficult to remedy a shortage of public spaces.

A final characteristic worth highlighting in the urban future without changed government policies is social instability. It is not unrealistic to suggest that in cities where the above trends continue, and which are ruled from above with the poor majority segregated in unserviced illegal settlements or deteriorated and overcrowded rented accommodation, the society will be increasingly violent and unstable. A failure today to develop competent representative local government which can work with community organizations also has damaging long term consequences. If the habits of democracy and participation become lost, they must be relearnt and this takes time. In many of the Third World nations which recently returned to democratic forms of government, citizen expectations exceeded government capacities to deliver improvements.

An alternative urban future

There is an alternative urban future, within each city, where government policies become rooted in making the best use of local skills, knowledge, culture and resources. This requires that governments turn to the capacities of the people who are already the most active city builders – individual citizens and the community organizations they form. The failure of government to support and help co-ordinate the actions of these people represents an enormous loss in what both government and these people can achieve.

For over 40 years, certain observers of urban developments have pointed to the dynamism shown by the people who organize the occupation of land illegally, who build their housing there (or manage the construction), who organize its defence against attempts to evict them, who mobilize to negotiate for secure tenure and for some government-provided infrastructure and services. It is within an informal and largely illegal market for real estate, building materials and builders that most new urban neighbourhoods have developed and a high proportion of new employment been created by their inhabitants. In recent years, more governments have shown greater tolerance to these activities and in some instances, have provided some support. But what is lacking in virtually all these instances is a realistic public framework for the future city.

We can hint at some characteristics of government action within an alternative urban future. The first is government support for a vast multiplication of successful small projects. The lessons coming from the leaders of successful community-based projects is that their projects cannot simply be scaled-up. It is not the aim of those involved in successful projects to replicate them. They are also well aware that the success was largely due to making best use of existing resources and working with existing institutions within a particular context. This makes it difficult to repeat them in different cities or districts under different circumstances.

What we learn from successful projects is that there are certain pre-conditions which allowed them to take place. They include the possibility for low-income groups to organize; they usually require technical help from outside agencies and collaboration between community organizations and local governments (or other agencies) in the installation of infrastructure and services. The lessons which must be sought from projects judged by their beneficiaries to be a success are those which create the pre-conditions to allow hundreds of other small-scale local success stories to develop – each rooted in its own particular context, addressing the priorities of the local populations and making best use of local resources.

This raises the question of the political structure needed to implement an alternative urban future. Government support for a participatory, bottom-up approach at local level can hardly be implemented within a non-representative top-down city or national government. The achievement of an alternative urban future depends on the extent to which poorer groups are able (or allowed) to organize not only within their district but also to become a greater political force within the city and the nation. Unless the needs of the poor majority acquire much greater influence within local and national governments, public sector investments financed by governments, banks and international development-finance institutions will continue to have little relevance to their needs. Governments (and aid agencies) will continue to give priority to a few major projects but in terms of area within the urban agglomeration and of people who benefit, these will prove relatively unimportant. Governments insulated from popular pressures are more likely to concentrate scarce resources on major highways, industrial estates, prestige buildings, airports and metro systems; their list of priorities bears little resemblance to those of most citizens. Poorer citizens' right to vote and so to influence new developments in their own city (and neighbourhood) is perhaps the only effective check against the exclusion of their needs in government decisions. But the possibilities open to more democratic local-governments will be very limited unless citizen pressure also succeeds in increasing the power and resources available to local government.

Perhaps the most important people in the future city will be a mix of community leaders and local politicians. At present, most are completely unknown within their own nation, let alone abroad. Yet these are likely to prove more important to the urban future than government ministers at the national level. It has been reported that in Latin America, the average term in office of a national minister is eight months; it is a hard task to influence and educate this level of policy maker.

Box 11.1 illustrates three different ways of spending $20 million to improve poorer groups' housing and living conditions. Option 1 was the most common approach during the 1960s and part of the 1970s; its high cost and narrow impact are evident. Option 2 represents one of the most common new approaches of the last 20 years; its limitations are also all too evident. Option 3 represents a far more effective model, as has been proven by hundreds of small projects implemented by community organizations with the help of NGOs or church groups over the last 30 years. What makes Option 3 unusual is that it is local government which supports it, and does so in a way which allows hundreds of small-scale locally-based actions which together powerfully address the problem.

Box 11.1: Different options for a government spending $20 million on improving housing and living environments

OPTION 1: $20 million spent on the construction of two-bedroom "low cost" housing units "for low-income groups". The cost of each unit is some $10,000, once the land has been purchased, the site prepared, the contractor paid for building the units and the infrastructure and the units allocated. Thus, 2,000 households or 12,000 people receive a good quality house – if we assume that on average, there are six persons per household. Cost recovery would

Box 11.1: (continued)

be difficult if these were from among the poorer households.

OPTION 2: $20 million is spent on a serviced-site project, so that more households can be reached than in public-housing projects. Knowing that poorer households need to live close to the main centres of employment, a relatively central site was purchased for $12 million with the other $8 million spent on site preparation and installing infrastructure and services. At a cost of $2,000 per plot, 10,000 households (or 60,000 people) could benefit. It would be easier to recover some costs than in the public-housing project but for the poorer households, $2,000 for a site on top of the cost of having to construct their own house would be too much.

OPTION 3: Local government makes available to any residents' organization formed by the majority of the inhabitants of an area the sum of $100,000 for site improvements. These residents' organizations have considerable flexibility as to how they choose to spend these funds and who they turn to for technical advice. For instance, they can use local NGOs for technical advice, as long as certain basic standards are met. Although what can be achieved with such a sum will vary greatly depending on site characteristics, local costs and the extent to which residents contribute their skills and labour free, within an area with 500 households, it should be possible to reblock the site to allow better, paved access roads and also to greatly improve site drainage, water supply and sanitation. Support could be given to local artisans to fabricate the materials, fixtures and fittings which are most cheaply and effectively made on site – for instance, a carpenter's co-operative to make doors and windows or cheap building block fabrication. Of the $100,000, an average of $150 is spent per household on improved infrastructure and services with $10,000 spent on technical advice and $15,000 on support for local businesses. The reblocking of the site also frees up sufficient land to allow 50 more housing plots to be developed within the existing site or on adjacent as yet undeveloped land, and the cost of providing these with infrastructure and services and of building a community health centre is paid for by selling them.

With $100,000 provided to 150 community organizations with an average of 500 households (3,000 people) the total cost was $15

Box 11.1: (continued)

million and the whole programme reached 150 X 3,000 people: 450,000 people. Since an average of 50 new housing plots were produced in each reblocking, not only did 450,000 people benefit from improved housing, infrastructure and services but 7,500 new plots with services were developed and new health centres constructed in each site. The possibility of cost recovery was much better than for Options 1 and 2 since most households could afford to pay $200 – or take out a loan which allowed repayment over a few years. Spending $15 million in this way still left $5 million from the original $20 million which could be used to improve some city-wide service – for instance, training community health workers to run health clinics and health campaigns in each settlement.

Source: Jorge E. Hardoy and David Satterthwaite, *Squatter Citizen: Life in the Urban Third World*, (London: Earthscan Publications, 1989).

Consider these options in the context of a city of one million inhabitants, growing at five per cent a year. Each would take several years to implement. Options 1 and 2 would do nothing to improve conditions in existing settlements. Option 1 would not produce sufficient new housing for one year's growth in population and Option 2's 12,000 units would only just do so. Option 3 would reach half the city's population with improved infrastructure and services and contribute much more than the other options to employment creation. It would support the development of local NGOs as centres of advice and support for low income organizations and would create almost as many new units as Option 2. Furthermore, $5 million would be left for investment in improving some city-wide service and prospects for cost recovery would be much better than for the other two options.

Approaches like those outlined in Option 3 in part save money because local residents contribute labour free. But many poor people have little or no free time to contribute because of very long working hours. Governments and international agencies may describe them as unemployed or under-employed because they have no registered employment but in reality, they work long hours, six or seven days a week.

But approaches like those outlined in Option 3 also mean major savings in the time of architects, planners, surveyors and other expensive professionals who would otherwise be involved in community-level consultations to resolve such issues as moving certain houses out of the way of access roads and collecting funds from households to pay for the improvements. There are also major savings as specialized equipment and materials can be used to install not only piped water but also sanitation, drainage and all weather roads and paths. The match between what is provided and the capacity to pay is much improved when local community organizations are fully involved in such decisions.

There is a critical need to ensure that there are local institutions from which community organizations can obtain loans and credits for these kinds of programme and funds to pay for technical advice. Here too, the role of local NGOs could be important. NGOs can serve as technical advisors to community organizations as has been documented in many case studies.[14] They could also act as supervisors of loans or credits. Many Third World NGOs have demonstrated new ways of working with low-income groups and their community organizations.[15] These are helping to develop new breeds of professionals; within the alternative urban future, there is less of a role for traditional planners and technocrats, but a great demand for social agents who work with community organizations and their leaders and for new types of project managers, architects, medical personnel, environmentalists, lawyers and sanitary engineers – of people skilled at managing programmes and projects which make best possible use of local knowledge, skills and enthusiasm and rely little or not at all on imported knowledge, machinery and skilled personnel.

New approaches will also demand changes among professionals and researchers in international organizations. Outside professionals often misunderstand community needs and priorities. Professionals discuss urban development in the Third World without taking into consideration the enormous variety of local circumstances within each nation and each city. Each district and neighbourhood is different; each city is heterogeneous and in constant change. If we think there is such a thing as a typical Third World city or a typical Asian, African or Latin American city, we fail to understand the diversity of cultures involved in these processes.

Many professionals also advocate urban policies to slow urban growth or change the spatial distribution of urban development, with little understanding of the particular social, economic and political factors which drive urbanization within any nation or region or the extreme cost to poor people if such policies were actually implemented. Many repressive, regressive policies have been advocated (and sometimes implemented) under the heading of "managing urban development". Virtually all are based on inaccurate stereotypes of the poor being passive and ignorant[16] – perhaps it is ironic that these may be characteristics more accurately applied to those who advocate such policies.

New approaches to urban problems will also demand more long-term historical perspectives for each city and its region, to understand the particular process of urban change better within that particular context. One among many reasons why so many urban policies have failed is that they were rooted in a very inaccurate understanding of urban change and its causes.

One pre-condition for implementing the alternative approach is greater public control over land use. Public authorities must provide broad physical guidelines for urban expansion to avoid the many problems associated with the uncontrolled urban expansion noted earlier. They must also ensure a great increase in supply and a reduction in cost for all the components of an adequate house including cheap, well-located sites, cheap building materials, and advice available to low-income groups on how to build healthy and safe houses at minimum cost. Increasing the supply and reducing the cost of land sites for low-income groups' housing is the most difficult problem. There have been so many examples in the last 30 years of government initiatives to increase the supply and reduce the cost of land for housing; virtually all claimed laudable social objectives and virtually all failed to achieve them.[17]

Mobilizing resources for the future city

One of the first questions directed to those who advocate a new direction in government policies is: how will it be funded? In regard to the suggestions above, how is it possible to produce the land, finance and technical know-how?

There are many unused or mis-used resources within most cities which could at least help initiate alternative approaches. Perhaps the most obvious are the large tracts of unused or under-utilized land in both central districts and suburban areas in most cities which belong to the state or to state-owned or controlled companies and institutions. A considerable proportion of these lands are in the hands of the armed forces, public railway companies, port authorities or border control authorities. Much of this land is vacant or under-utilized (such as land around railway stations and yards), or used for activities which are no longer appropriate for central locations (for example army barracks, training fields and sports grounds which could be relocated to less central areas). In many cities, religious authorities and religious orders are also important land owners.

There is also the misuse or under-utilization of local revenue bases. Local governments often collect only a small fraction of the theoretical yield of local taxes or revenues, as a result of inefficient collection systems or failures to update rates in line with inflation. Most urban authorities lack something as basic as an up-to-date cadastral survey. This is essential not only for regulating land uses but also as the information base for property taxes.

Local governments also often fail to charge those who benefit from publicly-funded infrastructure and services the full costs of their provision. The irony is that local and city governments often supply water, sewers, garbage collection and roads to middle and upper-income groups and to the main commercial and industrial enterprises at below their real cost, which contributes to their lack of capital to expand provision to poorer groups. They also fail to penalize polluters, which not only leads to major health problems but can also mean a loss of revenue.

Local governments also fail to make best use of existing infrastructure. As noted in Chapter 5, it makes little sense to make major investments in increasing the supply of water to a city by 30–40 per cent when improved maintenance in the existing water system to cut the number of leaks and improved billing to ensure major consumers pay the full cost would also increase the water available for new consumers by the same 30–40 per cent. Building, planning and infrastructure codes which set standards too high waste scarce resources.

But the most important resource for the future city, as suggested already, is the knowledge, ingenuity and organizational capacity of citizens themselves. Much could be achieved in terms of the direct improvement of living conditions and of services if governments no longer deemed illegal and repressed – but instead supported – the vast range of individual, household and community-based actions which are the most dynamic force within most cities. This great range of activities could be helped and co-ordinated by government actions to guarantee the availability of essential resources – land sites, technical advice, infrastructure networks and basic services. Such an approach also demands a legal system to protect the human environment from contamination by industrial production and to protect individuals from exploitation by employers, landlords and landowners. This approach cannot solve more fundamental problems which are rooted in unequal distribution of wealth and power both within nations and internationally. But it can support the efforts of the true builders of their cities, and would help initiate many effective responses to contemporary problems in Third World cities.

Chapter Twelve

NEW PARTNERSHIPS FOR HEALTHY CITIES

Sandy Cairncross, Jorge E. Hardoy and David Satterthwaite

Introduction

Earlier chapters have described the extent to which hundreds of millions of urban inhabitants suffer from disease, disablement and premature death. They have shown how most of the areas in which they live have little or no provision for piped water, sanitation, drainage, the removal of household wastes, all-weather roads, emergency life-saving services or the control of disease vectors. They have discussed the many factors behind this suffering and have described how new interventions could alleviate a very considerable proportion of this suffering.

Three themes in regard to such interventions have recurred constantly in earlier chapters and appear to be central to the promotion of more healthy cities – especially within nations where there are serious constraints on increases in public expenditure. These are a recognition that current approaches are not working; that new approaches demand action on many fronts; and that new approaches must be based on local knowledge, resources and institutional capacities.

On the first of these themes, chapters 1 and 11 described the scale of this failure of governments and international agencies to improve housing and health for low income urban populations. Chapters 2-4 were illustrations of the result of this failure and how low income groups coped, in the absence of effective government action. Chapters 5-10 gave more details of this failure for water, sanitation, drainage, garbage disposal, disease vector control and emergency services, while also describing new approaches. But most governments and aid agencies act as if they had a solution to urban (and rural) housing and health problems, if only they had sufficient funds. We do not believe that current approaches, even if scaled up severalfold, would have much positive impact.

Earlier chapters also stressed that inadequate housing and poor health are the result of many factors and that improved housing and health demanded action on many fronts. The factors which influence a person's health and housing conditions range from something as broad as the international context which affects each nation's economic performance and the possibility for each Third World government of receiving aid or access to export markets through to something as specific as each person's level of education and literacy and their relationship with others in their family. Social, economic, cultural and political factors are a powerful influence on health – as well as the presence of the pathogen, toxic substance or event which is the direct cause of ill-health. An effective "healthy cities" programme will have to address many factors such as inadequate incomes, inadequate provision for education, the non-availability of cheap and adequate accommodation and of legal house sites affordable to poorer groups.

The third theme, of each national society having to address their own housing and health problems making best use of their own resources, knowledge and institutional capacity, also recurred constantly. Chapter 5 on water supply pointed to the many inappropriate western norms, concepts and practices used in the Third World and gave examples of more appropriate "unconventional" solutions. Chapters 5 and 6, while recognizing low income households' limited capacity to pay, described how "unconventional" water and sanitation systems can be installed in a high proportion of low income settlements with most or all costs recovered. Chapters 7 and 8 described how municipal authorities, working with low income groups and their community organization, can design and put in place cheap and effective drainage and garbage collection systems although both pointed to some of the difficulties in doing so. Chapter 9 stressed that traditional house designs are often more appropriate to comfort, safety and the control of disease vectors than modern, imported designs and materials and that good design and construction based on local materials and knowledge can minimize the risk of pest infestation. Chapter 10's approach to life saving services is rooted in measures within low income settlements to reduce the inhabitants vulnerability and in partnerships between government agencies, NGOs and community organizations to cope more rapidly and effectively with emergencies. Chapter 11's outline of an alternative urban future is rooted in government policies whose principal aim is to support the knowledge, resources and capacities of low income groups and the community organizations they form.

Part of the reason for this stress on the use of local resources is the recognition that most Third World governments will not have growing public resources and most poorer groups will not have growing incomes. It is much easier for governments to address health problems when their national economies are buoyant enough to promote higher incomes for a substantial proportion of their lower-income groups. Higher incomes for poorer groups means reductions in malnutrition and better capacity to pay for housing and services. But within the context of the debt crisis and the economic stagnation evident in most Third World nations, this is an unrealistic hope.

It is within this context of limited government and individual capacity to pay that solutions must be found. New approaches outlined in this book do not preclude improvements in the future, if and when these can be afforded. In low-income settlements in cities in some of the poorest Third World nations, the most appropriate local solutions for water and sanitation may be improvements in water vendor services and ventilated, improved latrines. The long term goal can still be water supplies piped into the kitchens, bathrooms and toilets of each house, and sanitation systems incorporating running water and the removal of excreta. These are generally far more convenient and preferred by inhabitants. They are often more healthy. But at present, a refusal by government agencies to consider intermediate solutions means that nothing is done for the vast majority of those in need.

Most of the new approaches discussed in this book centre on professionals and public agencies working with low-income urban dwellers in identifying their needs and the best means to address them and then working together, in an inter-disciplinary way, to implement a solution. Ingenuity and partnership become the substitute for capital; a participatory community-based diagnosis of the main health problems and their causes a substitute for expensive medical surveys.

New partnerships between government and community organizations

Health-promoting actions have to start at the individual, household and community level. It may seem inappropriate to begin a discussion of public interventions to promote healthy cities with the role of individuals and community organizations. They include among them very few health professionals, if any, and may include many illiterate or semi-literate people. In most instances, between 40 and 50 per cent of them will be infants, children and adolescents. But at present, these are the people working hardest to solve health problems since these are their own health problems. Much as we dislike falling back on solutions which draw on their skills, knowledge, motivation and organizational capacity – upper income groups don't have to build their own houses, develop their own neighbourhoods and work with local authorities to install infrastructure and provide services – there is no other solution unless there is a reversal in the distribution of income within nations and internationally. It is obvious that the true achievement of healthy cities for all demands a more equal distribution of wealth nationally and globally. In this book, we seek only to emphasize ways of reducing the health problems of poor urban households within the existing structure of global and national income and wealth distribution. This should not detract from the need also to reduce the fundamental inequalities which underpin poverty and poor health.

As the report of a World Health Organization Expert Committee states:

> The key for governments is to provide the framework within which thousands of community actions can flourish – informed and guided by the latest knowledge about health promoting interventions and helped by new methodologies for rapid community based diagnoses. Such a framework must also ensure that these thousands of actions reinforce each other (and avoid conflicts as in one neighbourhood level drainage scheme dumping excess water into another area).[1]

Table 12.1 (see p. 266) outlines how health risks can be tackled with a combination of actions at different levels which support and reinforce each other. Most of these interventions are not beyond the means of most Third World governments. But they do demand a decentralized, multi-sectoral approach with government agencies' inputs guided by low income groups and the neighbourhood or community organizations that they form. More to the point, the community should participate in choosing priorities for the interventions listed in the Table.

This means co-operation between local government and community-based or neighbourhood-based citizen groups – for instance in joint programmes to drain stagnant pools to locate and destroy disease vectors within homes and their surrounds, and to set up emergency life-saving systems. In most instances, these cannot be provided at an affordable cost without the support of those living in low-income settlements. Box 12.1 illustrates how community organizations

Box 12.1: The urban community development programme in Rocinha, Rio de Janeiro

Rocinha is one of Rio's largest and oldest *favelas*, with at least 80,000 inhabitants. It is perched on steep slopes above prosperous residential and commercial areas which surround it. Before the upgrading programme, environmental conditions had been very poor; raw sewage and garbage accumulating in the settlement. The open areas where children played were usually contaminated both with garbage and with faecal matter. During the rainy season these were washed down along with domestic waste water, in open drains. These drains often flooded the lowest lying areas – which were also the poorest areas. Provision for garbage collection was very inadequate.

Research which formed part of a research/action project on women's health between 1983 and 1985 found that 30 per cent of the women had a child who had died (77 per cent of them during the first year of life), 27 per cent had experienced miscarriages and 85 per cent had suffered some health problems during pregnancy. More than half had received no anti-tetanus vaccine during any of their pregnancies and 63 per cent had no orientation on childbirth during the pre-natal period. The research also revealed the lack of information available to women about contraception.

Rocinha has a long history of community activity. For instance, residents set up a *mutirao* (mutual-aid group), in 1970, to work on Sundays and holidays to clean public areas and clear ditches; the municipal government supplied the basic tools. Since then, services have gradually improved; Rocinha has three day-care services, three health posts and two community schools run and supported by residents. In 1979, they initiated a project to construct a new sewer but this was never completed.

In 1980, Rio de Janeiro's Municipal Secretariat and UNICEF began an Urban Community Development Programme to develop Action Plans for *favelas* with organizations formed by their residents.

Box 12.1: (continued)

Together, they would tackle the most serious problems there and identify how best to do so, combining residents' own efforts with municipal inputs. This recognized that resident initiatives were underway within many *favelas* (often helped by NGOs) to provide some health care and to improve sanitation or water supply. In many instances, these could be made more effective or given more continuity with appropriate government support. Project staff also recognized that many *favelas* were so densely populated, especially in inner-city areas, that they needed to be incorporated into existing city networks for (for instance) water supply, sanitation, drainage and garbage disposal.

Rocinha was chosen as the site for a demonstration project because its inhabitants had already demonstrated their capacity to organize and work together. Residents' groups prepared an upgrading plan with UNICEF and staff from the newly formed Municipal Secretariat for Social Development. A survey was initiated to provide the basis for the plan to include improvements to water supply, sanitation, informal education and health services. A decision was made to concentrate on completing the sewer in "*Rua* 3" (Street 3) which had been begun three years previously but not completed. Certain residents were paid to work part time to liaise between residents and the engineers and to work with project staff in mobilizing residents to help in the construction work.

To prepare for construction, a seminar was organized on basic sanitation, attended by representatives of government agencies (including those responsible for water, sewerage and garbage) and Rocinha residents. Work began in late 1981 in *Rua* 3 on the main sewer trunk-system and five manholes; on laying household connections to the main which prepared *Rua* 3 houses for connection in the future to the city's water supply; on draining and paving the area around the water tap; on constructing a new collection post for garbage bins which would be regularly collected by the municipal sanitation company; and on the rehabilitation of sites adjacent to the sewer mains, and on those formerly used as garbage dumps, to make them suitable for recreation. By early 1982, the sewer had been completed, despite the steep slope and difficult terrain. Residents

Box 12.1: (continued)

contributed to the work by providing labour and equipment, and organized their own contributions.

This programme in Rocinha served as the model for similar schemes in nine other *favelas* where community organizations had demonstrated a capacity to organize mutual-aid works and were prepared to take responsibility for carrying out project assignments. These were also *favelas* where the issue of land ownership was not subject to court litigation. Residents' associations mobilized local labour to build sewerage and drainage systems, stairways and water distribution systems, while the Municipal Secretariat for Social Development provided technical advice and delivered construction materials. This reached 18,300 beneficiaries and the total cost was less than half that of the same work if it had been undertaken by a conventional contractor. Residents contributed labour, organization, administration, some basic equipment, construction materials and maintenance. Estimates suggest that the residents met around 25 per cent of the costs of purchasing materials. It is also interesting to note that salaries and administrative costs represented half of total costs; this implies that projects such as these, while making a major saving in capital costs, still demand a high level of involvement by local government and utility agency staff. In 1986, similar initiatives were launched in many other *favelas*.

Source: *Urban Examples* No.15, UNICEF, drawing largely on Shluger, Ephim, "Expanding Project Coverage – Review of Urban Basic Services Projects of Rio de Janeiro and Buenos Aires", paper produced for the UNICEF Inter-Agency Urban Meeting in Madras, India, March 1987.

worked with local government and an outside agency (UNICEF) in addressing housing and health problems in Rio de Janeiro.

Neighbourhood organizations and their federations can become a powerful force in tackling environmental health problems and may be the only ones which can deal effectively with such issues as domestic violence and drug and alcohol abuse; Box 12.2 gives one example of such a federation. Support and technical assistance to community organizations and their federations from municipal and city authorities, non-governmental organizations and aid agencies can greatly increase their effectiveness in dealing with environmental health problems.

Box 12.2: Federations of community organizations – the example of CONAMUP (Mexico)

The National Co-ordinating Body of Mexico's Urban Popular Movements (CONAMUP) is an umbrella organization for dozens of urban community organizations throughout Mexico. It seeks more realistic and participatory solutions to the severe urban problems which confront poorer groups in Mexico. Its members include tenants' movements, organizations representing the homeless, neighbourhood organizations and movements of women and street vendors. Its work (through its members) includes setting up nurseries and health workshops, controlling the use of drugs and alcohol abuse, and campaigns against rape and domestic violence and the promotion of community measures to deal with these. It has helped set up community-run kitchens and non-profit stores selling basic goods. It also fights on behalf of members for changes in government policies – for instance for lower-income groups to be given access to government-owned land which remains unused and for an elected authority for the Mexico City Metropolitan Area.

Source: "Mexico's urban popular movements – a conversation with Pedro Moctezuma", interview by Julio D. Davila, *Environment and Urbanization* Vol. 2, no. 1, April 1990, pp. 35–50.

Some pre-conditions for the new approach

A recent World Health Organization study on *Urbanization and its Implications for Child Health* noted some of the pre-conditions for new partnerships between governments and community organizations:

> Community or neighbourhood organizations and federations are generally more active wherever city and municipal authorities are elected and resources to deal with environmental health problems are readily forthcoming. Neighbourhood organizations can set priorities and join with local authorities and non-governmental organizations in surveys to identify the main health problems and the action needed to deal with them in the shape of environmental improvements and preventive measures. This can mean major savings in time and money. For instance, if access roads are to be introduced into squatter

settlements (so that ambulances and other emergency vehicles can enter), and this means that some houses have to be moved (to make space for the roads), the whole neighbourhood may be strongly opposed to the scheme. But the full involvement of neighbourhood organizations in determining priorities for health improvement – including the introduction of access roads – has been shown to minimize opposition to the measures proposed. In some cases, the professional staff taking part have recognized that neighbourhood organizations have actually improved their site plans.[2]

Chapter 11 elaborated on these and other pre-conditions. One of the most important is an understanding by government agencies of the constraints on poorer groups' capacity to contribute labour, materials and funds to community schemes. Chapter 2 illustrated the capacity of low-income groups to organize, to acquire land and build houses (when political circumstances allowed), but it also illustrated the limits on their capacity to set up their own health-care service and improve infrastructure. Without the right kind of technical advice, funding, specialist equipment and materials, communities' capacity to install or improve infrastructure and services is very limited. Chapter 11 stressed the need for local institutions from which low income households and the community organizations they form can obtain credit and technical advice. Chapter 11 also stressed that government action must also greatly increase the supply and reduce the cost of all the components of an adequate house including land sites within easy reach of jobs and building materials.

Another pre-condition for the new approach is accurate knowledge about the main health problems suffered by poorer groups, and their causes. Box 12.3 gives an example from Amman, Jordan's capital and largest city, where a survey to plan an upgrading programme in squatter settlements provided the means for a dialogue between government officials and low-income groups about their health problems and how these should be addressed.

An obvious pre-condition for joint action between local agencies and community organizations is the existence of a representative community organization. Little can be done if there is no community organization – or when existing community organizations represent particular factions or vested interests. The best way to overcome this will obviously vary greatly from settlement to settlement but there are certain means by which community participation can be promoted. The first, as noted in previous chapters, is representative governments; democratic practices in government interventions at settlement or neighbourhood level are hardly likely to develop within non-democratic municipal, city and national government structures.

Box 12.3: Health surveys in squatter settlements in Amman, Jordan

When a health survey was planned in certain squatter settlements prior to an upgrading programme, it was recognized that any outsider (especially someone from government) would be perceived as a threat. Squatter households live in fear of eviction and the demolition of their dwellings. Yet basic information about squatter households, their shelters and the site is needed to design the most appropriate interventions and allow the transfer of tenure to the occupants.

The health study proved to be the means by which project staff could gain the confidence of squatters. As interviewers went from house to house with scales to weigh children and kits to collect stool samples, neighbours gathered. The fact that children's health is perceived by the squatters as an issue of great importance and the weighing was an instant contribution (not a promise of some future action) helped allay their suspicions. A nurse who led the team carried a first aid kit and gave assistance where needed; burns from the kerosene stoves used in these crowded living quarters (4.5 persons per room) were a major complaint during the winter months. Survey personnel also gave advice on how to seek medical assistance.

The health survey was combined with the registration of beneficiaries and the physical survey. These also included information needed for the health assessment – for instance, questions to women on the number of children born and children surviving, which allow the calculation of infant and child mortality indices. The physical survey included questions and observations on food storage and toilet practices, water sources, storage and consumption. The health survey made the other surveys more acceptable; those doing the physical survey with their measuring tapes were so suspect to the

Box 12.3: (continued)

community that the women in the health team gradually took over many of their tasks as well.

The survey was to provide a baseline assessment of current health conditions and to define as far as possible how existing living conditions operate as determinants of infant and child mortality. It also sought to provide the details needed about the population and its growth in the areas to be upgraded. None of the squatter areas had been enumerated before and there were no reference points for project staff beyond arbitrarily-drawn boundaries to identify each dwelling.

This special concern proved important in integrating health with the more conventional upgrading works, which concentrate on physical aspects in a settlement. When stool samples taken for children under age three were examined, they revealed a high prevalence of intestinal parasite infections. Interviewers also found that all infants and small children had diapers or were swaddled at night; this was true for the youngest during the day as well. Defecation by toddlers in shared courtyard areas was rare. Most environmental contamination came from sources that the residents could not control such as sewage flushed down from the legal housing areas, above the settlement. Immediate action was obviously needed to treat the children and instruct the mothers on diagnosis, treatment and prevention. But it also led to the recognition that help was needed from the Ministry of Health to provide services in squatter areas. And, of course, action was needed to stop the flow of sewage down the hill. The findings from the analyses of young children's stool samples prompted immediate sewer construction as well as the first community-health sessions held by a doctor assigned from the Ministry of Health.

Source: Drawn from a case study in *Urban Examples* No 15, UNICEF, by Dr Leila Bisharart (see note 3 for more details).

A second factor which can encourage the development of community organizations is a degree of constancy and honesty in local government in their support and enablement; years or decades of unfulfilled promises from local politicians have hardly encouraged poorer people to believe in local governments' capacity to help solve their problems. The third is a re-orientation of existing government programmes towards a more community-based bottom-up approach. For instance, a public agency would find it easier to develop a community-based approach to identifying and destroying disease vectors if it already supported a successful community-based programme for ante- and post-natal care through midwives and community health workers. The fourth is the use of a new kind of professional – community facilitators – whose job it is to provide the links between communities and government agencies, and also other institutions such as church groups, charities, private voluntary agencies and labour unions.

The role of local government

The approach sketched above implies a different kind of local government – more activist, representative and decentralized. It also implies institutional changes which promote co-ordination between different sectoral agencies.

Government projects which are judged to be success stories often owe their achievements to *ad hoc* arrangements between different sectoral agencies where public-health specialists, doctors and paramedical personnel, engineers, architects and planners all work together. *Ad hoc* arrangements can overcome rigid sectoral divisions in one or two projects; they cannot serve as the basis for the enormous expansion needed in multi-sectoral actions within hundreds of projects. To return to the example of Rocinha described in Box 12.1, the report from which the box drew stated that the key to institutionalizing the innovative approach adopted for one project was to ensure that all the different municipal and state sectoral agencies whose responsibilities covered water, sanitation, drainage, health care and garbage disposal co-ordinated their efforts within each *favela*, guided and co-ordinated by local residents' associations.

> For a single or for several projects, this is relatively easy, given agreement on the worth of the work to be undertaken. For city-wide and continuous programmes, fundamental changes are needed in the way agencies operate. And ... changes are needed in the norms, codes and regulations which presently guide their actions.[4]

In most nations, there is talk in government circles about strengthening local government but there is little action towards this. City and municipal governments throughout the Third World lack the power, trained personnel and resources to address either health or housing problems adequately. However, it is at city level and below (the district, neighbourhood or borough) that governments must be able to support community action and to provide the planning and management framework within which to co-ordinate it. These lower levels of government hold most of the legal and institutional responsibilities for the planning and maintenance of urban areas, and for providing infrastructure, services and facilities to enterprises and inhabitants. They usually have responsibilities also for the provision of health-care centres and emergency life-saving services, and for the enforcement of health and safety standards in new residential developments.

In reality, as earlier chapters show, virtually all city and municipal governments in the Third World fail to meet these responsibilities. They lack the investment capability to make any impression on the huge backlog of needs for infrastructure and services. Even where infrastructure is expanded – very often through support from national government or works undertaken by a national government agency – local government lacks the resources to maintain the new facilities. Local governments' powers to increase revenues are usually highly constrained by national government. It is not uncommon for the richer income groups to be paying very little for publicly-provided piped water, sewers, drainage and household garbage collection while most of the poor majority receive no public service and no publicly-funded infrastructure. Instead, they often have to pay private water vendors and garbage collectors many times the price that the richer groups pay the city water authorities. A World Bank study went so far as to say that local governments are generally "fragmented, confused about their functions and all too often either invisible or largely ceremonial".[5]

Most local governments also have a legislative framework of codes and standards which is inappropriate to the tasks confronting them. In most of Africa and much of Asia, these are still largely based on colonial legislation and practices which were put in place to serve a tiny European minority with high standards of housing, infrastructure and services. In much of Latin America, they are based on European precedents put in place many decades ago. Contemporary institutions and agencies not only lack investment capacity, power and trained personnel. They also work within an outmoded and constraining legislative and normative framework.

National governments must take the lead in changing the legislative base and in strengthening city government. In most cities, building codes will have to be revised; the standards they demand are unaffordable for the poor majority. At present, codes often deem illegal the only building materials that lower-income groups can afford for instance mud or mud bricks, plastic sheeting and the cheapest wood based panels. Land sub-division standards may be too high; large minimum lot-sizes simply price people out of the market. What is needed are appropriate standards – not necessarily lower standards. In some instances, higher standards may be needed for capital projects to minimize maintenance needs.[6] Building and planning codes would achieve far more if the enforcement of standards was replaced by technical advice from centres, located throughout low-income areas, whose role would be to advise on how houses could be built or modified to improve health and safety. Government support for rapid expansion in the production of cheap building materials and building components, fixtures and fittings (lintels, roofs, doors, windows, shutters, screening, pipes, latrine covers, and so on) could do much to lower the cost of building or upgrading a house. This could be combined with advice on how house designs and materials can tackle problems of disease vectors. Support for workshops to produce such materials and fittings in each city district would also generate employment. Decentralized production lowers transport costs to the site; for large, heavy, relatively low-cost materials and components, the cost of transporting them to the house site is often a considerable proportion of total cost.

The private sector

Many governments and aid agencies have recently begun promoting privatization as a way to meet basic needs: safe and sufficient supplies of water, drains and excreta disposal, health care services, all-weather roads and regular collection of garbage. The idea that privatization can improve provision to low-income groups in most urban centres of the Third World is usually greatly overstated. However, within the specific context of each nation (and urban centre) there may be important specific roles for private sector enterprises, especially if this is understood to include informal enterprises, non-profit community enterprises and non-governmental organizations, as well as formal commercial enterprises.

The justification for privatization given by its proponents is usually that the government is short of capital. Their hope is that the private sector will provide the capital needed to expand and improve services, if offered the opportunity. In this instance, the private sector would be taking over some of the responsibilities of local government.

But in most Third World cities, many of the poorer inhabitants already use the private sector to obtain certain services and land for housing or rented accommodation. In most cities, it is the main source of rental accommodation; the high level of overcrowding and poor quality accommodation provided by landlords in Olaleye as described in Chapter 3 is not untypical of the standard of accommodation in many other Third World cities. The extent to which people depend on rented accommodation (usually whole families, or several individuals, in each room) and the extent to which such accommodation is located in illegal or informal settlements is rarely appreciated in the West.[7] Illegal sub-divisions are the largest source of land for new housing in hundreds of Third World cities: this too is the private sector taking on the task of supplying building plots outside government regulation, and usually obtaining good returns from doing so. In these two examples, the private sector can hardly be said to provide good quality goods and services. The lack of infrastructure and services supplied by the enterprises making illegal sub-divisions, the level of tenant exploitation and the poor conditions in most rental housing do not support the idea that privatization will necessarily improve standards for poorer groups. The supply of water in these settlements is also often privatized since in the absence of a piped-water system, water vendors provide the supplies. The high price – and often poor quality – of the water sold also suggests problems with privatization, although these sometimes relate more to an inefficient supply system than to exploitative practices.

An additional problem is that private companies are selective. In San Martin (Chapter 2), a basic garbage-collection service did develop, funded directly by user charges, but no private enterprise would consider the installation of water, sewers and drains. But the simultaneous installation of different kinds of infrastructure and services brings very substantial cost savings. In addition, as earlier chapters suggest, they complement each other. Water supplies piped to each house require drains connected to each house – and preferably sewers. Sewers need sufficient water to keep them unblocked. House-sites usually need drains for rain-water. Roads and other paved areas need drains. Drains need efficient garbage collection otherwise they become blocked with garbage; so too, on occasion, do sewers. Garbage collection costs are reduced if most or all houses are close to paved roads. The public good is served when all are installed together. This brings the greatest improvement in health; if only water supply is improved, this may increase health problems as waste-water forms stagnant pools which then serve as breeding grounds for insects which spread diseases.

It is difficult to conceive of private companies helping to improve and extend piped-water supplies, sewers, drains, roads and pavements as one package, especially to poorer households and poorly-located residential areas. Private companies will always be reluctant to extend services to poorer areas especially if this requires a large investment. For instance, it would not cost much for a private company to see if a new bus service to a squatter community would be profitable. If this does not prove profitable, the company loses no capital investment. But laying water pipes or sewers to a squatter community is a much greater risk, since it is far more expensive and the company can hardly dig up the whole system and try again elsewhere. Land developers may install all the infrastructure, but not in developments which poorer households can afford. This is why private companies concentrate on one or two items. Water supply is the most attractive because people pay as they consume and often pay for the initial cost of connection. Enforcing payment is easier because supplies can be cut off. Garbage collection may also be attractive since the capital investment to set up the service need not be high and again, services can be stopped if households do not pay. But a household's use of drains, roads and paths cannot be cut off when it cannot pay, unless the provider has the power to evict them.

In addition, the privatization of natural monopolies such as piped water, sewers and drains, presents governments with special problems, since there are no competitive pressures to help keep down price and encourage improved quality. Such natural monopolies require large capital investments to set up the supply but once in place, the cost of extending them to more people within a city is relatively low. Once a piped water supply or sewer system is built, it is virtually impossible for another business to compete by building another water or sewer system. It is also ridiculous to think of two or more companies, each with their own piped water, sewer and road system, competing against each other to serve the same households.

If a natural monopoly is privatized, it has to be carefully regulated both in regard to prices and to quality of service. If a private firm runs a city's water supply, residents have no other piped supply they can turn to, if prices get too high or quality too low. But if water supplies are privatized because local government is so weak, how can this same local government be strong enough to regulate the private firms? How can it fulfil its responsibility to ensure that quality of service is guaranteed and that prices are controlled? A company can use the threat of bankruptcy, abandonment or sale to an asset-stripper to extract a subsidy from the government or the municipality; in the small, poorer Third World nations, there are few competitors able to take over the running of a large system at short notice.[8]

Privatization does not remove the need for government intervention; it only changes the nature of this intervention. Government remains responsible for ensuring an adequate quality of service is maintained and that the public are not over-charged. For certain services, ensuring adequate quality is a problem even if there is a competitive market. Domestic water supply is the most important example because households cannot necessarily judge whether the water they use is safe to consume. If private enterprises provide water supplies, local government must not only control prices but also monitor quality and have in place an effective deterrent system to penalize companies which fail to maintain adequate standards.

There are instances where the arguments for privatization of certain services appear particularly convincing. In some cities (or parts of cities), government weakness or inefficiency may provide a strong case for the private supply of certain services or kinds of infrastructure. Public companies which fail to provide adequate services to businesses who can pay for such services constrain the growth in production and employment. As Lee has pointed out in his study of infrastructure provision in Nigeria, the failure of government to provide businesses with adequate standards of water supply, electricity, telephones and drains means that these businesses make very large investments to guarantee their own supplies – their own electricity generators, wells for water and microwave telephone systems. The costs to each business are enormous and any larger-scale supplier (public or private) could meet their demands far more cheaply.[9]

In other services, especially those which are not a natural monopoly, private enterprises can help improve quality and the range of choice available to the public. In city transport, private enterprises often provide a cheaper, more flexible service than public-sector bus companies; private buses, mini-buses, shared taxis, powered rickshaws and a whole host of other kinds of "paratransit" either replace or supplement public-sector buses in virtually all Third World cities. Large companies, whether private or public, may be poorly suited to running such services because they do not provide sufficient flexibility. Private enterprises might also improve garbage collection at an affordable cost to customers with appropriate encouragement and regulation by local government and in many instances, they do so. And as Chapter 5 described, where households' water comes mainly from vendors, and where the combination of very low household incomes and poor local government makes the installation of piped supplies impossible, water supplies should be cheaper and of better quality if different vendors compete with each other. Here, one option for local government would be to help vendors to improve services as well as to regulate quality.

One reason why private companies are claimed to operate more profitably than public enterprises is their greater efficiency in collecting payments for services provided. Public bodies which are lax about collecting payments often subsidize richer groups and penalize the poorest. For instance, a public water company's failure to collect payments for piped water or to increase tariffs to reflect rising costs has the effect of subsidizing those with piped water (often not among the poorer households) and penalizing those with no piped supply, since it lowers the returns to the company and thus inhibits new investment to expand the service. Improving cost recovery – in terms of reducing the proportion of households who do not pay the full cost of some service – is one important way to pay for better maintenance of the system and its expansion to reach new households. But improved cost recovery cannot be at the expense of the poorest households not receiving services.

In conclusion, allowing private enterprises to provide certain services which are provided inadequately or not at all by local government is worth considering, especially if the services are not natural monopolies. But for the services which are the main concern of this book, there will be problems with quality and provision if there is no competent local government to supervise levels of private service and charges. If local government is competent, it should be able to provide such services more cheaply and effectively itself. If local governments' lack of resources is the reason for privatization, it would be worth considering first whether strengthening local governments' capacity to raise capital would not be a more effective reform. Privatization must be considered within the more important, long-term goal of developing strong and representative local government. Effective local government can make choices as to where private-sector initiatives can contribute to improving housing and health. Choices can be made as to which components the private sector might most usefully supply: for instance the finance, the construction, the operation of a system, customer billing or maintenance. If privatization is to serve the public good, it always implies collaboration between public and private in some form. The question is – within each local context, in which functions are there advantages for private-sector involvement?

In the final analysis, the aim is to seek a compromise between guaranteeing a basic level of service to everyone and maximizing cost recovery to allow the service to maintain (or improve) its quality and increase its coverage. Earlier chapters have given examples of where new technologies and innovative institutional arrangements have greatly cheapened the cost of supplying a basic level of services – and narrowed the gap between a basic service cost and what people can afford. These arrangements can also make it easy for households to obtain better services once they can afford to pay more, for instance, in bringing piped water into the house itself from the yard outside.

The non-commercial private sector

A more relevant debate about privatization and improving environmental health for lower-income groups has to do not with private commercial enterprises but with non-profit organizations and with organizations set up by residents of particular areas. Such organizations can not only match private enterprise's record in cost recovery but also provide cheaper services (since no profit is made) and be more immediately accountable to their customers.

There is tremendous potential in new partnerships between local governments and local community organizations. This could be regarded as privatization in another form, but where control of some service rests largely with representatives of the consumers of that service.

The possibility of tackling the most serious health problems with limited resources needs co-operation between local government and community-based citizen groups. Joint programmes can be set up to drain stagnant pools, to reblock existing settlements so that pipes, drains and access roads can be installed and space made for schools and clinics, to locate and destroy disease vectors within homes and their surrounds, to design educational programmes on health prevention and personal hygiene, to set up emergency life-saving systems which can provide first aid in each neighbourhood and rapidly take seriously ill or injured persons to a hospital. There is no lack of examples of innovative joint government-community programmes to improve infrastructure and service provision; many examples of these have been given in earlier chapters. Other publications have many examples of similar partnerships for improving housing quality.[10]

Third World based non-government organizations have also demonstrated new participatory ways to work with community organizations in this area. Among those which have been documented are the work of FUNDASAL in El Salvador,[11] the work of SPARC in Bombay,[12] the new approaches in Mexico City pioneered by COPEVI and CENVI[13] and the work of the Human Settlements Foundation and the Asian Coalition for Housing Rights in Bangkok.[14] There are also examples of innovative NGOs working to improve sanitation as in the examples given in Chapter 6 of the Orangi Pilot Project in Karachi, and Shulabh International and Asha Sadan in India. Third World NGOs and Western private voluntary- organizations have also developed effective urban primary health-care systems.[15]

The problem is that these examples remain the exceptions; they are not currently the conventional approach and governments have not institutionalized them on a large scale. What is needed is a vast multiplication in the number of such innovative projects. This is not the same as replicating or "scaling up" successful projects, as Chapter 11 stresses; it is ensuring that tens of thousands of local solutions can be developed by local institutions which match local needs and resources. Supporting such a multiplication of projects demands that there are local institutions within each city (and preferably city district) from which community organizations can obtain loans or credits. External funding from national agencies or foreign sources could never fund directly the tens of thousands of such community initiatives which are needed; even if such agencies had the commitment, they lack the institutional structure to implement it. Nor is it viable for representatives of Third World NGOs working with community organizations to have to travel to Europe or North America every time they need to raise funds for a community-based project.

The promotion of healthy cities is about making the suppliers of health and environmental services more responsive to consumer demands. It is about local government giving the private sector more power in decision making, a bigger role in service provision and more rights in determining priorities. But this private sector is made up of low-income citizens and their community organizations, and the non-profit professional groups who pioneer new ways of working with them. These are the major actors in the construction and maintenance of Third World cities. Governments' success in curtailing ill-health, disablement and premature death in Third World cities will largely depend on the extent to which they work with this coalition, this sector, transforming the current atmosphere of indifference, or indeed repression, into one of partnership.

Table 12.1: Government-community partnerships in addressing housing and health problems in urban residential areas*

Health risks	*Action at individual and household level*	*Public action at neighbourhood or community level*	*Action at city or district level*	*Action at national level*
Contaminated water – typhoid, hepatitis, dysenteries, diarrhoea, cholera etc.	Protected water supply to house; promote knowledge of hygienic water storage	Provision of water supply infrastructure. Knowledge and motivation in community	Plans to undertake this and resources to do so	Ensure that local and city governments have the power, funding base and trained personnel to implement actions at household, neighbourhood, city and district level.
Inadequate disposal of human wastes – pathogens from excreta contaminating food, water or fingers leading to faecal – oral diseases or intestinal worms (e.g. hookworm, roundworm, tapeworm, schistosomiasis)	Support for construction of easily maintained latrine/WC matching physical conditions; social preferences and economic resources; washing facilities; promote hand washing	Mix of technical advice, equipment installation and its servicing and maintenance (mix dependent on technology used)	Plans to undertake this plus resources. Trained personnel and finances to service and maintain	Review and where appropriate change legislative framework and norms and codes to allow and encourage actions at lower levels and ensure infrastructure standards are appropriate to needs and the resources available.
Waste water and garbage – water-logged soil ideal to transmit diseases like hookworm; pools of contaminated standing water, conveying enteric diseases and providing breeding ground for mosquitoes spreading filariasis, malaria and other diseases. Garbage attracting disease vectors	Provision of storm/surface water drains on plot and spaces for storing garbage that are rat, cat, dog and child proof	Design and provision of storm and surface water drains. Advice to households on materials and construction techniques to make houses less damp	Regular removal or provision for safe disposal of household wastes and plan framework and resources for drains	Support for training courses and seminars for architects, planners, engineers etc on the health aspects of their work
Insufficient water for domestic hygiene – diarrhoeal diseases, eye infections (including trachoma), skin diseases, scabies, lice, fleas	Adequate water supply for washing and bathing. Provision for laundry at household or community level	Health and personal hygiene education for children and adults. Facilities for laundry at this level, if not within individual houses	Support for health education and public facilities for laundry	Technical and financial support for educational campaigns. Coordination of housing, health and education ministries

Table 12.1 (continued)

Health risks	*Action at individual and household level*	*Public action at neighbourhood or community level*	*Action at city or district level*	*Action at national level*
Disease vectors or parasites in house structure with access to occupants/food/water e.g. rats, cockroaches and other insects (including vector for Chagas disease)	Support for improved house structure – e.g. tiled floors, protected food storage areas, roofs/walls/ floors protected from disease vectors	Technical advice and information; part of adult/child education programme	Loans for upgrading house. Guarantee supply of cheap and easily available materials, fixtures and fittings	Ensure building codes and official procedures to approve house construction/improvement are not inhibiting individual, household and local government actions. Support for nationwide availability of building loans, cheap materials (where possible based on local resources) and building advice centres. Produce technical and educational material to support this
Inadequate size house/ ventilation – helps spread diseases such as TB, influenza and meningitis (aerosol drop transmission) especially when many households share premises. Risks of household accidents increased with overcrowding; it becomes impossible to safeguard children from poisons and open fires or stoves	Technical advice and financial support for house improvement or extension and provision of cheap sites with basic services in different parts of the city to offer low income groups alternatives to their current shelter	Technical advice on improving ventilation; education on overcrowding related diseases and accidents	Loans (including small ones with flexible repayment); support for building advice centres in each neighbourhood	
Children playing in and around house site constantly exposed to dangers from traffic, unsafe sites or sites contaminated with faeces or pollutants	Organization of child care services to allow care for children in households where all adults work	Provision within each neighbourhood of well drained site separated from traffic, kept clean and free from garbage and easily supervised. Ensure first aid services are to hand	Support given to neighbourhood level play, sport and recreation facilities.	
Indoor air pollution through open fires or poorly designed stoves – exacerbate respiratory illness, especially in women and children	Posters/booklets on improved stove design and improving ventilation etc	Ensure availability of designs and materials to build improved designs and investigate possibilities of promoting use of alternative fuels		
House sites subject to landslides or floods as result of no other land being affordable to lower income groups	Regularize each household's tenure if dangers can be lessened; relocation through offer of alternative sites as last resort	Action to reduce dangers and encourage upgrading or offer alternative sites	Ensure availability of safe housing sites that lower income groups can afford	National legislation and financial and technical support for interventions by local and city governments in land markets to support lower level action. Training institutions to provide needed personnel at each level

Table 12.1 (continued)

Health risks	*Action at individual and household level*	*Public action at neighbourhood or community level*	*Action at city or district level*	*Action at national level*
Illegal occupation of house site or illegal subdivision with disincentive to upgrade, lack of services and mental stress from fear of eviction	Regularize each household's tenure and provision for piped water, sanitation and storm and surface water drainage	Local government working with community to provide basic infrastructure and services and incorporation into 'official city'	Support for incorporating illegal subdivisions and for providing tenure to squatter households	
Nutritional deficiencies and low income	Action to reduce intestinal worm burden and worm transmission. Support for income generating work within the house	Food supplements/school meals. Support for enterprises in low income settlements or set up by their inhabitants. If land is available, promote its use for growing vegetables. If malnutrition is serious, consider most appropriate programme to reach most seriously affected groups		Structural reforms, funds for food supplement or other emergency nutrition programmes and other measures to improve poorer groups' real income
No or inadequate access to curative/preventive health care and advice	Widespread availability of simple primer on first aid and health in the home with home visits by health workers to promote its use	Primary health care centre; emphasis on child and maternal health, preventive health and support for community action and for community volunteers	Small hospital (first referral level) and resources and training to support lower level services and volunteers	Technical and financial support for nationwide system of hospitals and health care centres. Preventive health campaigns (e.g. immunization) and nationwide availability of drugs and equipment. Set up training system for paramedics/community health workers. Provide guidelines for setting up emergency services and planning and risk minimization in risk prone areas to minimize injuries and damage if disaster occurs.
No provision for emergency life saving services in event of injury or serious illness	Widespread availability of simple primer on first aid and health in the home with educational programmes on minimizing risks	Basic equipment (e.g. stretchers, first aid) available and accessible 24 hours a day. Community volunteers with basic training on call and arrangements for rapid transfer of sick person to hospital. Equipment to rescue and treat people saved from burning houses	Support for neighbourhood level equipment plus organization of training programmes for community volunteers. Fire fighting equipment, contingency plans for emergencies	
	Discussions with individuals and community organizations about some minimum charges in site layout to improve emergency vehicle access and create fire breaks			

* Many of the above actions to improve or extend houses or to improve the quality of the services and facilities that the house contains will often be constrained for houses, flats, rooms or house sites which are rented. One should recall that a high proportion of the lowest income individuals and households rent their accommodation in most Third World cities and improving their quality and reducing health risks will need government programmes and actions which are not summarized in this Table.

Source: This is a slightly revised version of a table which appeared in Jorge E. Hardoy and David Satterthwaite, "Housing and health – do architects and planners have a role?", *Cities* vol. 4, No. 3, 1987.

NOTES AND REFERENCES

Introduction

1. Morley, David and Hermione Lovel, *My Name is Today: an Illustrated Discussion of Child Health, Society and Poverty in Less Developed Countries*, Macmillan Publishers, London, 1986.
2. For more details, see World Health Organization, *World Health Statistics 1989*, Publications Unit, WHO, Geneva, 1989.
3. Tabibzadeh, I., A. Rossi-Espagnet and R. Maxwell, *Spotlight on the Cities: Improving Urban Health in Developing Countries*, World Health Organization, Geneva, 1989.
4. World Health Organization, *Urbanization and its Implications for Child Health: Potential for Action*, Geneva, 1989.
5. Stambouli, Fredj, "Born Underprivileged" *World Health*, World Health Organization, Geneva, March 1990.
6. UNICEF and WHO estimates quoted in *The State of the World's Children 1987*, UNICEF, Oxford University Press, 1987.
7. Morley and Lovel 1986, see note 1.
8. Morley and Lovel 1986, see note 1. See also Beverley A. Carlson and Tessa M. Wardlaw , *A Global, Regional and Country Assessment of Child Malnutrition*, Staff Working Papers no. 7 UNICEF, New York, 1990.
9. Michal Jancloes, "More than a billion ... ", *World Health*, World Health Organization, Geneva, March 1990. Dr Jancloes of WHO suggests that there are close to 2.2 billion people living in a state of severe poverty and among these, more than 700 million live in extreme poverty.
10. Jancloes 1990, see note 9.
11. UN Population Division, UN Statistical Office and WHO estimates quoted in UNICEF, *The State of the World's Children 1987*, Oxford University Press, 1987.
12. Morley and Lovel 1986, see note 1.
13. World Health Organization, *Global Estimates for Health Situation Assessment and Projections, 1990*, Division of Epidemiological Surveillance and Health Situation and Trend Assessment, Geneva, April 1990.
14. See for instance Dr Akira Shimouchi, "Controlling pneumonia in children", *World Health*, November 1989.
15. World Health Organization 1990, see note 13.

16. Rohde, Jon E., "Why the other half dies: the science and politics of child mortality in the Third World", *Assignment Children* vol. 61/62, 1983. To support this statement, he quotes from Thomas McKeown, "The role of medicine: dream, mirage or nemesis?", Nuffield Provincial Hospitals Trust, London, 1976 and from Walsh McDermott, "Modern medicine and the demographic disease pattern of overly traditional societies: a technologic misfit" in "Manpower for the World's Health" edited by Henry van Zile Hyde, *The Journal of Medical Education* vol. 41, no. 9, September 1966.
17. For a discussion of the most common housing sub-markets in Third World cities and the factors which influence the form they take in any particular city, see Hardoy, Jorge E. and David Satterthwaite, *Squatter Citizen: Life in the Urban Third World*, Earthscan Publications, London, 1989 and the special issue of *Environment and Urbanization* vol. 1, no. 2, October 1989, which was on the theme of "Beyond the Stereotype of Slums: How poor people find accommodation in Third World cities".

Chapter 1.

Later sections of this chapter develop and expand on sections of a paper entitled "Housing and Health: What Role for Architects and Planners" by Jorge E. Hardoy and David Satterthwaite, *Cities* vol. 4, no. 3, 1987.

1. Calculated from statistics in United Nations, *The Prospects for World Urbanization: Revised as of 1984-5*, ST/ESA/SER.A/101, New York, 1987.
2. In many regions in Europe, North America and Australia in the last two decades or so, increases in the proportion of population living in urban centres has slowed, halted or even, in some instances, reversed. But this is essentially due to what might be termed the "urbanization" of rural areas as industries and commercial and financial enterprises develop in greenfield sites or rural settlements where inhabitants enjoy a quality of infrastructure and services (including piped water, sewers, collection of solid wastes and connection to transport and communications networks) previously associated with urban areas. Comparable trends towards a decentralization of industry, commerce and finance out of major cities or metropolitan areas to smaller urban centres and rural areas is also evident in some Third World nations and regions for similar reasons; see for instance Daniel R. Vining Jr., "The growth of Core Regions in the Third World", *Scientific American* vol. 252, no. 4, April 1985, and Chapter 8 of Jorge E. Hardoy and David Satterthwaite, *Squatter Citizen: Life in the Urban Third World*, Earthscan Publications, London, 1989. There are some indications that certain regions in Europe and North America which have experienced this phenomenon of "counter-urbanization" or "counter-metropolitanization" in recent decades are now experiencing, once again, population growth centring in certain cities. But it will probably need a new round of census data for censuses taken in 1989, 1990 and 1991 to verify its extent and importance.
3. Chapters 2, 3 and 4 are case studies of Buenos Aires, Lagos and Allahabad. Some examples of other case studies:

For Alexandria, see Mounir Soliman, "Informal land acquisition and the urban poor in Alexandria", *Third World Planning Review* vol. 9, no. 1, February 1987.

For Guayaquil, see Caroline O.N. Moser, "A Home of One's Own: Squatter Housing Strategies in Guayaquil, Ecuador", in Alan Gilbert, Jorge E. Hardoy and Ronaldo Ramirez (eds.) *Urbanization in Contemporary Latin America*, John Wiley and Sons, 1982.

For Karachi, see Jan van der Linden, "Squatting by organized invastion - a new reply to a failing housing policy?", *Third World Planning Review* vol. 4, no. 4, November 1982.

For Khartoum, see Omer M.A. El Agraa, Adil M. Ahmad, Ian Haywood and O.M. El Kheir, *Popular Settlements in Greater Khartoum*, Sudanese Group for Assessment of Human Settlements, Khartoum, the Sudan, 1985.

For Lima, see Lisa Peattie, "Participation: a case study of how invaders organize, negotiate and interact with government in Lima, Peru", *Environment and Urbanization* vol. 2, no. 1, April 1990.

For Lusaka, see Ann and Thomas Schlyter, *George – the Development of a Squatter Settlement in Lusaka, Zambia*, The Swedish Council for Building Research, Stockholm, 1980.

For Mexico City, see Priscilla Connolly, "Uncontrolled Settlements and Selfbuild: What kind of solution? The Mexico City Case", in Peter Ward (ed.), *Self Help Housing: A Critique*, Mansell, London, 1982.

For Nairobi, see Philip Amis, "Squatters or Tenants: the Commercialization of Unauthorized Housing in Nairobi", *World Development* vol. 12, no. 4, 1984, pp. 87-96.

For Recife, see Alexandrina Sobreira de Moura, "Brasilia Teimosa – the organization of a low income settlement in Recife, Brazil", *Development Dialogue* 1, 1987, pp. 152-169.

For Sao Paulo, see N.G. Bonduke and R. Rolnik, "Loteo Clandestino – Jardin Flor da Primavera", *Medio Ambiente y Urbanizacion* Year 3, no. 9, IIED-America Latina, Buenos Aires, 1984 and Celine Sachs, "The growth of squatter settlements in Sao Paulo: a study of the perverse effects of the State Housing Policies", *Man and his Environment*, Social Science Information 22, 4/5, 1983.

4. Examples include the case study in Buenos Aires (Chapter 2) and Sobreira de Moura 1987, Peattie 1990 and Moser 1982, see note 3,
5. Hardoy and Satterthwaite, 1989, see note 2.
6. McAuslan, Patrick, *Urban Land and Shelter for the Poor* (Revised Edition), Earthscan Publications, London (forthcoming).
7. These are figures quoted in UNICEF, *The State of the World's Children 1990*, Oxford University Press, 1990.
8. The governments of many poor Third World nations claim that more than 90 per cent of their urban populations had access to health services in the mid 1980s including Mozambique (100 per cent), Niger (99 per cent), the Sudan (90 per cent), Tanzania (99 per cent), Bolivia (90 per cent), Pakistan (99 per cent) and Myanmar – formerly Burma (100 per cent). These are figures quoted in UNICEF 1990, see note 7.
9. Hardoy and Satterthwaite 1989, see note 2.
10. Cointreau, Sandra J., *Environmental Management of Urban Solid Wastes in Developing Countries: a Project Guide*, Urban Development Technical Paper no. 5. the World Bank, Washington DC, June 1982.
11. Sources for Box 1.1. For information on Asian cities: K.C. Sivaramakrishnan,

and Leslie Green, *Metropolitan Management – The Asian Experience*, Oxford University Press (for the World Bank), 1986. For additional information on Bangkok: Dhira Phantumvanit and Wanai Liengcharernsit "Coming to terms with Bangkok's environmental problems", *Environment and Urbanization* vol. 1, no 1, IIED, April 1989, pp. 31-39; and United Nations, Population Growth *Population Growth and Policies in Mega-Cities: Bangkok*, Population Policy Paper No 10, Department of International Economic and Social Affairs, ST/ESA/SER.R/72, New York, 1987. For additional information on Karachi: Sahil, "Marine pollution and the Indus Delta", Volume 1 (House journal of National Institute of Oceanography, Karachi, Pakistan), 1988, pp. 57-61; and United Nations, *Population Growth and Policies in Mega-Cities: Karachi*, Population Policy Paper No 13, Department of International Economic and Social Affairs, ST/ESA/SER.R/77, New York, 1988. For additional information on Manila: Rosario D. Jimenez and Sister Aida Velasquez "Metropolitan Manila: a framework for its sustained development", *Environment and Urbanization*, vol.1, no 1, IIED-London, April 1989, pp. 51-58. Information on African cities drawn from chapters in Richard E. Stren and Rodney R. White (eds.), *African Cities in Crisis*, Westview Press, USA, 1989, especially: Thiecouta Ngom, "Appropriate standards for infrastructure in Dakar", pp. 176-202; Saitiel Kulaba, "Local government and the management of urban services in Tanzania", pp. 203-245; Mohamed O. El Sammani, Mohamed El Hadi Abu Sin, M. Talha, B.M. El Hassan and Ian Haywood, "Management problems of Greater Khartoum", pp. 246-275; and Kankonde Mbuyi, "Kinshasa: problems of land management, infrastructure and food supply", pp. 148-175. For Sao Paulo: Vilmar Evangelista Faria, chapter on Sao Paulo, in Mattei Dogon and John D. Casada (eds), *The Metropolis Era Volume 2*, Sage Publications, Beverly Hills, London and New Delhi, 1988, pp. 294-309.

12. Murphy, Denis, "Hong Kong: Some are left out" in *Housing by People in Asia*, newsletter published by Third World Network and the Asian Coalition for Housing Rights, April 1990.
13. UNICEF 1990, see note 7, drawing from Teresa Albanez, Eduardo Bustelo, Giovanni Andrea Coma and Eva Jespersen, *Economic Decline and Child Survival: the Plight of Latin America in the Eighties*, UNICEF, International Child Development Centre, Florence, Innocenti Occasional Papers no. 1, March 1989.
14. Figures given in David Morley and Hermione Lovel, *My Name is Today: an Illustrated Discussion of Child Health, Society and Poverty in Less Developed Countries*, Macmillan Publishers, London, 1986, drawing from World Bank, *Health Sector Policy Paper*, Washington DC, 1980.
15. Tabibzadeh, I., A. Rossi-Espagnet and R. Maxwell, *Spotlight on the Cities: Improving Urban health in Developing Countries*, World Health Organization, Geneva, 1989.
16. UNICEF 1990, see note 7.
17. UNICEF 1990, see note 7 and Albanez et al. 1989, see note 13.
18. Hardoy and Satterthwaite 1989, see note 2.
19. See Introduction, note 17.
20. Tabibzadeh, Rossi-Espagnet and Maxwell 1989, see note 15.
21. For details and examples, refer to Hardoy and Satterthwaite 1989, see note

2.

22. Tabibzadeh, Rossi-Espagnet and Maxwell 1989, see note 15.
23. Basta, Samir S., "Nutrition and health in low income urban areas of the Third World", *Ecology of Food and Nutrition* vol. 6, 1977, pp. 113-124.
24. World Health Organization, *Urbanization and its Implications for Child Health: Potential for Action*, Geneva, 1989 and Tabibzadeh, Rossi-Espagnet and Maxwell 1989, see note 15.
25. Bangladesh: Das, Ananda Mohan, A. Mannan Bangali, Shabbir Ahmed and M.D. Shahidullah, *An Overview of Health Scenario in Slums and Hazaribag area of Dhaka* Directorate General of Health Services, Government of Bangladesh, Dhaka, May 1990.
    Karachi: Agha Khan University students 1986 (unpublished) quoted in Trudy Harpham, Tim Lusty and Patrick Vaughan (eds.), *In the Shadow of the City: Community Health and the Urban Poor*, Oxford University Press, 1988.
    Manila: Republic of the Philippines, City of Manila Health Department Statistics Division of Preventable Diseases, Manila, 1973; Food and Nutrition Research Center Survey for four regions and Greater Manila, 1973; and unpublished survey of 6,000 households by the Nutrition Foundation of the Philippines and Tondo Foreshore Development Authority, May 1975. All three sources quoted in Basta 1977, see note 23.
    Panama City: M. Kouray and M.A. Vasquez, "Housing and certain socio-environmental factors and prevalence enteropathogenic bacteria among infants with diarrhoeal disease in Panama, *American Institute of Tropical Medicine and Hygiene* 18, pp. 936-41 quoted in Harpham, Lusty and Vaughan 1988, see above.
    Port-au-Prince: J.E. Rohde, "Why the other half dies: the science and politics of child mortality in the Third World", *Assignment Children* vol. 61/62, 1983.
    Porto Alegre: J.J. Guimaraes and A. Fischmann, "Inequalities in 1980 infant mortality among shantytown residents and non-shanty town residents in the municipality of Porto Alegre, Rio Grande do Sul, Brazil", *Bulletin of the Pan American Health Organization* 19, 1985, pp. 235-251.
    Sao Paulo: World Bank, *Staff Appraisal Report: Brazil Second Health Project*, Sao Paulo basic health care and national health policy studies, Population, Health and Nutrition Department, Washington DC, 1984.
26. Ghosh, S., T.K. Ramanujacharyulu, V. Hooja and S. Madhaven, "Mortality patterns in an urban birth cohort", *Indian Journal of Medical Research* vol. 69, pp. 616-623, quoted in Morley and Lovel 1986, see note 13.
27. Basta 1977, see note 23.
28. Arden Miller, C., "Setting Priorities for Health Care", Chapter 5 in *Habitat, Health and Development*, Joseph S. Tulchin (ed.), Lynne Reinner Publishers Inc., Boulder, Colorado, USA, 1986.
29. A paper on the impact of urbanization and industrialization on mortality in different regions of Brazil documents an increase in infant mortality in Sao Paulo during an economic boom between 1965 and 1973 and a decline in infant mortality during a period of recession between 1973 and 1983. "During the recession, deliberate policy interventions .. reduced the number of deaths from causes related to sanitation, eventually overcoming adverse socio-economic conditions" – see Diana Oya-Sawyer, Rogelio Fernandez-Castilla and Roberto Luis de Melo Monte-Mor, "The impact of urbanization

and industrialization on mortality in Brazil", *World Health Statistics Quarterly* vol. 40, 1987, pp. 84-95.

30. Many empirical studies have demonstrated an inverse relationship between mother's education and child mortality; for an overview and discussion as to why, see John C. Caldwell and Pat Caldwell, "Education and literacy as factors in health" in Scott B. Halstead, Julia A. Walsh and Kenneth S. Warren (eds.), *Good Health at Low Cost*, Conference Report, the Rockefeller Foundation, October 1985.
31. John Briscoe, "Water Supply and Health in Developing Countries: Selective primary health care revisited" in *Habitat, Health and Development*, see note 28.
32. World Health Organization, *Intersectoral Action for Health – the Role of Intersectoral Cooperation in National Strategies for Health for All*, background document for the technical discussions, 39th World Health Assembley, May 1986, A39/86-832/1.
33. M. Bapat and N. Crook, "The environment, health and nutrition: an analysis of interrelationships from a case study of hutment settlements in the city of Poona" *Habitat International* vol. 8, no. 3/4, 1984.
34. See for instance, Caroline O.N. Moser,"Gender planning in the Third World: meeting practical and strategic gender needs", *World Development* vol. 17, no. 11, 1989, pp. 1799-1825.

Chapter 2

The information for this chapter is drawn from a pilot study of habitat and health conditions undertaken in 1984/5 as part of a research project organized by the Instituto Internacional de Medio Ambiente y Desarrollo (IIED-America Latina) with funding from the International NGO Division of the Canadian International Development Agency and from the Dutch Ministry of Housing, Physical Planning and the Environment. It drew on various information sources: a survey of population, housing and health characteristics for just over one third of the population of San Martin; an examination of clinical records and physical and laboratory tests for a small sample of families; physical examinations of the site and structures on the site; and interviews both with people within the settlement and those living outside but with knowledge of particular aspects of relevance to the study. The parish priest of the area provided a lot of the background information to the invasion and how it was organized.

The researchers undertaking this work, from the Centro de Estudios Urbanos y Regionales (CEUR) based in Buenos Aires, also organized a course on "Health Promotion for the Community" for the inhabitants of San Martin and for those living in neighbouring settlements. Most of the documentation about this case study and its findings are in Spanish; for more details, write to Beatriz Cuenya, CEUR, Piso 7, Cuerpo A, Corrientes 2835, (1193) Buenos Aires,Argentina. For more details on the way in which the land invasion was organized, see Beatriz Cuenya, Diego Armus, Maria Di Loreto and Susana Penalva, "Land invasions and grassroots organization: the Quilmes settlements in Greater Buenos Aires, Argentina" in *Environment and Urbanization* vol. 2, no. 1, April 1990, pp 61-73.

1. *Villa miseria* is the Argentine term for a squatter settlement; the literal translation is "misery settlement" or "misery village". These are illegal settlements which usually developed on vacant land sites in central zones and on the urban periphery. Housing and living conditions in such settlements are very poor. Usually, the vacant site is occupied gradually as different households come to the site and begin building. The first *villas miserias* date from the 1930s although the number of people living in them only became significant during the 1960s.
2. Llovet, Juan Jose, "El sector salud durante el regimen militar", *Medio Ambiente y Urbanizacion* no. 5, December 1983, pp. 31-34.
3. Interview with the president of one of the area's Development Centres.
4. A delegate from San Martin, quoted in an interview in *El Porteño* no. 10, Buenos Aires, October 1982
5. Quoted from the article "Toma de tierras", *Al Sur*, April 1982.
6. Testimony of one of the Quilmes Oeste settlement dwellers published in the article "Las tierras para el hombre", *El Porteño* no. 10, Buenos Aires, October 1982.

7-8. Interview with *barrio* leaders from San Martin

9. *Linea* magazine, January 1982.
10. Reported in the newspaper *Clarin*, 12 February, 1982
11. Testimony of a resident reported in *El Porteño* see note 4.
12. Reported in *El Sol*, a daily newspaper, December 29th, 1981.
13. Interview with a *barrio* leader.
14. *Nuestra Esperanza* no. 3.

Chapter 3

This chapter is drawn from a longer and more detailed report: see Akin Aina, Tade, *Health, Habitat and Underdevelopment in Nigeria with special reference to a low income settlement in Metropolitan Lagos*, IIED Human Settlements Programme Technical Report, London, 1990. Available from IIED, 3 Endsleigh Street, London WC1H ODD, UK.

1. Aradeon, David, Tade Akin Aina and Joe Umo, "South West Nigeria" in: Hardoy J. and Satterthwaite D. (eds.) *Small and Intermediate Urban Centres: Their Role in National and Regional Development*, Hodder and Stoughton/IIED, London, 1986.
2. Estimated by the Lagos State Development and Property Company
3. Marris, Peter, *Family and Social Change in an African City: A Study of Rehousing in Lagos*, Routledge and Kegan Paul, London, 1961, p. 8.
4. Perhaps the most direct health and habitat study available is F.O. Okediji and O. Aboyade, "Social and economic aspects of environmental sanitation in Nigeria: a tentative report", *NISER Reprint Series, no. 47, Ibadan*, 1967.
5. Ejiogu, C.N. "Metropolitanization: the growth of Lagos" in J.C. Caldwell (ed.) *Population Growth and Socio-Economic Changes in West Africa*, Columbia University Press, New York, 1975.
6. Ejiogu 1975, see note 5.
7. Marris 1961 pp. 82-83, see note 3.

8. Marris 1961 p. 83, see note 3.
9. Okediji and Aboyade 1967 p. 12, see note 4.
10. Nigeria, Federal Republic of, *Third National Development Plan 1975-80*, Lagos, 1975.
11. Nigeria, Federal Republic of, *Fourth National Development Plan 1981-1985*, The National Planning Office, Federal Ministry of National Planning, Lagos, 1981.
12. Okoye, T.O., "Historical development of Nigerian housing policies with special reference to housing the urban poor" in Philip Amis and Peter Lloyd (eds.), *Housing Africa's Urban Poor*, Manchester University Press, 1990.
13. Lagos State Ministry of Economic Development, *Statistical Survey of Lagos State*, November/December 1976, p. 76.
14. Lagos State of Nigeria, *Lagos State Interim Regional Plan (1980-2000)*, Ministry of Economic Planning and Land Matters, Urban and Regional Planning Division, Lagos State Secretariat, Ikeja, 14 January, 1980.
15. Marris 1961 pp. 82-3, see note 3.
16. For 1967 figures, see F.O. Okediji, "Socio-economic status and attitudes to public health problems in the Western State: a case study of Ibadan" in J.C. Caldwell (ed.) *Population Growth and Socio-Economic Change in West Africa*, published for the Population Council of New York, Columbia University Press, New York and London, 1975 p. 279; for 1958 figures, see Marris 1961 p. 83, see note 3.
17. Akin Aina, Tade, *Health, Habitat and Underdevelopment in Nigeria with special reference to a low income settlement in Metropolitan Lagos*, IIED Human Settlements Programme Technical Report, London, 1990.
18. For more details, see Akin Aina, Tade "Many routes enter the market place - housing submarkets for the urban poor in Metropolitan Lagos, Nigeria", *Environment and Urbanization*, vol. 1, no. 2, 1990, pp. 38-49.
19. This is from an unpublished and undated report from the main physical planning authority in Metropolitan Lagos, the Lagos Executive Development Board entitled *The Abule-Nla Redevelopment Scheme*, p. 3.
20. Okpala, D.C.I., *Institutional Problems in the Management of Nigerian Urban Environment*, NISER Monograph Series, no. 16, Ibadan, 1986, p.13 and Okediji 1975 p. 279, see note 16.
21. These figures for Olaleye Village were obtained from another unpublished report prepared by the Department of Urban and Regional Planning, Governor's Office, Lagos entitled *The Olaleye Villages Neighbourhood Upgrading Scheme*, September 1982, p. 1.
22. See note 21.
23. See note 21.
24. Abrams, Charles et al. "Metropolitan Lagos" edited selection of the UN 1963 Report, *Habitat International*, vol. 5, nos. 1/2, 1980, pp. 55-83.
25. 'Junior employees' is a term used to denote the lower echelons of the hierarchy in the public sector in Nigeria. The hierarchy includes, top management, middle management, supervisory categories, and the junior employees or junior workers. Incomes, responsibility and other benefits match the designation.
26. Governors Office, Lagos State (undated) *The Olaleye – Iponri Upgrading Scheme Report*, Department of Urban and Regional Planning, Lagos.

27. This information is drawn from a similar survey carried out for Olaleye-Iponri by the Department of Urban and Regional Planning, Office of the Governor, Lagos State. The unpublished report of this study provided a breakdown and analysis of the pattern of land-use in Olaleye-Iponri – see note 26.
28. For more details, refer to Akin Aina 1990, see note 18 and Akin Aina, Tade "The construction of housing for the urban poor of Lagos" *Habitat International*, vol. 12, no. 1, 1988, pp. 37-39.
29. *The Olaleye – Iponri Upgrading Scheme Report*, see note 26.
30. The phenomenon of private water-hawkers either using water-tankers or carrying buckets and other containers has become a major feature of the supply of water in Metropolitan Lagos and other major Nigerian urban centres where there are shortages of water.
31. This was the study carried out by the Department of Urban Renewal of the Lagos State Government with the support and assistance of Habitat (UNCHS) before Olaleye – Iponri was selected as a pilot project.

Chapter 4

This chapter is based on the findings of research undertaken by staff from the International Institute for Development Research in Allahabad, India, under the direction of Dr H.N. Misra. A slightly longer version was printed in *Cities* vol. 5, no. 2, May 1988 (Butterworth Press) and this chapter is printed with their kind permission.

The research on which it is based is part of a wider programme of research and training and of the provision of technical and legal advice to low income inhabitants in squatter settlements undertaken in four different Third World cities – Allahabad, Buenos Aires, Khartoum and Lagos. Comparable studies to this were undertaken by the Centro de Estudios Urbanos y Regionales (Centre for Urban and Regional Studies) in Buenos Aires, the Sudanese Group for Assessment of Human Settlements in Khartoum and the Lagos Group for the Study of Human Settlements in Lagos. The work took place under the direction and co-ordination of the Human Settlements Programme of the International Institute for Environment and Development.

The author is grateful to the International NGO Division of the Canadian International Development Agency for support for the research and indeed for the long term support given to research undertaken by the International Institute for Development Research in recent years. Gratitude is also due to the Ministry of Housing, Physical Planning and Environment of the Netherlands for their support of the health survey and to the United Nations Centre for Human Settlements for their general support. Special thanks are due to many people for their help and support in this work. These include Dr Jorge E. Hardoy and David Satterthwaite from IIED's Human Settlements Programme, Dr Rama Misra (Reader in Gynaecology) and Dr G.J. Gupta (lecturer in Health Education) at M.L.N. Medical College in Allahabad, and Dr H.N. Ganguli, a local medical practitioner for their expert advice. Professor R.P. Misra, Vice Chancellor of Allahabad University has also helped greatly in supporting IIDR's work and in helping to arrange seminars and symposia to allow the presentation and discussion of the findings of the research.

Dr S.C. Sharma (Medical officer in charge) and Savitri Srivastava (Social Educator) at the City Welfare Bureau have been a great help in the preparation of the report while Professor R.L. Dwivedi, an expert in urban planning, has also given valuable advice. Thanks are also due to Jais Raj Shukla and Anata Misra both for help in preparing this report and in data collection and to Indra Raj Singh, Ram Kishore and Poonam Pandey for collecting information and data.

1. Harrison, J.B., "Allahabad: A Sanitary History" in Kenneth Ballhatchet and John Harrison (eds.), *The City in South Asia: pre-Modern and Modern*, Curzon Press, London, 1981.
2. Backward castes are those from the bottom of the hierarchic Indian caste structure. The scheduled caste were formerly known as untouchables and in rural areas are usually landless agricultural labourers, working for very low wages.
3. In 1857, a rebellion began against British rule in India which is known by Indian historians as the First War of Independence but referred to by British historians as the Indian Mutiny. The first outbreak started in Meerut in Uttar Pradesh and spread to Allahabad among other urban centres; it was in the aftermath of this that the administration of Uttar Pradesh passed from the East India Company to the British Crown.
4. Harrison 1981, see note 1.
5. The jurisdiction of Allahabad Development Authority is within the 82 square kilometre area defined by the boundaries and a further eight kilometres beyond the boundary.

Chapter 5

1. World Health Organization, *The International Drinking Water Supply and Sanitation Decade; Review of Mid-Decade Progress*, Geneva, 1987.
2. Esrey, S.A. and J.P. Habicht, "Epidemiologic evidence for health benefits from improved water and sanitation in developing countries", *Epidemiologic Reviews* vol. 8, 1986, pp. 117-128.
3. West, S., M. Lynch, V. Turner, B. Munoz, P. Rapoza, B. Mmbaga and H. Taylor, "Water availability and trachoma", *Bulletin of the World Health Organization* (in press).
4. White, G.F., D.J. Bradley and A.U. White, *Drawers of Water*, Chicago University Press, Chicago, 1972.
5. Pinnewala, S.K. and H.M.D.R. Herath, "Study of Water Collection and Use in Selected Communities of Kurunegala District", Department of Sociology, University of Peradeniya, Sri Lanka, 1986.
6. White et al 1972, see note 4.
7. Adrianzen, T. and G.G. Graham, "The high cost of being poor; water", *Archives of Environmental Health*, vol. 28, 1974, pp. 312-315.
8. Zaroff, B. and D.A. Okun, "Water vending in developing countries", *Aqua* vol. 5, 1984. pp. 289-295.
9. Briscoe, John, *Water Supply and Sanitation in the Health Sector in the Asia Region: Information Needs and Program Priorities*, report to USAID, Chapel Hill, University of North Carolina, 1985.
10. Laugeri, L., *Cost Recovery in Community Water Supply and Sanitation;*

Report of the Second Informal Consultation on Institutional Development, World Health Organization, Geneva, WHO/CWS/87.5, 1987.

11. Whittington, D., D. Lauria, D.A. Okun and X. Mu, *Water Vending Activities in Developing Countries*, WASH Technical Report no. 45, US Agency for International Development, Washington DC, 1987.
12. Goudy, A.P. and F.M. Law, "Bombay water supply project: demand and resource planning" *Proceedings of the Institution of Civil Engineers* part 1, vol. 80, 1986. pp. 945-967.
13. Bachmann, G. and M. Hammerer, "80 per cent of losses come from 20 per cent of leaks", *World Water*, October 1984, pp 48-50.
14. Lewis, M.A. and T.R. Miller, "Public-private partnership in water supply and sanitation in sub-Saharan Africa", *Health Policy and Planning*, vol. 2, no. 1, pp. 70-79.
15. World Bank, *Water Supply and Waste Disposal*, Poverty and Basic Needs Series, World Bank, Washington DC, 1980.
16. World Bank 1980, see note 15.
17. Warford, J. and R. Turvey, "Lahore water supply – tariff study", Public Utilities Report no. PUN 12, World Bank, Washington DC, 1974.
18. Habib, R. "Expensive Air", *Jordan Times*, 15-16 January 1987, p.5.
19. Shipman, H.R. "Water metering practices", *Agua*, vol. 2, 1978, pp. 2-12.
20. Metcalf and Eddy, *Draft final report on water distribution and tariff study: Rangoon, Burma* vols. 1 and 2, 1981.
21. Bachmann and Hammerer 1984, see note 13.
22. Yassuda, E.R., J.V. Kochen and E.F. Borba, "Reduction of losses and costs in water distribution systems through appropriate technology", SABESP, Sao Paulo, 1981.
23. White et al, 1972 see note 4.
24. Cairncross, S. and R.G. Feachem, *Environmental Health Engineering in the Tropics: an Introductory Text*, John Wiley & Sons, Chichester, 1983.
25. Hebert, P.V., "Impact of design criteria and standards on water supply costs in the Philippines", Symposium on Water Resources Research in the 1980s, Quezon City, Philippines, 1983.
26. See Zaroff and Okun 1984, note 8 and Briscoe 1985, note 9.
27. Okun, D.A. "Financing water supply systems" in E.J.Schiller and R.L.Droste (eds.) *Water Supply and Sanitation in Developing Countries*, Ann Arbor Science, 1982, pp. 251-267.
28. Cairncross, S. and J. Kinnear, "Measurement of the elasticity of domestic water demand; a study of water vendors and their clients, in urban Sudan", report to UK Overseas Development Administration, London School of Hygiene and Tropical Medicine, 1988.

Chapter 6

1. Pasternak, S., "Las favelas del municipio de san pablo : Resultados de una investigacion", *Revista Interamericana de Planification*, vol. XIV, no. 34., 1980.
2. Basta, S.S., "Nutrition and health in low-income urban areas of the Third World", *Ecology of Food and Nutrition*, vol. 6, 1977, pp 113-124.

3World Health Organization, *Health Survey Report*, Report to the Government of Afghanistan (Ministry of Public Health) and WHO, Kabul, 1978.

4. Rodhe, J. E. "Why the other half dies: the science and politics of hild mortality in the Third World", *Assignment Children* vol. 61/62, pp. 35-67.
5. Ruiz, W., "Poverty's children – understanding disease in a Peru in shantytown", *IDRC Reports* vol. 17, no. 4, Ottawa, 1988.
6. Benyoussef, A. *et al.*, "Sante, migration et urbanization: una etude collectiva au Senegal", *Bulletine WHO* vol. 49, 1973, pp 517-537.
7. Kleens, J. W. L., "Rehousing and infections by soil transmitted helminths in Singapore", *Singapore Medical Journal*, vol. 7, 1966, pp 12-29.
8. Feachem, R. G. *et al. Sanitation and Disease: Health Aspects of Excreta and Wastewater Management*, John Hopkins University Press, Baltimore, 1983; J.M. Kalbermatten *et al.*, *Appropriate Sanitation Alternatives – A Planning and Design Manual*, Johns Hopkins University Press, Baltimore, 1982; and Cairncross, S. and R.G. Feachem, *Environmental Health Engineering in the Tropics – an Introductory Text*, John Wiley & Sons, Chichester, 1983.
9. UNCHS, *Water Supply and Waste Disposal Management; Impact-Evaluation Guidelines* Nairobi, Kenya, 1987,
10. Chauhan, S. K. and K. Gopalakrishnan, "A million villages, a million decades *Ekistics* vol.. 303, November/December 1983, pp 488-498.
11. Latham, L *el al.*, *The Nutritional and Economic Implications of Ascaris Infection in Kenya*, World Bank Staff Working paper no. 271, Washington DC, 1977.
12. These are reviewed in J.M. Kalbermatten *et al.*, *Appropriate Sanitation Alternatives – A Planning and Design Manual*, Johns Hopkins University Press, Baltimore, 1982 and World Bank, *Water Supply and Waste Disposal*, Poverty and Basic Needs Series, Washington DC, 1980.
13. Kalbermatten 1982, see note 12 and D.D. Mara, *The Design of Ventilated Improved Pit Latrine*, TAG Technical Note no. 13, World Bank, Washington DC, 1984.
14. Carroll, R. F., "Affordable sanitation for Developing Countries", Note no. N147/80, Building Research Establishment, Garston, England; and J. Van Nostrad, and J.G. Wilson, *The Ventilated Improved Double-pit Latrine; A Construction Manual for Botswana*, TAG Technical Note no. 13, World Bank, Washington, D. C., 1983.
15. Sources for Box 6.3. Mozambique: B. Brandberg, "The latrine project, Mozambique", IDRC Manuscript Report – MR58e, Ottawa, 1985; H. Paqui, "Low cost sanitation in Mozambique", *Waterlines* vol. 7, no 1. Ghana: D.D. Mara, *The Design of Ventilated Improved Pit Latrine*, TAG Technical Note no. 13, World Bank, Washington, D. C., 1984. Malawi: B. Brandberg, "Low cost sanitation in Malawi – the urban to rural approach", *Developing World Water*, Grosvenor Press International, Hong Kong, 1988.
16. UNCHS, *The Conservation of Drinking Water Supplies: Techniques for Low-Income Settlements*, Nairobi, Kenya, 1990.
17. Roy, A. K. *et al.*, *Manual on the Design, Construction and Maintenance of Low-cost, Pour-flush, Waterseal Latrines in India*, TAG Technical Note no. 10, World Bank, Washington, D. C., 1984 and D.D. Mara, *The Design of Pour Flush Latrines*, TAG Technical Note, World Bank, Washington DC, 1986

18. Sources for Box 6.4. India: "Low cost options for urban sanitation", *Urban Edge* vol. 11, no. 10, World Bank, Washington DC, 1987; UNCHS, *Low Cost Sanitation Project in Bihar, India*, Project Monograph, Nairobi, 1986; and P. Wan, "Sanitation: a People's Programme", *Developing World Water*, Grosvenor Press, Hong Kong, 1987. For Indonesia: G.J. de Kruijff, "A feasible sanitation alternative", *Developing World Water*, Grosvenor Press, Hong Kong, 1987. For Pakistan: Q.A. Bakhtiaci, "Community management for sanitation: a case study on the UNICEF sponsored Baldia Soakpit Project", *Developing World Water*, Grosvenor Press, Hong Kong, 1987.
19. Kalbermatten et al. 1982, see note 8.
20. Sinnatamby, G. S. *Low-cost Sanitation Systems for Urban Peripheral Areas in Northeast Brazil*, Ph.D. Thesis, Department of Civil Engineering, The University, Leeds, 1983
21. Mara, D. D. and S.G. Sinnatamby, "Rational design of septic tanks in warm climates", *The Public Health Engineer* vol. 14, no. 4, 1986, pp 49-55.
22. Otis, R. J. and D.D. Mara, *The Design of Small Bore Sewer Systems*, TAG Technical Note no. 14, World Bank, Washington, D.C., 1985.
23. UNCHS, *The Design of Shallow Sewer Systems*, Nairobi, Kenya, 1986.
24. World Health Organization 1978, see note 3.

Chapter 7

This chapter is a slightly edited version of Chapter 1 in *Surface Water Drainage for Low-Income Communities* by Sandy Cairncross and E.A.R. Ouano, to be published by the RUD Programme, World Health Organization, 1990. Chapter 2 of this report considers the technical aspects of drainage design and construction and includes a section on how a community can plan its own drainage improvements without external support. This will be of interest to an engineer making a first approach to a local drainage problem. Chapter 3 discusses the rehabilitation and maintenance. Most of the chapter is technical, but lay readers will not find it difficult to follow. Chapter 4 considers participation by the community in drainage schemes.

1. Moser, Caroline O.N., "A home of one's own: squatter housing strategies in Guayaquil, Ecuador" in Alan Gilbert, Jorge E. Hardoy and Ronaldo Ramirez (eds.), *Urbanization in Contemporary Latin America*, John Wiley and Sons, Chichester, 1981.
2. See note at the beginning of this chapter.

Chapter 8

Stenio Cuentro, author of the case study in Recife, wishes to thank his friend Edjar Rocha Lima, present director of the Waste Management Departments of Paulista and Olinda, who very kindly provided updated information and edited the final text, and Eliana Barboza for her excellent typing. The text for this case study was translated from Portuguese into English by Julio D. Davila, of the Human Settlements Programme, International Institute for Environment and Development. The case study by Dri Malla Gadgi was translated from French by Jane Bicknell.

1. Cointreau, Sandra J., *Environmental Management of Urban Solid Wastes in*

Developing Countries: a Project Guide, Urban Development Technical Paper No 5. World Bank, Washington DC, June 1982.

2. Cointreau 1982, see note 1; also see chapter 10 for more details.
3. Cairncross, Sandy and Richard G. Feachem, *Environmental Health Engineering in the Tropics – an Introductory Text*, John Wiley and Sons, Chichester (UK), 1983.
4. Cointreau 1982, see note 1. This document draws on various World Bank city studies (for instance of Tunis and Onitsha) which document how poor areas receive much poorer levels of service and discuss why and how this can be resolved.
5. United Nations Centre for Human Settlements (Habitat), *Refuse Collection Vehicles for Developing Countries*, Nairobi, Kenya, 1988.
6. Furedy, Christine, "Social considerations in solid waste management in Asian cities", *Regional Development Dialogue* vol. 10, no. 3, Autumn 1989 and Cointreau 1982, see note 1. The United Nations Centre for Human Settlements (Habitat) also has a research and technical assistance programme on "small-scale, cottage based waste recycling industries".
7. See sources listed in note 6 and also Christine Furedy, "Appropriate technology for urban wastes in Asia", *Biocycle*, July 1989.
8. For one example in Manila where some 20,000 people live in or close to a major garbage dump known as "Smokey Mountain", see Rosario D. Jimenez and Sister Aida Velasquez, "Metropolitan Manila: a framework for its sustained development", *Environment and Urbanization* vol. 1, no. 1, April 1989.
9. Frank Flintoff quoted in Cointreau 1982, p. 42, see note 1.
10. Furedy 1989, see note 6.
11. Olinda Municipality, *Triangulo de Peixinhos: Projeto Piloto de Urbanizacao*, 1985.
12. The criticisms of the World Bank-funded project involved questioning the convenience and high costs of centralization and of wasting 2,000 tonnes of garbage by depositing it in large sanitary landfills rather than recycling the material and partially recovering costs. Pernambuco State authorities requested officials in Olinda to prepare a document presenting their ideas and defending their arguments for recycling and composting of refuse through integrated and participatory planning (see Rodolfo Aureliano, Ruy Rego and Ivan Mauricio, "Limpeza urbana integrada ao ecossistema", Olinda Municipality, mimeo, 1984).
13. Recife city centre, with a population of some 200,000, generates 170 tonnes of rubbish every day, or an average of 0.85 kg/day per person. The city's richest neighbourhoods, on the other hand, produce between 1.2 and 1.8 kg/day per person.
14. In 1983, Recife's local authorities recognised only 72 settlements as *favelas* or low-income settlements. The figures used in this text were arrived at by De Moura and Souza through their own research entitled "Land ownership conflicts in Greater Recife", supported by the Federal University of Pernambuco and the Joaquim Nabuco Foundation.
15. This is a slightly shortened version of a paper prepared by Dji Malla Gadgi for OXFAM; the full version is printed in *Baobab* no. 4, Alin, Oxfam, 1990.

Chapter 9

This is a condensed version of a chapter printed in C.F. Curtis (ed.), *Appropriate Technology in Vector Control*, CRC Press, Boca Raton, Florida, 1990 and we are grateful to Dr Curtis and to the publishers for allowing it to be included in this volume.

1. World Health Organization, *Uses of Epidemiology in Housing Programmes and in Planning Human Settlements*, Technical Report Series no. 544, Geneva, 1974.
2. Agarwal, Anil, *Mud, Mud; The Potential of Earth-based Materials for Third World Housing*, Earthscan Publications, London, 1981.
3. Oliver, Paul (ed.), *Shelter and Society*, Barrie and Jenkins, London, 1969.
4. Oliver, Paul (ed.), *Shelter in Africa*, Barrie and Jenkins, London, 1971.
5. Kroeger, Alex, "Housing and health in the process of cultural adaptation: a case study among jungle and highland natives of Ecuador", *Journal of Tropical Medicine and Hygiene* vol. 83, p.53, 1980.
6. Dethier, J., *Des Architectures de Terre*, Centre Georges Pompidou, Paris, 1981.
7. Schofield, C.J. and G.B. White, "House design and domestic vectors of disease" *Transactions of the Royal Society for Tropical Medicine and Hygiene* vol. 78, no. 285, 1984.
8. Lea, R.G., *Reducing the Risk of Pest Infestations: Design Recommendations and Literature Review*, Building Research Establishment Digest, Princes Risborough, 1980.
9. Mason, D., *Hospitals can Damage your Health*, British Pest Control Association, London, 1985; A.R. Norman, "Hygiene in hospital kitchens" *The Lancet* vol. 8480, 561, March 1986; and Lea 1980, see note 8.
10. Schofield and White 1984, see note 7.
11. Schofield, C.J., "Population dynamics and control of Triatoma infestans" Annales de la Société Belge de Médicine Tropicale volo 65 (supplement 1), 149, 1985.
12. Schofield, C.J. "The behaviour of Triatominea (Hemiptera:Reduviidae) – a review" *Bulletin of Entomological Research*, vol. 69, 363, 1979.
13. Schofield, C.J. and G.B. White, "Density dependent feeding success in triatomine bugs and other vectors" in N.H.R. Burgess, G.R. Port and R.N. Titchener (eds.), *Ecoparasites of Veterinary and Medical Importance in Temperate Areas*, Royal Army Medical College, London, 1982.
14. Deobhanker, P.B. "Malaria control in Bombay by legislative measures and other non-insecticidal methods of vector control" in V.P. Sharma, Y.H. Bang, P. Rosenfield and C.P. Pant (eds.), *Community Participation for Disease Vector Control*, Indian Malaria Research Centre, 1986, p. 101.
15. Lok, Chan Kai, *Singapore's Dengue Haemorrhagic Fever Control Programme: a Case Study on the Successful Control of Aedes aegypti and Aedes Albopictus using Mainly Environmental measures as a Part of Integrated Vector Control*, South East Asian Medical Centre Publication no. 45, Tokyo, 1985.
16. Reiter, P. and D. Sprenger, "The used tyre trade: a mechanism for the worldwide dispersal of container breeding mosquitoes" *Journal of the American Mosquito Control Association* vol. 3, 494, 1987.

17. SUCAM, *Doenças e Migracão Humana*, Ministerio da Saude, Brasilia, 1982; and A. Cruz Marques, "Human migration and the spread of malaria in Brazil" *Parasitology Today* vol. 3, no. 166, 1987.
18. World Health Organization, *Ten Years of Onchocerciasis Control in West Africa*, WHO document OCP/GVA/85.1B, Geneva, 1985.
19. World Health Organization, *Manual on Environmental Management for Mosquito Control with special emphasis on Malaria Vectors*, WHO offset publications no. 66, Geneva, 1982.
20. Cranson, P.S., R.D. Tee, P.F. Credland and A.B. Kay, "Chironomid haemoglobins: their detection and role in allergy to midges in the Sudan and elsewhere" *Mems American Entomology Society* vol. 34, p.71, 1984; and P.S. Cranson, "Allegens of non-biting midges (Diptera:Chironomidae): a systematic survey of chironomid haemoglobins" *Medical and Veterinary Entomology* vol. 2, p.117, 1988.
21. Cruz Marques 1987, see note 17 and C.J. Schofield, *Malaria and its Anopheline Vectors in the Amazon Region of Brazil*, unpublished report to the World Bank, Washington DC, 1986.
22. Deobhanker 1986, see note 14.
23. Coluzzi, M., A. Sabatini, V. Petrarca and M.A. Di Deco, "Chromosomal differentiation and adaptation to human environments in the Anopheles gambiae complex", *Transcripts of the Royal Society for Tropical Medicine and Hygiene*, vol. 73, 483, 1979.
24. White, G.B., "Factors influencing densities of mosquitoes resting indoors" *Annual Report of the East African Institute of Malaria and Vector Borne Diseases* 1969.
25. Hooper, C., *Design for Climate; Guidelines for the Design of Low-cost Houses for the Climates of Kenya*, Housing Research and Development Unit, University of Nairobi, Kenya, 1975; and O.H. Koenigsberger, T.G. Ingersoll, A. Mayhew and S.V. Szokalay, *Manual of Tropical Housing and Building Part One: Climatic Design*, Longman, London, 1973.
26. Kolstrup, N., *Studies on the Transmission and Control of Wucheria bancrofti in North East Tanzania*, PhD thesis, University of London, 1980.
27. Kolstrup 1980, see note 26.
28. Lehane, M.J. and C.J. Schofield, "Flight initiation in Triatoma infestans (Klug) (Hemiptera:Reduviidae)", *Bulletin of Entomology Research*, vol. 72, no. 497, 1982; and C.J. Schofield and J.N.S. Matthews, "Theoretical approaches to active dispersal and colonisation of houses by Triatoma infestans", *Journal of Tropical Medicine and Hygiene* vol. 88, p.211, 1985.
29. Forattina, O.P., E.O. da Rocha e Silva, O.A. Ferreira, E.X. Rabello and D.G.B. Pattoli, "Aspectos ecológicos da tripanossomose americana; III-dispersão local de triatomineos, com especial referencia ao Triatoma sordida" *Revista da Saude Publica*, vol. 5, 193, 1971.
30. Soler, C.A., H. Schenone and H. Reyes, "Problemas derivadas de la reaparación de Triatoma infestans en viviendas desinsectadas y el concepto de reinfestación" *Boletin Chileno de Parasitologia* vol. 24, 83, 1969; and C.J. Schofield, unpublished data, 1985.
31. Schofield, C.J., unpublished data 1985.
32. Mellanby, K., *Scabies*, E.W. Classey, London, 1972; and J.R. Busvine, *Insects and Hygiene*, Methuen, London, 1966.

33. Cairncross, Sandy, "Low cost sanitation technology for the control of intestinal helminths" *Parasitology Today* vol. 3, p.94, 1987; and Sandy Cairncross and Richard G. Feachem, *Environmental Health Engineering in the Tropics – An Introductory Text*, John Wiley and Sons, Chichester (UK), 1983.
34. Bucher, E.H. and C.J. Schofield, *Uso de la Tierra y Enfermedad de Chagas* Centro de Zoologia Aplicada, Cordoba Publ. no. 8, 1984; and R.A. Ronderos, J.A. Schnack and R.A. Mauri, "Resultados preliminares respecto de la ecologia de Triatoma infestans (Klug) y especies congenericas con referencia especial a poblaciones peridomiciliares" *Medicina Buenos Aires* 40 (suppl. 1), 187, 1980.
35. Schofield 1985, see note 11; and C.J. Schofield, "Control of Chagas disease vectors" *British Medical Bulletin*, vol.41, p.187, 1985.
36. Lane, R.P., "Chicken house reservoirs of sandflies" *Parasitology Today* 2, 248, 1986,
37. Cranston 1988, see note 20; J.D. Charlwood, "Observations on the bionomics of Anopheles darlingi root (Diptera:Culicidae) from Brazil" *Bulletin of Entomological Research* vol. 70, 685, 1980; and J.E. Hudson, "Anopheles darlingi Root (Diptera:Culicidae) in the Surinam rain forest" *Bulletin of Entomological Research*, vol. 74, 129, 1984.
38. Barlow F., "Physical processes associated with formulations", *British Crop Protection Council Monographs*, 17, 127, 1976; and F. Barlow, A.B. Hadaway, L.S. Flower, J.E.H. Gross and C.R. Turner, "Some laboratory investigations relevant to the possible use of new pyrethroids in control of mosquitoes and tsetse flies" *Pesticide Science* 8, 291, 1977.
39. Zeledon, R. and L.G. Vargas, "The role of dirt floors and of firewood in rural dwellings in the epidemiology of Chagas' disease in Costa Rica" *American Journal of Tropical Medicine and Hygiene*, vol. 33, 232, 1984.
40. Kalshoven, L.G.E., "Observations on the blood-sucking reduviid Triatoma rubrofasciata (De Geer) in Java" *Ent Berichten* 30, 41, 1970.
41. Gorla, D.E. and C.J. Schofield, unpublished data, 1982.
42. Gorla, D.E. and C.J. Schofield, unpublished data, 1982.
43. Briceno-Leon, R., "Rural housing for control of Chagas' disease in Venezuela" *Parasitology Today* 3, 384, 1987; M.G. Lunt, "Stabilized soil blocks for building" *Overseas Building Notes* no. 184, 1980; A. Vildoso, F.M. Monzon, A. Hays, S. Matuk and F. Vitoux, *Seguir Construyendo con Tierra*, CRATERRE, France, 1984; D.J.T. Webb, "Construction en terre stabilisee au Kenya" Proceedings of the International Conference on Economical Housing in Developing Countries: Materials Construction Techniques Components, Paris, 1983; D.J.T. Webb, "Low cost housing and parasite vectors" *Parasitology Today* 1, 65, 1985; D.J.T. Webb and A.J. Lockwood , *BREPAK Operators Manual*, Building Research Establishment Client Report CR21/87, 1987; and I.L.O., *Small Scale Manufacture of Stabilised Soil Blocks*, Technical memorandum no. 12, Geneva, 1987.
44. Briceño Leon 1987, Webb 1983, and Webb and Lockwood 1987, see note 43.
45. Webb 1983, see note 43.
46. Webb and Lockwood 1987, see note 43.
47. White, G.B., C.J. Schofield, N.G. Williams, D.J.T. Webb and C.J. Boase, "The role of compressed soil blocks in low-cost housing for the control of

vector borne diseases" *Transcripts of the Royal Society of Tropical Medicine and Hygiene*, vol. 79, 282, 1985.
48. I.L.O. 1987, see note 43.
49. Omer, S.M. and J.L. Cloudsley-Thompson, "Survival of female Anopheles gambiae Giles through a nine-month dry season in Sudan" *WHO Bulletin* 42, 319, 1970.
50. Gamboa, C.J., "El proceso modificador de la vivienda en el medio rural des estado Miranda (Venevuela). Su relación con la infestación por Rhodnius prolixus" Archivos Venezolanos de Medecina Tropical y Parasitologia Medica vol.5, 353, 1973.
51. Bruce-Chwatt, L.J. and J. de Zulueta, *The Rise and Fall of Malaria in Europe: a Historico-epidemiological Study*, Oxford University Press, 1980.
52. Briceno Leon 1987 see note 43; and R. Briceno-Leon, "Aspectos psicosomaticos de la enfermedad de Chagas" *Boletin Asociacion Venezuela Psicologica Sociedad* 9, 37, 1986.
53. Agarwal 1981, see note 2; Dethier 1981, see note 6; and T. Hongvivatana, "Human behaviour and malaria", 29th SEAMEDTROPMED Seminar: Social and economic research in tropical diseases, Kuala Lumpur, 1986.
54. Linsdsay, S. and M. Gibson, "Bednets revisited; old idea, new angle" *Parasitology Today* 4, 237, 1988.
55. Manson, P., "Experimental proof of the mosquito-malaria theory" *British Medical Journal* ii, 949, 1900.
56. Wilson, D.B., "Construction, irrigation and malaria" *East African Medical Journal* 34, 479, 1957.

Chapter 10

The assistance of many individuals in the preparation of this chapter is acknowledged. The document by the World Health Orgaqnization's RUD Programme on "Access to Life-Saving Services in Urban Areas" has provided a wealth of material, and the contribution of Luiz Edmundo Costa Leite, Secretary of Municipal Public Works, Rio de Janeiro, E A R Ouano, Consulting Engineer, Manila, the Philippines, W A Hassouna, Health Planning Advisor, Ministry of Public Health, Kuwait, and James Lewis of Datum International, UK, is gratefully acknowledged.

Chapter 11

1. For a discussion of this, see chapters 8 and 9 in Jorge E. Hardoy and David Satterthwaite, *Squatter Citizen: Life in the Urban Third World*, Earthscan Publications, London, UK, 1989.
2. See for instance: Daniel R. Vining Jr, "The growth of core regions in the Third World" *Scientific American* vol. 252, no. 4, April 1985; Nigel Harris, "Some trends in the evolution of big cities: studies of the USA and India" *Habitat International* vol. 8, no. 1, 1984, pp 7-28; A.B. Rofman, "Argentina: a mature urban pattern" *Cities* vol. 2, no. 1 Butterworth Press, 1985; P.M. Townroe and D. Keen , "Polarization reversal in the State of Sao Paulo", *Regional Studies* vol. 18.1, 1984, pp 45-54; and Martha Schteingart, "The environmental problems associated with urban development in Mexico City" *Environment and Urbanization* vol. 1, no. 1, April 1989,

3. See note 2 for Chapter 1.
4. See report of the seminar organized by IIED-America Latina on *Funding Community Level Initiatives*, September 1990 (available from IIED, 3 Endsleigh Street, London WC1H ODD, UK). See also A. Harth Deneke and M. Silva, "Mutual help and progressive housing development: for what purpose? Notes on the Salvadorean experience" in Peter Ward (ed.), *Self Help Housing: a Critique*, Mansell, London, 1982.
5. Tabibzadeh, I., A. Rossi-Espagnet and R. Maxwell, *Spotlight on the Cities – Improving Urban Health in Developing Countries* World Health Organization, Geneva, 1989, 174 pages.
6. Asian Coalition for Housing Rights, "Evictions in Seoul, South Korea" *Environment and Urbanization* vol. 1, no. 1, April 1989, pp. 89-94.
7. Calculated from the Aid Project Database compiled by the Human Settlements Programme, International Institute for Environment and Development – write IIED, 3 Endsleigh Street, London WC1H ODD, UK for list of publications derived from this database.
8. Bartone, Carl R. and Stephen K. Mayo, *Economic Trends and Macroeconomic Policies Affecting Urban Development in the Third World*, background paper to WHO Expert Committee on Environmental Health in Urban Development World Health Organization, RUD/WP/90.15, Geneva, 1990.
9. See for instance the widespread use of child labour within London in the early nineteenth century as described in Christopher Hibbert, *London: a Biography of a City*, Penguin Books, London, 1980.
10. Hardoy, Jorge E. and David Satterthwaite, *Environmental Problems in Third World Cities: a Global Issue Ignored?* IIED Issue Paper, London, 1989.
11. Hardoy and Satterthwaite 1989, see note 10.
12. Hardoy and Satterthwaite 1989, see note 10; and Jeffrey H. Leonard and David Morell, "Emergence of environmental concern in developing countries: a political perspective; *Stanford Journal of International Law*, vol. 17, issue 2, 1981, pp 281-313.
13. Angel, Shlomo and Somsook Boonyabancha, "Land sharing as an alternative to eviction: the Bangkok experience" *Third World Planning Review* vol. 10, no. 2, May 1988; and Yap Kioe Sheng, "Some low income housing delivery sub-systems in Bangkok, Thailand" *Environment and Urbanization* vol. 1, no. 2, October 1989, pp. 27-37.
14. See for instance case studies in Bertha Turner (ed.), *Building Community – A Third World Case Book*, Habitat International Coalition, London, 1988; SINA, *NGOs and Shelter*, Mazingira Institute, Nairobi, 1988; and Czech Conroy and Miles Litvinoff (eds.), *The Greening of Aid*, Earthscan Publications, London, 1988.
15. For one example, see "NGO Profile: SPARC – Developing new NGO lines", *Environment and Urbanization* vol. 2, no. 1, April 1990, pp. 91-104 and also case studies in the publications listed in note 14.
16. These were reviewed in Caroline O.N. Moser and David Satterthwaite, "The characteristics and sociology of poor urban communities", paper presented to the workshop on Community Health and the Urban Poor, Oxford, July 1985.
17. Hardoy and Satterthwaite 1989, see note 1.

Chapter 12

1. World Health Organization, "Report of the WHO Expert Committee on Environmental Health in Urban Development", Geneva, 23 April, 1990.
2. World Health Organization, *Urbanization and its Implications for Child Health: Potential for Action*, Geneva, 1988.
3. For more information, see Leila Bisharat and Hisham Zagha, *Health and Population in Squatter Areas of Amman: a Reassessment After Four Years of Upgrading*, Urban Development Department, the Hashemite Kingdom of Jordan, June 1986; and Leila Bisharat and Magdy Tewfik, "Housing the Urban Poor in Amman: Can Upgrading Improve Health?", *Third World Planning Review* vol. 7, no 1., February 1985.
4. *Urban Examples* No 15, UNICEF, drawing largely on Ephim Shluger, "Expanding Project Coverage – Review of Urban Basic Services Projects of Rio de Janeiro and Buenos Aires", paper produced for the UNICEF Inter-Agency Urban Meeting in Madras, India, March 1987.
5. Cochrane, G. *Policies for Strengthening Local Government in Developing Countries*, World Bank Staff Working Paper No 582, Washington DC, 1983.
6. Gakenheimer, Ralph and Carlos Enrique Jorge Brando, "Infrastructure Standards" in Lloyd Rodwin (ed.), *Shelter, Settlement and Development*, Allen and Unwin, London, 1987.
7. See for instance: Anne Schlyter, "Commercialization of Housing in Upgraded quatter Areas: a Preliminary Presentation of the Case of George, Lusaka", paper presented in the International Research Conference on Housing Policy, Sweden, June, 1986; Omer M.A. El Agraa and M.Y. Shaddad, *Housing Rentals in the Sudanese Capital*, Sudanese Group for Assessment of Human Settlements, Khartoum University Press, 1988; E.A. Wahab, *The Tenant Market of Baldia Township*, Urban Research Working Papers no. 3, Amsterdam Free University, 1984; Urban Poor Institute, *Information Packet on the Urban Poor of Korea* (mimeo), 1988; Michael Edwards, "Cities of Tenants: renting among the urban poor in Latin America", in Alan Gilbert, Jorge E. Hardoy and Ronaldo Ramirez (eds.) *Urbanization in Contemporary Latin America*, John Wiley and Sons, Chichester, 1982; and Philip Amis, "Squatters or tenants: the commercialization of unauthorized housing in Nairobi", *World Development* vol. 12, no. 1, 1984.
8. Cairncross, Sandy "The private sector and water supply in developing countries: Partnership or profiteering?", *Health, Policy and Planning*, vol. 2, no. 2, 1987, pp. 180-184.
9. Lee, Kyu Sik, *Infrastructure Investment and Productivity: the case of Nigerian Manufacturing – a framework for policy study*, discussion paper, Water Supply and Urban Development Division, the World Bank, 1988.
10. See case studies in Bertha Turner (ed.), *Building Community – A Third World Case Book*, Habitat International Coalition, London, 1988; SINA, *NGOs and Shelter*, Mazingira Institute, Nairobi, 1988; and Czech Conroy and Miles Litvinoff (eds.), *The Greening of Aid*, Earthscan Publications, London, 1988.
11. Harth Deneke, A. and M. Silva, "Mutual help and progressive housing development: for what purpose? Notes on the Salvadorean experience" in Peter Ward (ed.), *Self Help Housing: a Critique*, Mansell, London, 1982. For two case studies of FUNDASAL's work with low income groups, see Alfredo

Stein, "The tugurios of San Salvador: a place to live, work and struggle", *Environment and Urbanization* vol. 1, no. 2, October 1989.

12. SPARC, "NGO Profile: SPARC – Developing new NGO lines", *Environment and Urbanization* vol. 2, no. 1, April 1990, pp. 91-104.
13. For english language descriptions, see case studies on COPEVI and CENVI projects in Turner 1988, see note 10.
14. For additional information on the Asian Coalition for Housing Rights, see "NGO Profile – Habitat International Coalition" *Environment and Urbanization* vol. 2, no. 1, April 1990.
15. Tabibzadeh, I., A. Rossi-Espagnet and R. Maxwell, *Spotlight on the Cities – Improving Urban Health in Developing Countries* World Health Organization, Geneva, 1989.

SUGGESTED FURTHER READING

Below are suggestions for further reading for those who want to follow up points raised in this book.

1. Urban Context

Stren, Richard E. and Rodney R. White (eds.), *African Cities in Crisis: Managing Rapid Urban Growth*, Westview Press, Boulder, USA, 1989, 335 pages, available through bookshops or from Westview, 5500 Central Avenue, Boulder, Colorado 80301, USA or 13 Brunswick Centre, Lodnon WC1N 1AF, UK.

Hardoy, Jorge E. and David Satterthwaite, *Squatter Citizen: Life in the Urban Third World*, Earthscan Publications, 374 pages, 1989, available through bookshops or from Earthscan, 3 Endsleigh Street, London WC1H ODD, UK.

UNCHS (Habitat), *Global Report on Human Settlements 1986*, Oxford University Press, Oxford, 1987.

2. Health and nutrition – general

Basta, Samir S. "Nutrition and Health in low income urban areas of the Third World", *Ecology of Food and Nutrition* vol. 6, 1977, pp 113-124.

Carlson, Beverley A. and Tessa M. Wardlaw , *A Global, Regional and Country Assessment of Child Malnutrition*, Staff Working Papers no. 7 UNICEF, New York, 1990, 128 pages. Available from UNICEF, 3 UN Plaza, New York, NY 10017, U. S. A. There is also a short summary by these same authors entitled *An Assessment of Child Malnutrition: a Summary* available from the same address as above.

Hardoy, Jorge E. and David Satterthwaite, "Housing and Health: What Role for Architects and Planners", *Cities* vol. 4, no. 3, 1987.

Harpham, Trudy, Tim Lusty and Patrick Vaughan (eds.), *In the Shadow of the City: Community Health and the Urban Poor*, Oxford University Press, 1988.

Harpham, Trudy, Patrick Vaughan and Susan Rifkin, *Health and the Urban Poor in Developing Countries; a Review and Selected Annotated Bibliography*, EPC Publications no. 5, available from the London School of Tropical Medicine and Hygiene, Keppel Street, London WC1E 7HT, UK.

Morley, David and Hermione Lovel, *My Name is Today: an illustrated discussion of child health, society and poverty in less developed countries*, Macmillan

Publishers, London, UK, 1986, 359 pages. Available from TALC, Box 49, St Albans, Herts AL1 4AX, U.K.

Pryer, Jane and Nigel Crook, *Cities of Hunger: Urban Malnutrition in Developing Countries*, OXFAM, 1988, 110 pages. Available from OXFAM, 274 Banbury Road, Oxford OX2 7DZ, UK.

Rohde, J.E., "Why the other half dies: the science and politics of child mortality in the Third World" *Assignment Children* vol. 61/62, 1983, pp. 35-67.

Rosenfield, P.L., C.G. Widstrand and A.P. Ruderman, "How tropical diseases impede social and economic development of rural communities: A research agenda" *Rural Africana* (8-9), Fall-Winter, 1980.

RUD Network, a quarterly newsletter published by the World Health Organization's programme on "Environmental health in rural and urban development in housing", includes articles on housing and health and gives details of new projects and publications. Available from the RUD programme, Division of Environmental Health, WHO, 1211 Geneva 27, Switzerland.

Tabibzadeh, I., A. Rossi Espagnet and R. Maxwell, *Spotlight on the Cities: Improving Urban Health in Developing Countries*, World Health Organization, Geneva, 1989. Available from Publications Division, WHO, 1211 Geneva 27, Switzerland.

Tulchin, Joseph S. (ed), *Habitat, Health and Development: a New Way of Looking at Cities in the Third World*, Lynne Reinner Publishers, Boulder, USA, 1986, especially chapters by John Briscoe on "Water supply and health in developing countries: selective primary health care revisited" and C. Arden Miller on "Setting priorities for health care." Available from Reinner, 948 North Street, Boulder, Colorado, USA.

United Nations Children's Fund, *The State of the World's Children 1990* (and other years – the report is published annually), Oxford University Press, 1990.

World Health Organization, *Urbanization and its Implications for Child Health: Potential for Action*, World Health Organization, Geneva, 1989. Available from Publications Division, WHO, 1211 Geneva 27, Switzerland or through WHO national/regional offices

3. Urban Health – country or case studies

Bapat, Meera and Nigel Crook, "The environment, health and nutrition: an analysis of interrelationships from a case study of hutment settlements in the city of Poona" *Habitat International* vol. 8, no. 3/4, 1984.

Bisharat, Leila and Magdy Tewfig, "Housing the Poor In Amman – Can Upgrading Improve Health?", *Third World Planning Review* vol. 7, no. 1, 1985.

Environment and Urbanization vol. 2, no. 2, October 1990 which is on the theme of "Children and the environment" includes three case studies which consider links between health and housing and living conditions:

- Harpham, Trudy, Paul Garner and Charles Surjadi, "Planning for child health in a poor urban environment: the case of Jakarta, Indonesia"
- Jacobi, Pedro, "Habitat and health in the municipality of Sao Paulo"
- Omer, Mohamed I.A., "Child health in the spontaneous settlements around Khartoum"

Available from IIED, 3 Endsleigh Street, London WC1H ODD, UK.

Halstead, Scott B., Julia A. Walsh and Kenneth S. Warren (eds), *Good Health at*

Low Cost, Conference Report, the Rockefeller Foundation, 1985. This includes country case studies and discussions of interventions to improve health status. Available from the Rockefeller Foundation, 1133 Avenue of the Americas, New York, NY 10036, USA.

UNICEF, "Universal child immunization: reaching the poor", *Urban Examples* no. 16, February 1990 and "Improving environment for child health and survival", *Urban Examples* no. 15, UNICEF, New York, 1988. Other issues of *Urban Examples* also have valuable case studies including Issue 13 ("Starting up with basic services"), Issue 12 ("Child survival and development of basic services") and Issue 4 ("Urban primary health care – health services the for urban poor – a process and a product"). These are available in English, Spanish and French from the Urban Advisor, UNICEF, 3 UN Plaza, New York, NY 10017, U. S. A.

4. Water, Sanitation, Drainage and Garbage Collection

Briscoe, John, "Water supply and health in developing countries: selective primary health care revisited" in Joseph S. Tulchin (ed), *Habitat, Health and Development: a New Way of Looking at Cities in the Third World*, Lynne Reinner Publishers, Boulder, 1986.

Cairncross, Sandy, Small Scale Sanitation, *Ross Bulletin no. 8*, 1988. Available from LSHTM, Keppel Street, London WC1E 7HT.

Cairncross, Sandy and E.A.R. Ouano, *Surface Water Drainage in Low-income Communities*, WHO, Geneva, 1990, Available from Publications, WHO, 1211 Geneva 27, Switzerland.

Cairncross, Sandy and Richard G. Feachem, *Environmental Health Engineering in the Tropics – An Introductory Text*, John Wiley and Sons, Chichester (UK), 1983.

Cointreau, Sandra, *Environmental Management of Urban Solid Waste in Developing Countries*, Urban Development Technical Paper no. 5, the World Bank, Washington DC, 1982. Available from World Bank Publications, 1818 H Street NW, Washington DC 20433, U.S.A.

Feachem, R., D.J. Bradley, H. Garelick and D.D. Mara, *Sanitation and Disease: Health Aspects of Excreta and Wastewater Management*, John Wiley and Sons, Chichester, UK, 1988.

Flintoff, F., *Management of Solid Wastes in Developing Countries*, W.H.O (SEARO), New Delhi, India, 1976.

Furedy, Christine, "Social considerations in solid waste management in Asian Cities" *Regional Development Dialogue* vol. 10, no. 3, Autumn 1989, pp. 13-40

Furedy, Christine, "Appropriate technology for urban wastes in Asia" *Biocycle* July 1989.

Kalbermatten, J.M., D.S. Julius and C.G. Gunnerson, *Appropriate Technology for Water Supply and Sanitation: A Review of the Technical and Economic Options*, World Bank, Washington DC, 1980, available from The World Bank, 1818 H Street NW, Washington DC 20433, USA.

Hasan, Arif, "Orangi pilot project, Karachi", in Czech Conroy and Miles Litvinov (eds.), *The Greening of Aid*, Earthscan Publications, London, 1988.

UNCHS (Habitat), *Delivery of Basic Infrastructure to Low Income Settlements: Issues and Adoptions*, U.N. Centre for Human Settlements (Habitat), Nairobi, Kenya, 1986, Available from Publications, UNCHS, P. O. Box 30030, Nairobi,

Kenya
UNCHS (Habitat), Low Cost Sanitation Project in Bihar, India, Project monograph for the International Year of Shelter for the Homeless, January 1986. Write to Publications, UNCHS, P. O. Box 30030, Nairobi, Kenya
UNCHS (Habitat), *Refuse Collection Vehicles for Developing Countries*, Nairobi, Kenya, 1988, 50 pages. Available from Publications Division, UNCHS, P.O. Box 30030, Nairobi, Kenya.
UNCHS (Habitat), *The Design of Shallow Sewer Systems*, Nairobi, Kenya, 1986. Available from Publications Division, UNCHS, P. O. Box 30030, Nairobi, Kenya.

5. Housing in urban areas

Angel, Shlomo, Raymon W, Archer, Sidhijai Tanphiphat and Amiel A. Wegelin (eds.), *Land for Housing the Poor*, Select Books, Singapore, 556 pages, 1983. Available from Select Books, 03-15 Tanglin Shopping Centre, 19 Tanglin Road, Singapore 1024.
Environment and Urbanization, vol. 1, no. 2, October 1989 which has papers on different Third World cities and a guide to the literature on "Beyond the stereotype of slums: how poor people find accommodation in Third World cities". Available from IIED, 3 Endsleigh Street, London WC1H ODD, UK.
Moser, Caroline O.N. and Linda Peake (eds.), *Women, Human Settlements and Housing*, Tavistock Publications, London and New York, 1987, 222 pages Available from International Thompson Publishing Services, North Way, Andover, Hants SP10 5BE, UK.

6. NGOs working in shelter, health and the environment.

Agarwal, Anil Darryl d'Monte and Ujwala Samarth (eds.), *The Fight for Survival: People's Action for Environment*, Centre for Science and Environment, New Delhi, India, 1987, 361 pages Available from CSE, 807 Vishal Bhawan, 95 Nehru Place, New Delhi 110019, India.
Hasan, Arif, "Community groups and non-government organizations in the urban field in Pakistan", *Environment and Urbanization* Vol 2, no. 1, April 1990. This issue of the journal has several other papers on community organizations and their role in housing. Available from IIED, 3 Endsleigh Street, London WC1H ODD.
SINA and Mazingira Institute, *NGOs and Shelter*, 1987. This is a package of case studies, feature articles and national overviews about the work of non-government organizations working in shelter in Africa and can be ordered from Mazingira Institute, P. O. Box 14550, Nairobi, Kenya.
Turner, Bertha (ed.), *Building Community: A Third World Case Book*, Habitat International Coalition. 1988. Available from BCB, P. O. Box 28, Dumfries DG2 ONS, Scotland.
UNICEF, *Urban Examples* as described under section 3 – many of the issues include case studies of Third World NGOs working in shelter, basic services and health.
UNCHS (Habitat), *Shelter for the Homeless: the Role of Non Governmental Organizations*, UNCHS (Habitat), Nairobi, 1987. Available from UNCHS (Habitat), P. O. Box 3003, Nairobi, Kenya

Contributors

The Editors

Sandy Cairncross is a Senior Lecturer in Tropical Public Health Engineering at the London School of Hygiene and Tropical Medicine. With a Ph.D in Civil engineering, he worked on water supply and sanitation for the governments of Lesotho and Mozambique for nearly ten years. His research interests include the health impacts of water supply and sanitation in Third World nations as well as innovative, cost effective approaches to the provision of urban infrastructure. His recent publications include: "Low cost sanitation technology for the control of intestinal helminths" *Parasitology Today* vol. 3, no. 94, 1987; *Environmental Health Engineering in the Tropics – An introductory text* (with Richard G. Feachem), John Wiley and Sons, Chichester (UK), 1983; and *Guidelines for the Safe Use of Wastewater and Excreta in Agriculture and Aquaculture* (co-authored with D.D. Mara), World Health Organization, Geneva, 1990.

Jorge E. Hardoy is President of the Instituto Internacional de Medio Ambiente y Desarrollo (IIED-América Latina) in Buenos Aires and President of the National Commission for Historical Monuments in Argentina. Qualifying as an architect in 1950 with a Masters and a Ph.D from Harvard University in city and regional planning, he has written widely on both historical and contemporary urban issues. He is a former President of the Inter-American Planning Society, twice a former Guggenheim Fellow and an advisor to the World Commission on Environment and Development (the Brundtland Commission). He also advises the World Health Organization and in 1990, chaired an Expert Committee for the World Health Organization on "Environmental Health in Urban

Development". Recent publications include two books written with David Satterthwaite – *La Ciudad Legal y la Ciudad ilegal*, GEL Publications, Buenos Aires, 1988 and *Squatter Citizen: Life in the Urban Third World*, Earthscan Publications, London, 1989 and *Repensando la Ciudad de America Latina* (edited with Richard M. Morse). GEL Publications, Buenos Aires, 1988. He is also editor of the journals *Medio Ambiente y Urbanizacion* and *Environment and Urbanization* and edits a series of books on urban history in Latin America, the latest of which is *Nuevas Perspectivas en Los Estudios sobre Historia Urbana Latinoamericana* (edited with Richard P. Morse) Ediciones GEL, Buenos Aires, 1989.

David Satterthwaite is a researcher who works both at IIED-America Latina and at its sister institution, the International Institute for Environment and Development in London. Trained as a development planner at University College, London with a first degree in history, recent publications include the books noted above written with Jorge E. Hardoy, "Improving Environment for Child Health" (Editor), *Urban Examples 15*, UNICEF, New York, 1989 and *Small and Intermediate Urban Centres: their Role in Regional and National Development in the Third World* (edited with Jorge E. Hardoy), Hodder and Stoughton, 1986. He is also editor of the journal *Environment and Urbanization* and on the advisory board of *Cities*. He was an advisor to the World Commission on Environment and Development and is currently an advisor to the World Health Organization and the United Nations Centre for Human Settlements (Habitat).

Chapter Authors

Chapter 1: Sandy Cairncross, Jorge E. Hardoy and David Satterthwaite – see above.

Chapter 2: Beatriz Cuenya, Hector Almada, Diego Armus, Julia Castells, María di Loreto and Susana Peñalva are the team based at the Centro de Estudios Urbanos y Regionales in Buenos Aires which undertook the housing and health study on which this chapter is based. Beatriz Cuenya, the team leader, is an architect who has been working on issues concerned with low income housing and housing sub-markets since 1977. Her recent publications include *De La Villa*

Miseria al Barrio Autoconstruido: Cuatro Experiencias Organizadas de Produccion del Habitat Popular co-authored with Oscar Yujnovsky and Ernesto Pastana, Ediciones CEUR, 1984 and *Habitat Popular: Experiencias y Alternativas en Paises de America Latina* (co-edited with Nora Clichevsy and Susana Peñalva), Cuadernos del CEUR 16, Buenos Aires, 1986. Beatriz Cuenya, Diego Armus, María di Loreto and Susana Peñalva also recently published "Land invasions and grassroots organization: the Quilmes settlement in Greater Buenos Aires, Argentina", *Environment and Urbanization* vol. 2, no. 1, April 1990.

Chapter 3: Dr Tade Akin Aina is a lecturer at the Department of Sociology, University of Lagos and convenor of the Lagos Group for the Study of Human Settlements – an interdisciplinary research and training group. Dr Aina is also a research fellow of the International Institute for Environment and Development and an editor of *Environment and Urbanization.* With a masters in Sociology from the London School of Economics and a Ph.D from the University of Sussex, his recent publications include *Health, Habitat and Underdevelopment in Nigeria with special reference to a low income settlement in Metropolitan Lagos*, IIED, London, 1990; "Petty landlords and poor tenants in a low-income settlement in Metropolitan Lagos, Nigeria" in Philip Amis and Peter Lloyd (eds.), *Housing Africa's Urban Poor*, Manchester University Press, 1990; and "Many routes enter the market place – housing submarkets for the urban poor in Metropolitan Lagos, Nigeria", *Environment and Urbanization*, vol. 1, no. 2, 1990, pp. 38-49.

Chapter 4: Dr Harikesh Misra is a reader in Geography at the University of Allahabad and a Senior Research Fellow of the International Institute for Development Research in Allahabad, India. He directed the team which investigated housing and health conditions in different squatter settlements in Allahabad. Recent publications include *Urban System of a Developing Economy*, IIDR, Allahabad, 1984, *Rural Geography* (Editor), Heritage Press, New Delhi, 1985, and "Rae Bareli, Sultanpur and Pratapgarh Districts, Uttar Pradesh State" in Jorge E. Hardoy and David Satterthwaite (eds.), *Small and Intermediate Urban Centres: their Role in National and Regional Development in the Third World*, Hodder and Stoughton, London, 1986.

Chapter 5: Dr Sandy Cairncross – see above.

Chapter 6: Dr Gehan Sinnatamby has been working with the United Nations Centre for Human Settlements (Habitat) since 1983 as a sanitation expert. With a Masters from Imperial College, London and a Ph.D in public health engineering from Leeds University, he has a special interest in finding cheap and effective ways of improving sanitation, solid waste collection and recycling in Third World cities and improving government performance in the maintenance of basic services. Recent publications include "Shallow systems offer hope to slums" (co-author), *World Water*, January-February 1986; "Shallow sewer system – a low-cost sanitation option", *Developing World Water*, Grosvenor Press International, Hong Kong, 1987 and "Rational design of septic tanks in warm climates" (co-authored with D.D. Mara) *The Public Health Engineer* vol. 14, no. 4, 1986, pp. 49-55. He has also produced a series of papers for UNCHS (Habitat) on water, sanitation and garbage disposal including *The Design of Shallow Sewer Systems*, Nairobi, Kenya, 1986.

Chapter 7: Sandy Cairncross – see above. Dr E.A.R. Ouano is a Filipino water engineer who was formerly on the staff of the Asian Institute of Technology in Bangkok. He has acted as advisor to many organizations, including the World Health Organization and now runs an engineering consultancy in Manila. He is the co-author (with Sandy Cairncross) of *Surface Water Drainage for Low-Income Communities*, the World Health Organization, Geneva, 1990.

Chapter 8: Stenio de Coura Cuentro is a Brazilian civil engineer who, since 1981, has been a partner of the firm Mogno Engenharia e Tecnologia Alernativa where he is presently Administrative and Financial Manager. He has worked on several projects in the areas of road surfacing, drainage, sewers and urban waste management. In 1983 he advised the municipality of Olinda on the "Triangulo de Peixinhos" project described in Chapter 8. In 1984-85, he helped design and manage the municipality of Paulista's waste management system and between 1986 and 1987 he was a Director of Recife's Waste Management Department. Since March 1987 he has been a Director of Operations of the Road Department of Pernambuco State. Since 1985 he has also been a researcher for the Department of Applied Research of Brazil's

National Housing Agency (BNH). Dji Malla Gadgi was working with the OXFAM office in Chad on the Ambassatna Nadif garbage collection scheme described in the chapter and is now working with the United Nations Development Programme in Chad. He has recently published a longer account of this project in the journal published by the Arid Lands Unit at OXFAM, *Baobab* no. 4, 1990.

Chapter 9: Dr Chris Schofield is with the World Health Organization in Geneva, working in the Special Programme for Research and Training in Tropical Diseases (TDR). He has a special interest in the best means to control diseases, with a particular interest in the control of Chagas' disease. He was also the founding editor of the journal *Parasitology Today*. Dr R. Briceño-Leon is Director of the Social Research Laboratory of the Central University of Venezuela and has a special interest in the sociology of disease vector control; he has been working with low income communities on how best to improve housing conditions and, through housing improvements to contribute to improved health. Dr N. Kolstrup has worked in Tanzania with a special interest in controlling malaria and improving ceilings as a means to limit the entry of disease vectors into homes; he is currently practising as a doctor in Norway. Dr David Webb is a civil engineer, working at the Building Research Establishment in the United Kingdom and has a special interest in improving building and housing design and improving the use made of local materials for building construction. Dr Graham White is an entomologist and an authority on malaria; he worked for many years in Africa and was formerly with the Department of Medical Parasitology at the London School of Hygiene and Tropical Medicine. He is currently senior public health entomologist at I.C.I. in Fernhurst, United Kingdom.

Chapter 10: Dr Gregory Goldstein is a physician and scientist working with the World Health Organization's Programme on Environmental Health in Rural and Urban Development and Housing (the RUD Programme). He is also Editor of *RUD Network*, a newsletter produced by the RUD Programme to keep institutions and professionals working in environmental health issues related to housing in touch with each other. Prior to joining the World Health

Organization, he was a lecturer at the Department of Public Health in the University of Sydney, Australia. He has a particular interest in the health aspects of housing.

Chapters 11 and 12 are by the editors.

Index